Causes, Symptoms and Management of Anemia

Causes, Symptoms and Management of Anemia

Editor: Martha Pratt

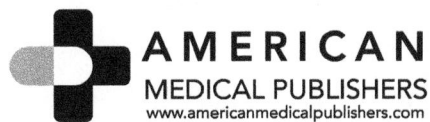

AMERICAN
MEDICAL PUBLISHERS
www.americanmedicalpublishers.com

AMERICAN
MEDICAL PUBLISHERS
www.americanmedicalpublishers.com

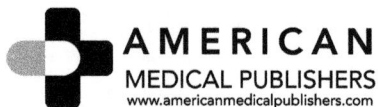

Cataloging-in-Publication Data

Causes, symptoms and management of anemia / edited by Martha Pratt.
   p. cm.
Includes bibliographical references and index.
ISBN 978-1-63927-181-8
1. Anemia. 2. Anemia--Etiology. 3. Anemia--Treatment. 4. Anemia--Diagnosis. 5. Blood--Diseases. I. Pratt, Martha.
RC641 .C38 2022
616.152--dc23

American Medical Publishers,
41 Flatbush Avenue,
1st Floor, New York,
NY 11217, USA

ISBN 978-1-63927-181-8 (Hardback)

Contents

Preface

Anemia is a disease that occurs due to the decreased amount of total red blood cells in the blood. Due to the deficiency of hemoglobin which carries oxygen, the person often experiences shortness of breath on exertion. It can also exhibit symptoms of a heart failure. The most common cause of anemia is blood loss. Several reasons can lead to blood loss such as severe trauma or surgery, menstruation, and gynecological disturbances. Other causes of anemia include fluid overload, which decreases the hemoglobin concentration, and certain gastrointestinal disorders. The common treatment of anemia includes oral and injectable iron, blood transfusions, erythropoiesis-stimulating agent and hyperbaric oxygen. This book discusses the fundamentals as well as modern approaches for management of anemia. It presents researches and studies performed by experts across the globe. It will serve as a valuable source of reference for graduate and post graduate students.

This book is a comprehensive compilation of works of different researchers from varied parts of the world. It includes valuable experiences of the researchers with the sole objective of providing the readers (learners) with a proper knowledge of the concerned field. This book will be beneficial in evoking inspiration and enhancing the knowledge of the interested readers.

In the end, I would like to extend my heartiest thanks to the authors who worked with great determination on their chapters. I also appreciate the publisher's support in the course of the book. I would also like to deeply acknowledge my family who stood by me as a source of inspiration during the project.

Editor

Prevalence and Predictors of Maternal Anemia during Pregnancy in Gondar, Northwest Ethiopia

Mulugeta Melku,[1] Zelalem Addis,[2] Meseret Alem,[3] and Bamlaku Enawgaw[4]

[1] Department of Hematology, School of Biomedical and Laboratory Sciences, College of Medicine and Health Sciences, University of Gondar, P.O. Box 196, 6200 Gondar, Ethiopia

[2] Department of Medical Microbiology, School of Biomedical and Laboratory Sciences, College of Medicine and Health Sciences, University of Gondar, 6200 Gondar, Ethiopia

[3] Department of Immunology and Molecular Biology, School of Biomedical and Laboratory Sciences, College of Medicine and Health Sciences, University of Gondar, 6200 Gondar, Ethiopia

[4] Department of Hematology, School of Biomedical and Laboratory Sciences, College of Medicine and Health Sciences, University of Gondar, 6200 Gondar, Ethiopia

Correspondence should be addressed to Mulugeta Melku; mulugeta.melku@gmail.com

Academic Editor: Aurelio Maggio

Background. Anaemia is a global public health problem which has an eminence impact on pregnant mother. The aim of this study was to assess the prevalence and predictors of maternal anemia. *Method.* A cross-sectional study was conducted from March 1 to April 30, 2012, on 302 pregnant women who attended antenatal care at Gondar University Hospital. Interview-based questionnaire, clinical history, and laboratory tests were used to obtain data. Bivariate and multivariate logistic regression was used to identify predictors. *Result.* The prevalence of anemia was 16.6%. Majority were mild type (64%) and morphologically normocytic normochromic (76%) anemia. Anemia was high at third trimester (18.9%). Low family income (AOR [95% CI] = 3.1 [1.19, 8.33]), large family size (AOR [95% CI] = 4.14 [4.13, 10.52]), *hookworm* infection (AOR [95% CI] = 2.72 [1.04, 7.25]), and *HIV* infection (AOR [95% CI] = 5.75 [2.40, 13.69]) were independent predictors of anemia. *Conclusion.* The prevalence of anemia was high; mild type and normocytic normochromic anemia was dominant. Low income, large family size, *hookworm* infection, and HIV infection were associated with anemia. Hence, efforts should be made for early diagnosis and management of *HIV* and *hookworm* infection with special emphasis on those having low income and large family size.

1. Background

Anaemia is a global public health problem affecting both developing and developed countries with major consequences for human health as well as social and economic development which results in a loss of billions of dollars annually [1–3]. According to the 2008 World Health Organization (WHO) report, anaemia affected 1.62 billion (24.8%) people globally [2]. It had an estimated global prevalence of 42% in pregnant women and is a major cause of maternal mortality [4, 5]. In Africa, 57.1% of the pregnant women were anemic. Moreover, anemia in pregnant women is a severe public health problem in Ethiopia; 62.7% of pregnant women were anemic [2]. Although the prevalence varies widely in different settings and accurate data are often lacking, in resource-limited areas terribly significant proportions of women of childbearing age particularly pregnant are anaemic [3]. Geographically, those living in Asia and Africa are at the greatest risk [1].

The effect of anemia during pregnancy on maternal and neonatal life ranges from varying degrees of morbidity to mortality. As many studies elucidated, severe anemia (Hg < 7 g/L) during pregnancy has been associated with major maternal and fetal complications. It increases the risk of preterm delivery [6, 7], low birth weight [6–9], intrauterine fetal death [7], neonatal death [10], maternal mortality [11], and infant mortality [12].

Anemia is multifactorial in etiology; the disease is thought to be mainly caused by iron deficiency in developing countries. In sub-Saharan Africa where iron deficiency is common, the prevalence of anemia has often been used as a proxy for iron deficiency anemia (IDA) [3]. Other micronutrient deficiency (vitamins A and B12, riboflavin, and folic acid) has also been a cause of anemia during pregnancy [13]. Likewise, Infectious diseases such as malaria, helminthes infestations, and HIV are also implicated with high prevalence of anemia in sub-Saharan Africa [14, 15]. There was also a considerable variation in the prevalence of pregnancy anemia because of the differences in socioeconomic conditions, lifestyles, and health seeking behaviors of different population across different countries and cultures and obstetrics and gynecological related condition of pregnant mothers [16–41].

Since anaemia during pregnancy has a deleterious consequences, WHO adopted reducing maternal mortality as one of the three health-related millennium development goals so that international community is committing within this framework to reduce maternal mortality by three quarter at the end of 2015 [42]. Anemia prevalence data remains an important indicator of public health since anemia is related to morbidity and mortality in the population groups usually considered to be the most vulnerable like pregnant women. At a global level, anemia prevalence is a useful indicator to assess the impact of widespread or highly effective interventions and to track the progress made towards the goal of reducing anemia during pregnancy [43]. Anemia prevalence study is also useful to monitor the progress of reproductive health [2]. Despite the efforts made to reduce the burden, its prevalence has not been studied yet comprehensively in developing countries. Thus, the objective of this study was to determine the prevalence and predictors of anemia among pregnant women who attended ANC in Gondar University Hospital.

2. Methods

2.1. Study Population, Sample Size, and Sampling Procedure.
The study population was pregnant mothers attending antenatal care (ANC) at Gondar University Teaching Hospital. The hospital is found in Gondar town under Amhara regional state of Ethiopia which is located at 750 Km far from Addis Ababa, the capital city of Ethiopia, to the Northwest part of the country. The town is situated at an altitude of 2100 to 2870 meters above the sea level. According to the 2007 Ethiopian census report, Gondar has a total population of 206 and 987 and more than half (108, 902) of them are females [44].

A single population proportion formula, $[n = (Z\alpha/2)^2 p(1 - p)/d^2]$, was used to estimate the sample size. However, due to the lack of previous studies about the prevalence of anemia during pregnancy in this particular area, 50% prevalence was used for calculation. By reviewing the records of daily flow of pregnant women for ANC utilization, about 1410 pregnant women were estimated

to visit ANC clinic during the study period. Since the population during the study period was below 10,000, the sample correction formula was applied. Then, a total of 302 pregnant women who attended ANC service were selected using systematic random sampling technique from their sequence of ANC visit in the period between March and April, 2012, for two months.

2.2. Data Collection.
A face-to-face interview using structured pretested questionnaire was employed to obtain data about sociodemographic, obstetric, and gynecological, dietary intake, and medical conditions of pregnant mothers. As for the current pregnancy, intake of haematinics, gestational age, ante partum hemorrhage, and dietary intake were documented. Blood pressure, weight, and height were measured and body mass index (BMI) was calculated as (weight (kg)/height (m^2)). Women were then categorized into four groups according to their BMI as follows: underweight (BMI ≤ 20 kg/m^2), normal (20 kg/m^2 ≤ BMI ≤ 24.9 kg/m^2), overweight (BMI of 25 kg/m^2 ≤ BMI ≤ 29.9 kg/m^2), and obese (BMI ≥ 30 kg/m^2) [23]. A total of 6 mL venous blood sample was obtained from each participant. Of this, 3 mL of it was drawn into ethylene diamine tetraacetic acid tube for complete blood count whereas the remaining 3 mL was drawn to plane tube for serological tests. Participants were also requested to give fresh stool sample for parasitological examination of intestinal parasitosis.

2.3. Laboratory Analysis.
Complete blood count including red blood cell count, hemoglobin concentration (Hgb), mean cell volume (MCV), mean cell hemoglobin (MCH), and mean cell hemoglobin concentration (MCHC), platelet count, and white blood cell count were carried out using SYXMEX KX-21 haematology analyzer (Sysmex Corporation Kobe, Japan). A thin and thick blood film had been prepared and stained with Giemsa stain for the detection and speciation of Plasmodium parasite species. Stool wet mount was prepared using saline and/or iodine and examined microscopically for identification of intestinal helminthes and protozoa parasitosis. All stool samples were processed within 30 minutes of collection. Serum and/or plasma samples were tested for HIV following the current HIV1/2 testing algorism using KHB (Shanghai Kehua bio-engineering Co., LTD., China), Statpack (Chembio Diagnostic Systems, Inc., New york, USA), and Uni-gold (Trinity Biotech Plc, Bray, Ireland). Syphilis reactivity was also tested using RPR test (Human GmbH-Wiesbaden, Germany) as per the manufacturer's instruction and recommendation.

2.4. Assessment of Anemia.
Hgb cutoff value adjusted to sea level altitude was used to define anemia on the basis of gestational age and to classify the degree of severity using WHO criteria. The Hgb value less than 11.0 g/dL at first and third trimesters and less than 10.5 g/dL at second trimester was used to define anemia. Based on the severity, women with Hgb value of (10 g/dL ≤ Hgb < 11 g/dL) at first and third trimesters and (10 g/dL ≤ Hgb < 10.5 g/dL) at second trimester were classified as mild anemic. Pregnant

women who had a Hgb value of $(7 \, \text{g/dL} \leq \text{Hgb} < 10 \, \text{g/dL})$ and $(\text{Hgb} < 7 \, \text{g/dL})$ were categorized as moderate and severe anemic, respectively, regardless of their gestational age [45]. Manufacturer references were used to define the normal ranges for MCV (80.0–100.0 fl), MCH (27.0–33.5 pg), and MCHC (32.0–36.0 g/dL).

2.5. Data Processing and Analysis. Data were entered to EPI info version 3.5.3 and then transferred to SPSS version 20 statistical package for analysis. Descriptive and summary statistics were carried out using percentages and mean ± SD and were presented in tables and graphs. Binary logistic regression analysis was conducted to evaluate the difference in anemia prevalence across the relevant variables. Odds ratio, Chi-square, and 95% CI for odds ratio were computed to assess the strength of association and statistical significance in bivariate analysis. Independent variables having P less than or equal to 0.2 in univariate analysis were included in multivariate analysis to control confounders in regression models. Variables having P value less than 0.05 in multivariate binary logistic regression model were considered to be statistically significant.

2.6. Ethical Clearance. The study was approved by institutional review board of University of Gondar. The purpose and importance of the study were explained to each study participants. Written consent was obtained from each woman. To ensure confidentiality of participants, information, anonymous typing was used whereby the name of the participants and any participants' identifier were not written on the questionnaire, and, also during the interview to keep the privacy, they were interviewed alone. Results were communicated with clinicians working in ANC unit for appropriate management.

3. Result

3.1. Characteristics of the Study Participants. A total of 302 pregnant women with a mean (±SD) age of 26.47 ± 5.24 years were included in the study. The majority 242 (80.1%), 284 (94%), 250 (82.8%), and 194 (64.2%) were urban dwellers, married, had attended primary school and above, and house wives by occupation, respectively. The average monthly income of the participants was 1860 Ethiopian Birr (EB) and 147 (48.7%) were living with three to four family members (Table 1).

Concerning obstetrical history, 57.3% were multigravida, of whom 52.7% had an interpregnancy interval of more than or equal to 24 months and 23.7% experienced abortion. Nearly 70% of the study participants were at third trimester. Assessment of medical condition of the participant revealed that 72.5% had a normal BMI, 95.4% had no history of chronic diseases, and 4.6% had history of previous surgery. Laboratory investigation showed that 10.3% and 26.5% of the participants were reactive for HIV and infected with one or more than one intestinal parasites, respectively. *A. lumbricoides* (34.1%), *hookworm* (25.3%), and *E. histolytica/dispar* (17.2%) were the predominant parasites found (Table 2).

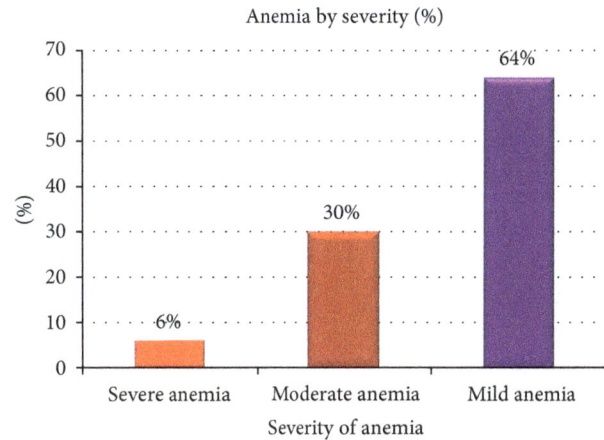

FIGURE 1: Percentage of anemia by severity among anemic pregnant women ($n = 50$).

The dietary habit and nutritional assessment revealed 19.8% did not take animal products in their current pregnancy, and 42.4% had a habit of eating green vegetables on monthly and above basis. About 80.1% had a habit of drinking coffee and tea after meal (data not shown). In their current pregnancy, 44.7%, 41.4%, and 7.3% took iron sulfate, folic acid, and multivitamin tables as nutritional supplement, respectively (Table 3).

3.2. Prevalence and Predictors of Anemia. The mean Hgb level of pregnant women was 11.96 ± 1.37 g/dL (range: 5.85–17.05 g/dL) and the overall prevalence of maternal anemia was 16.6% ($n = 50$). Of the anemic women, 6%, 30%, and 64% were severely, moderately, and mildly anemic, respectively (Figure 1).

Based on red blood cell morphologic classification of anemia, of the total anemic pregnant mothers, 76% had normocytic normochromic anemia and 14% had microcytic hypochromic type of anemia (Table 4).

High prevalence of anemia was observed in those pregnant women who were living with more than four family members (36.4%), illiterate (25.7%), and whose monthly family income < 1000EB (22%) (Table 1). In addition, high prevalence rate of anemia was found among mothers who were HIV seropositive (38.7%), infected with *hookworm* (34.8%), underweighted (30%), with more than four gravidae (32.3%), having chronic disease (27.3%), and at 3rd trimester (18.9%) (Table 2).

The prevalence of anemia among those who had a habit of eating animal products in their food stuff, not having a habit of eating vegetable, and who take tea/coffee after meal was 17.8%, 22.4%, and 15.3%, respectively. About 18.6% and 17.5% pregnant women who did not take iron sulphate and folate as nutritional therapy, respectively, were anemic (Table 3).

In bivariate analysis illiteracy, low monthly family income, large family size, underweight, gravidity, *hookworm* infection, and HIV seropositivity were significantly associated with maternal anemia. But in multivariate logistic regression analysis controlling the possible cofounders, only

TABLE 1: Sociodemographic characteristics of pregnant women and prevalence of anemia by sociodemographic characteristics (n = 302).

Variable	Anemia		Total (%)	COR (95% CI)
	Yes	No		
Age				
year	23 (15.8)	123 (84.2)	146 (48.3)	1
25–29 years	13 (15.9)	69 (84.1)	82 (27.2)	1.01 (0.48, 2.11)
≥30 years	14 (18.9)	60 (81.1)	74 (24.5)	1.25 (0.6, 2.60)
Residence				
Rural	11 (18.3)	49 (81.7)	60 (19.9)	1.17 (0.56, 2.45)
Urban	39 (16.1)	203 (83.9)	242 (80.1)	1
Marital status				
Married	47 (16.5)	237 (83.5)	284 (94)	1
Others*	3 (16.7)	15 (83.3)	18 (6)	1.01 (0.28, 3.62)
Maternal educational status				
Illiterate	18 (25.7)	52 (71.3)	70 (23.2)	3.31 (1.29, 8.54)*
Primary school	5 (9.4)	48 (90.6)	53 (17.5)	0.997 (0.30, 3.33)
Secondary school	20 (19)	85 (81)	105 (34.8)	2.25 (0.89–5.65)
Tertiary	7 (9.5)	67 (90.5)	74 (24.5)	1
Occupation				
House wife	38 (19.6)	156 (80.4)	194 (64.2)	2.27 (0.91, 5.67)
Government employed	6 (9.7)	56 (90.3)	62 (20.5)	1
Other**	6 (13)	40 (87)	46 (15.2)	1.4 (0.42, 4.65)
Family monthly income				
EB	30 (21.9)	107 (78.1)	137 (45.4)	3.22 (1.28, 8.13)*
1000–2575 EB	14 (15.6)	76 (84.4)	90 (29.8)	2.12 (0.77, 5.81)
EB	6 (8)	69 (92)	75 (24.8)	1
Family size				
≤2	16 (13.10)	106 (86.9)	122 (40.4)	
3-4	22 (15)	125 (85)	147 (48.7)	1.17 (0.58, 2.34)
≥5	12 (36.4)	21 (63.6)	33 (10.9)	3.79 (1.56, 9.17)*

Significant (P < 0.05) in bivariate analysis; other include single, divorced, and widowed; other** include private employed, farmers, merchants, and students.

low monthly family income (AOR = 3.15, 95% CI: 1.19, 8.33), large family size (AOR = 4.13, 95% CI: 1.62, 10.52), *hookworm* infection (AOR = 5.75, 95% CI: 2.40, 13.69), and HIV seropositivity (AOR = 2.72, 95% CI: 1.014, 7.25) remained being independent predictors of pregnancy anemia (Table 5).

4. Discussion

The overall prevalence of anemia was 16.6% (95%CI (12.6, 20.6)). This prevalence was comparable to studies conducted in Trinidad and Tobago (15.3%) [16], Thailand (20.1%) [17], Zurich (18.5%) [45], Hawassa (15.3%) [39], and Gondar town (22%) [46].

The prevalence is considerably lower than previous study reports from Malaysia (35%), Jordan (34.7%), Vietnam (43.2%), Southeastern Nigeria (76.9%), Eastern Sudan (62.6%), and Jimma, Ethiopia (38.2%) [22, 23, 25, 35, 38, 41]. The possible reason for the difference may be resulted from geographical variation of factors across different areas. In addition, lower prevalence can be attributed to gradual improvement of life style and living standards and health seeking behavior by the effort of government to achieve the

Millennium development goal aimed to reduce the maternal mortality by three-quarter by year 2015. In support of this argument, the prevalence of anemia in women of age 15–49 years had decreased from 27% in 2005 to 17% by the year 2011 in Ethiopia [47].

In this study, mild anemia was common followed by moderate anemia. This is consistent with reports from Africa and elsewhere in the world [23, 25, 29, 31, 39]. This study tried to demonstrate the common morphological characteristic of anemia among pregnant mothers. Of the total anemic pregnant women, 76% had normocytic normochromic anemia followed by microcytic hypochromic type which is in agreement with a report from Turkey [18] and Azezo, Gondar town [46].

This study demonstrated that mothers who have low monthly family income were three times more likely to be anemic as compared to those with high monthly family income. This is in agreement with some studies [24, 29] and contradicted to other reports [22, 23, 40, 41]. According to the 2007 Ethiopian central statistical agency household income consumption and expenditure survey, more than 57% of the total expenditure is spent on food [48]. Moreover, in

TABLE 2: The prevalence of anemia according to the obstetrics and medical factors ($n = 302$).

Variable	Anemic		Total (%)	COR (95% CI)
	Yes (%)	No (%)		
Gravidity				
Primigravidae	15 (11.6)	114 (88.4)	129 (42.7)	1
Secundigravidae	11 (14.3)	66 (85.7)	77 (25.5)	1.27 (0.55, 2.92)
3-4 gravidae	14 (21.5)	51 (78.5)	65 (21.5)	2.09 (0.94, 4.65)
≥5 gravidae	10 (32.3)	21 (67.7)	31 (10.3)	3.62 (1.43, 9.17)*
History of abortion				
Yes	8 (19.5)	33 (80.5)	41 (23.7)	0.94 (0.391, 2.27)
No	27 (20.4)	105 (79.6)	132 (76.3)	1
Interpregnancy interval				
1st pregnancy	15 (11.6)	114 (88.4)	129 (42.7)	1
	2 (14.3)	12 (85.7)	14 (4.6)	1.27 (0.26, 6.21)
≥24 months	33 (20.8)	126 (79.2)	159 (52.7)	2 (1.03, 3.86)
Gestational age				
1st trimester	1 (12.5)	7 (87.5)	8 (2.6)	1
2nd	12 (12.2)	86 (87.8)	98 (32.5)	0.98 (0.11, 8.62)
3rd	37 (18.9)	159 (81.1)	196 (64.9)	1.63 (0.19, 13.65)
Body mass index				
Underweight	9 (30)	21 (70)	30 (10)	2.42 (1.03, 5.64)*
Normal and above	41 (15.1)	231 (84.9)	272 (90)	1
Presence of chronic disease				
Yes	4 (27.3)	11 (72.7)	14 (4.6)	1.4 (0.38, 5.21)
No	47 (16.3)	241 (83.7)	288 (95.4)	1
Presence of peptic ulcer disease				
Yes	20 (18.3)	89 (81.7)	109 (36.1)	1.22 (0.66, 2.27)
No	30 (15.5)	163 (84.5)	193 (63.9)	1
History of previous surgery				
Yes	2 (14.3)	12 (85.7)	14 (4.6)	0.83 (0.181, 3.84)
No	48 (16.7)	240 (83.3)	288 (95.4)	1
Malaria attack in current pregnancy				
Yes	3 (20)	12 (80)	15 (5)	1.28 (0.347, 4.7)
No	47 (16.4)	240 (83.6)	287 (95)	1
Hookworm infection				
Yes	8 (34.8)	15 (65.2)	23 (7.6)	3.01 (1.20, 7.52)*
No	42 (15.1)	237 (84.9)	279 (92.4)	1
HIV infection				
Reactive	12 (38.7)	19 (61.3)	31 (10.3)	3.87 (1.74, 8.62)*
Nonreactive	38 (14)	233 (86)	271 (89.7)	1
Syphilis				
Reactive	3 (27.3)	8 (72.7)	11 (3.6)	1.95 (0.5, 7.61)
Nonreactive	47 (16.2)	244 (83.8)	291 (96.4)	1

*Significant ($P < 0.05$) in bivariate analysis. Chronic disease comprises hypertension, kidney disease, cardiac problems, and diabetes mellitus.

this study, 80% of study participants were from urban area suggesting that they are food net buyers. As income is low, the expenditure for food becomes low. Besides, due to food price inflation, the purchasing power of income is low. So, low income groups did not get adequate nutrition and thereby low family income groups were at risk of anemia.

According to the results of our study, pregnant mothers who had been living within a family of more than four members were more likely to be anemic compared to those living with ≤ 2 family members. Nevertheless, in Jordan [23], there was no significant difference of anemia prevalence between groups of pregnant mothers living with varying family sizes. This difference may be attributed as in Jordan case; the study was undertaken in rural district where there was not great variation in family size and income. But, in this study, 80% of pregnant women were in urban areas having

TABLE 3: Prevalence of anemia in relation to dietary habit, ANC followup, and nutrient supplementation at their current pregnancy period ($n = 302$).

Variable	Anemia Yes	Anemia No	Total ($N = 302$)	COR (95% CI)
Eating meat and animal products				
Yes	43 (17.8)	199 (82.2)	242 (80.1)	1
No	7 (11.7)	53 (88.3)	60 (19.9)	0.61 (0.26, 1.44)
Eating green leafy vegetables				
Yes	39 (15.4)	214 (84.6)	253 (83.8)	1.00
No	11 (22.4)	38 (77.6)	49 (16.2)	1.6 (0.75, 3.372)
Taking fruit after meal				
Yes	34 (16.6)	172 (83.5)	206 (68.2)	1
No	16 (16.7)	80 (83.3)	96 (31.8)	1.012 (0.53, 1.94)
Taking coffee or tea immediately after meal				
Yes	37 (15.3)	205 (84.7)	242 (80.1)	0.65 (0.32, 1.32)
No	13 (21.7)	47 (78.3)	60 (19.9)	1
ANC followup during current pregnancy				
Yes	28 (16.1)	146 (83.9)	174 (57.6)	1
No	22 (17.2)	106 (82.8)	128 (42.4)	1.08 (0.59, 1.99)
Iron sulphate table intake in current pregnancy				
Yes	19 (14.1)	116 (85.9)	135 (44.7)	1
No	31 (18.6)	136 (81.4)	167 (55.3)	1.39 (0.75, 2.59)
Folic acid intake in current pregnancy				
Yes	19 (15.2)	106 (84.8)	125 (41.4)	1
No	31 (17.5)	146 (82.5)	177 (58.6)	1.19 (0.64, 2.2)
Multivitamin intake in current pregnancy				
Yes	3 (13.6)	19 (86.4)	22 (7.3)	1
No	47 (16.8)	233 (83.2)	280 (92.7)	1.28 (0.36, 4.49)

TABLE 4: Distribution of morphologic type anemia among study participants.

Morphologic type of cells	Anemic status Anemic n (%)	Not anemic n (%)	Total n (%)
Microcytic hypochromic (MCV < 80 fl, MCH < 27 pg)	8 (16%)	1 (0.4%)	9 (3.0%)
Normocytic Normochromic (MCV and MCH within the normal value)	38 (76%)	235 (93.2%)	273 (90.4%)
Macrocytic normochromic (MCV > 100 fl, MCH (27 pg < MCH < 33.5 pg))	2 (4%)	5 (1.98%)	7 (2.3%)
Other combinations	2 (4%)	11 (4.37%)	13 (4.3%)
Total	50 (16.6%)	252 (83.4%)	302 (100%)

varying income levels and 20% in rural areas with varying family size.

This study also showed that the proportion of anemia among pregnant women who had been infected with HIV was significantly higher compared to those noninfected that is six times at higher risk. This is in line with previous studies [29, 31–33, 35]. This increased prevalence of anemia among HIV seropositive pregnant women may be explained by the fact that HIV infection is associated with lower serum folate, vitamin B12, and ferritin in pregnancy [31]. In addition, Anemia in HIV/AIDS patients may arise from a number of causes, including deregulation of the host immune system leading to destruction or inhibition of hematopoietic cells [49].

In our study, *hookworm* has increased the risk of being anemic and this finding was consistent with other studies [26, 41, 46]. This is because adult *hookworm* parasites attach and injure upper intestinal mucosa and also ingest blood. This brings about gastrointestinal blood loss and induces depletion of iron, folic acid, and vitamin B12 that ultimately anemia [13, 50].

Even though it was not statistically significant in multivariate logistic regression (but significant in bivariate analysis), multigravida and grand gravida had high odds for anemia as compared to primigravidae. Likewise, studies in Malaysia [22], Burkina Faso [29], Sudan [38], and Jimma [41] reported that gravidity did not have statistically significant contribution for difference in anemia prevalence.

TABLE 5: Multivariate binary logistic regression analysis of pregnancy anemia with predictor variables ($n = 302$).

Variables	Anemia		Total	OR (95% CI)	
	Yes	No		COR (95% CI)	AOR (95% CI)
Maternal educational status					
Illiterate	18 (25.7)	52 (74.3)	70	**3.31 (1.29, 8.54)**	0.61 (0.14, 2.68)
Primary	5 (9.4)	48 (90.6)	53	0.997 (0.30, 3.33)	0.37 (0.08, 1.73)
Secondary	20 (19)	85 (81)	105	2.25 (0.89–5.65)	0.99 (0.30, 3.22)
Tertiary	7 (9.5)	67 (90.5)	74	1	1
Family income/month					
Low (<1000 birr)	30 (21.9)	107 (78.1)	137	3.22 (1.28, 8.13)	3.15 (1.19, 8.33)*
Medium (1000–2575 birr)	14 (15.6)	76 (84.4)	90	2.12 (0.77, 5.81)	1.80 (0.62, 5.18)
High (>2575 birr)	6 (8)	69 (92)	75	1	1
Family size					
≤2	16 (13.1)	106 (86.9)	122	1	1
3-4 members	22 (15)	125 (85)	147	1.17 (0.58, 2.34)	1.03 (0.49, 2.13)
≥5 members	12 (36.4)	21 (63.6)	33	3.78 (1.56, 9.17)	4.13 (1.62, 10.52)**
Body mass index					
Underweight (<20 kg/m^2)	9 (30)	21 (70)	30	**2.42 (1.03, 5.64)**	2.27 (0.83, 6.21)
Normal and above (≥20 kg/m^2)	41 (15.1)	231 (84.9)	272	1	1
Gravidity					
Primigravidae	15 (11.6)	114 (88.4)	129	1	1
Secungravidae	11 (14.3)	66 (85.7)	77	1.27 (0.55, 2.91)	1.1 (0.37, 3.08)
3-4 gravidae	14 (21.5)	51 (78.5)	65	2.09 (0.94, 4.65)	2.19 (0.68, 6.99)
≥5 gravidae	10 (32.3)	21 (67.7)	31	**3.62 (1.43, 9.17)**	1.87 (0.31, 11.36)
Hookwarm					
Yes	8 (34.8)	15 (65.2)	23	3.01 (1.2, 7.52)	2.72 (1.01, 7.25)*
No	42 (15.1)	237 (84.9)	279	1	1
HIV					
Yes	12 (38.7)	19 (61.3)	31	3.9 (1.74, 8.62)	5.75 (2.4, 13.69)***
No	38 (14)	233 (86)	271	1	1

Bold numerical values indicate significant in bivariate but not in multivariate analysis. *Significant ($P < 0.05$), **significant ($P < 0.01$), and ***highly significant ($P < 0.001$) in multivariate analysis.

Despite this, a study from Trinidad and Tiago, multigravida had significantly increased likelihood of being anemic than primigravidae [16]. The disparity may be as a result of sociodemographic characteristic difference between study participants. In this study, participants who were multigravida had the following characteristics. 90% had normal and above BMI, 78% were urban residents, and 50% of them had middle and high monthly family income. These situations may reduce the risk of anemia in multigravida pregnant mothers participated in this study.

In this study, supplementation of iron sulphate, folic acid, and multivitamin during the current pregnancy period did not significantly reduce the prevalence of anemia as compared to those who did not take these supplementations. The finding was in contradiction with other studies [19–21, 25, 26, 28]. The possible reason may be that, in anemic pregnant women, these nutritional supplements were more likely to be prescribed as an intervention for management of anemia in their previous ANC visit. This needs a further study to explicitly explain how much effective the current WHO nutritional supplementation recommendation program is being implemented for prevention and control of anaemia in pregnant women [51].

4.1. Limitations of the Study. One of the limitation of this study is the nature of the study design its self, being as a cross-sectional study design, it does not show which preceded anemia or risk factors. Due to constraint of time and resource, stool concentration technique and parasite density were not done so we could not assess the impact of parasite load on the severity of anemia. In addition to this, the low sensitivity of wet mount to detect parasite in patient with low parasite load may underestimate the prevalence of intestinal parasite and alter odds ratio. The other limitation is that this study was conducted at tertiary care hospital located at Gondar town and majority of the study participants were urban residents. But many of the pregnant women in that district were living in rural areas where access to antenatal facilities is limited, so the prevalence of anemia would have been even more if the study was done in the general population.

5. Conclusion

In conclusion, the prevalence of anemia among pregnant women was high especially at third trimester. Mild type of anemia was the commonest one. Morphologically, the predominant type of anemia was normocytic normochromic, followed by microcytic hypochromic anemia. Low family income, high family size, *hookworm* infection, and living with HIV/AIDS were the main predictors of maternal anemia. To reduce the prevalence, there is a need to strengthen health care seeking behavior of women to ensure early diagnosis and management of HIV, hookworm, anemia, and other medical conditions. There is also a need to encourage family planning, and design policies and strategies pertinent to reduction of anemia in low income groups. A large community based study needs to be done to determine the prevalence and predictors of anemia in the general population of pregnant women. Besides, further studies using micronutrient assay techniques which are sensitive for the detection of latent anemia before the change of RBC morphology and indices takes place have to be conducted.

Conflict of Interests

The authors declare that there is no conflict of interests regarding the publication of this paper.

Authors' Contribution

Mulugeta Melku participated in designing the study, performed the data collection and statistical analysis, and was a lead author of the paper. Zelalem Addis, Meseret Alem, and Bamlaku Enawgaw participated in designing the study and helped in drafting the paper. All authors read and approved the final paper.

Acknowledgments

The authors thank all midwives and laboratory staffs who heartfully participated during data collection and laboratory analysis activities. The authors are also grateful to thank pregnant women for their voluntary participation in our study. Lastly, they would like to thank the University of Gondar and Gondar University Hospital for financial and logistics supports.

References

[1] E. McLean, M. Cogswell, I. Egli, D. Wojdyla, and B. De Benoist, "Worldwide prevalence of anaemia, WHO Vitamin and Mineral Nutrition Information System, 1993–2005," *Public Health Nutrition*, vol. 12, no. 4, pp. 444–454, 2009.

[2] WHO, *Worldwide Prevalence of Anaemia 1993–2005: WHO Global Database on Anaemia*, WHO, Geneva, Switzerland, 2008.

[3] WHO and UNICEF, *Focusing on Anaemia: Towards an Integrated Approach for Effective Anaemia Control*, WHO, Geneva, Switzerland, 2004.

[4] Y. Balarajan, U. Ramakrishnan, E. Özaltin, A. H. Shankar, and S. V. Subramanian, "Anaemia in low-income and middle-income countries," *The Lancet*, vol. 378, no. 9809, pp. 2123–2135, 2011.

[5] WHO, UNICEF, UNFPA, and World Bank, *Maternal Mortality in 2005: Estimates Developed by WHO, UNICEF, UNFPA and World Bank*, WHO, Geneva, Switzerland, 2007.

[6] F. W. Lone, R. N. Qureshi, and F. Emanuel, "Maternal anaemia and its impact on perinatal outcome," *Tropical Medicine and International Health*, vol. 9, no. 4, pp. 486–490, 2004.

[7] F. W. Lone, R. N. Qureshi, and F. Emmanuel, "Maternal anaemia and its impact on perinatal outcome in a tertiary care hospital in Pakistan," *Eastern Mediterranean Health Journal*, vol. 10, no. 6, pp. 801–807, 2004.

[8] H. S. Lee, M. S. Kim, M. H. Kim, Y. J. Kim, and W. Y. Kim, "Iron status and its association with pregnancy outcome in Korean pregnant women," *European Journal of Clinical Nutrition*, vol. 60, no. 9, pp. 1130–1135, 2006.

[9] F. Bodeau-Livinec, V. Briand, J. Berger et al., "Maternal anemia in Benin: prevalence, risk factors, and association with low birth weight," *The American Journal of Tropical Medicine and Hygiene*, vol. 85, no. 3, pp. 414–420, 2011.

[10] T. Kousar, Y. Memon, S. Sheikh, S. Memon, and R. Sehto, "Risk factors and causes of death in Neonates," *Rawal Medical Journal*, vol. 35, no. 2, pp. 205–208, 2010.

[11] B. J. Brabin, M. Hakimi, and D. Pelletier, "An analysis of anemia and pregnancy-related maternal mortality," *Journal of Nutrition*, vol. 131, no. 2, pp. 604S–615S, 2001.

[12] T. Marchant, J. A. Schellenberg, R. Nathan et al., "Anaemia in pregnancy and infant mortality in Tanzania," *Tropical Medicine and International Health*, vol. 9, no. 2, pp. 262–266, 2004.

[13] Sight and Life, "Nutritional Anemia," SIGHT AND LIFE Press, 2007, http://www.sightandlife.org/fileadmin/data/Books/Nutritional_anemia_book.pdf.

[14] S. Ouédraogo, G. K. Koura, K. Accrombessi, F. Bodeau-Livinec, A. Massougbodji, and M. Cot, "Maternal anemia at first antenatal visit: prevalence and risk factors in a malaria-endemic area in Benin," *The American Journal of Tropical Medicine and Hygiene*, vol. 87, no. 3, pp. 418–424, 2012.

[15] K. Tolentino and J. F. Friedman, "An update on anemia in less developed countries," *The American Journal of Tropical Medicine and Hygiene*, vol. 77, no. 1, pp. 44–51, 2007.

[16] E. O. Uche-Nwachi, A. Odekunle, S. Jacinto et al., "Anaemia in pregnancy: associations with parity, abortions and child spacing in primary healthcare clinic attendees in Trinidad and Tobago," *African Health Sciences*, vol. 10, no. 1, pp. 66–70, 2010.

[17] B. Sukrat and S. Sirichotiyakul, "The prevalence and causes of anemia during pregnancy in Maharaj Nakorn Chiang Mai Hospital," *Journal of the Medical Association of Thailand*, vol. 89, supplement 4, pp. S142–S146, 2006.

[18] L. Karaoglu, E. Pehlivan, M. Egri et al., "The prevalence of nutritional anemia in pregnancy in an east Anatolian province, Turkey," *BMC Public Health*, vol. 10, article 329, 2010.

[19] M.-J. A. Brian, S. D. Leary, G. D. Smith, H. J. McArdle, and A. R. Ness, "Maternal anemia, iron intake in pregnancy, and offspring blood pressure in the avon longitudinal study of parents and children," *The American Journal of Clinical Nutrition*, vol. 88, no. 4, pp. 1126–1133, 2008.

[20] E. Fujimori, A. P. S. Sato, S. C. Szarfarc et al., "Anemia in Brazilian pregnant women before and after flour fortification with iron," *Revista de Saude Publica*, vol. 45, no. 6, pp. 1027–1035, 2011.

[21] S. Thirukkanesh and A. M. Zahara, "Compliance to vitamin and mineral supplementation among pregnant women in urban and rural areas in Malaysia," *Pakistan Journal of Nutrition*, vol. 9, no. 8, pp. 744–750, 2010.

[22] J. Haniff, A. Das, L. T. Onn et al., "Anemia in pregnancy in Malaysia: a cross-sectional survey," *Asia Pacific Journal of Clinical Nutrition*, vol. 16, no. 3, pp. 527–536, 2007.

[23] L. Al-Mehaisen, Y. Khader, O. Al-Kuran, F. Abu Issa, and Z. Amarin, "Maternal anemia in rural Jordan: room for improvement," *Anemia*, vol. 2011, Article ID 381812, 7 pages, 2011.

[24] R. Ayub, N. Tariq, M. M. Adil, M. Iqbal, T. Jaferry, and S. R. Rais, "Low haemoglobin levels, its determinants and associated features among pregnant women in Islamabad and surrounding region," *Journal of the Pakistan Medical Association*, vol. 59, no. 2, pp. 86–89, 2009.

[25] Q. Zhang, Z. Li, and C. V. Ananth, "Prevalence and risk factors for anaemia in pregnant women: a population-based prospective cohort study in China," *Paediatric and Perinatal Epidemiology*, vol. 23, no. 4, pp. 282–291, 2009.

[26] R. Aikawa, N. C. Khan, S. Sasaki, and C. W. Binns, "Risk factors for iron-deficiency anaemia among pregnant women living in rural Vietnam," *Public Health Nutrition*, vol. 9, no. 4, pp. 443–448, 2006.

[27] A. J. Rodríguez-Morales, R. A. Barbella, C. Case et al., "Intestinal parasitic infections among pregnant women in Venezuela," *Infectious Diseases in Obstetrics and Gynecology*, vol. 2006, Article ID 23125, 2006.

[28] D. A. Khan, S. Fatima, R. Imran, and F. A. Khan, "Iron, folate and cobalamin deficiency in anaemic pregnant females in tertiary care centre at Rawalpindi," *Journal of Ayub Medical College, Abbottabad*, vol. 22, no. 1, pp. 17–21, 2010.

[29] N. Meda, L. Mandelbrot, M. Cartoux, B. Dao, A. Ouangré, and F. Dabis, "Anaemia during pregnancy in Burkina Faso, West Africa, 1995-96: prevalence and associated factors," *Bulletin of the World Health Organization*, vol. 77, no. 11, pp. 916–922, 1999.

[30] D. Geelhoed, F. Agadzi, L. Visser et al., "Severe anemia in pregnancy in rural Ghana: a case-control study of causes and management," *Acta Obstetricia et Gynecologica Scandinavica*, vol. 85, no. 10, pp. 1165–1171, 2006.

[31] C. C. Dim and H. E. Onah, "The prevalence of anemia among pregnant women at booking in Enugu, South Eastern Nigeria," *Journal of Obstetrics and Gynaecology*, vol. 26, no. 8, pp. 773–776, 2006.

[32] O. Adesina, A. Oladokun, O. Akinyemi, T. Akingbola, O. Awolude, and I. Adewole, "Risk of anaemia in HIV positive pregnant women in Ibadan, South West Nigeria," *African Journal of Medicine and Medical Sciences*, vol. 40, no. 1, pp. 67–73, 2011.

[33] M. D. Dairo and T. O. Lawoyin, "Socio-demographic determinants of anaemia in pregnancy at primary care level: a study in urban and rural Oyo State, Nigeria," *African Journal of Medicine and Medical Sciences*, vol. 33, no. 3, pp. 213–217, 2004.

[34] D. J. VanderJagt, H. S. Brock, G. S. Melah, A. U. El-Nafaty, M. J. Crossey, and R. H. Glew, "Nutritional factors associated with anaemia in pregnant women in northern Nigeria," *Journal of Health, Population and Nutrition*, vol. 25, no. 1, pp. 75–81, 2007.

[35] C. J. Uneke, D. D. Duhlinska, and E. B. Igbinedion, "Prevalence and public-health significance of HIV infection and anaemia among pregnant women attending antenatal clinics in southeastern Nigeria," *Journal of Health, Population and Nutrition*, vol. 25, no. 3, pp. 328–335, 2007.

[36] E. A. Achidi, A. J. Kuoh, J. T. Minang et al., "Malaria infection in pregnancy and its effects on haemoglobin levels in women from a malaria endemic area of Fako Division, South West Province, Cameroon," *Journal of Obstetrics and Gynaecology*, vol. 25, no. 3, pp. 235–240, 2005.

[37] T. Marchant, J. R. M. Armstrong Schellenberg, T. Edgar et al., "Anaemia during pregnancy in southern Tanzania," *Annals of Tropical Medicine and Parasitology*, vol. 96, no. 5, pp. 477–487, 2002.

[38] I. Adam, A. H. Khamis, and M. I. Elbashir, "Prevalence and risk factors for anaemia in pregnant women of eastern Sudan," *Transactions of the Royal Society of Tropical Medicine and Hygiene*, vol. 99, no. 10, pp. 739–743, 2005.

[39] S. Gies, B. J. Brabin, M. A. Yassin, and L. E. Cuevas, "Comparison of screening methods for anaemia in pregnant women in Awassa, Ethiopia," *Tropical Medicine and International Health*, vol. 8, no. 4, pp. 301–309, 2003.

[40] S. Desalegn, "Prevalence of anaemia in pregnancy in Jima town, Southwestern Ethiopia," *Ethiopian Medical Journal*, vol. 31, no. 4, pp. 251–258, 1993.

[41] T. Belachew and Y. Legesse, "Risk factors for anemia among pregnant women attending antenatal clinic at Jimma University Hospital, southwest Ethiopia," *Ethiopian Medical Journal*, vol. 44, no. 3, pp. 211–220, 2006.

[42] United Nation, *United Nations Millennium Declaration: Resolution Adopted By the Geneal Assembly*, United Nation, Newyork, NY, USA, 2000.

[43] World Health Organization, "The World Health Report 2002: Reducing risks, promoting healthy life," 2002, http://www.who.int/whr/2002/en/whr02_en.pdf.

[44] CSA, *Summary and Statistical Report of the 2007 Population and Housing Census: Population Size By Age and Sex*, CSA, Addis Ababa, Ethiopia, 2008.

[45] WHO, *Haemoglobin Concentrations For the Diagnosis of Anaemia and Assessment of Severity, Vitamin and Mineral Nutrition Information System*, WHO, Geneva, Switzerland, 2011.

[46] M. Alem, B. Enawgaw, A. Gelaw, T. Kena, M. Seid, and Y. Olkeba, "Prevalence of anemia and associated risk factors among pregnant women attending antenatal care in Azezo Health Center Gondar town, Northwest Ethiopia," *Journal of Interdisciplinary Histopathology*, vol. 1, no. 3, pp. 137–144, 2013.

[47] CSA, *Ethiopia Demographic and Health Survey: Preliminary Report*, CSA, Addis Ababa, Ethiopia, 2011.

[48] CSA, *Household Income, Consumption and Expenditure (HICE) Survey 2004/5. Volume I: Analytical Report*, CSA, Addis Ababa, Ethiopia, 2007.

[49] D. H. Henry and J. A. Hoxie, "Hematologic manifestation of AIDS," in *Hematology: Basic Principles and Practices*, R. Hofman, E. Benz, S. Shattil et al., Eds., pp. 2585–2628, Churchill Livingstone, New York, NY, USA, 5th edition, 2008.

[50] S. Brooker, P. J. Hotez, and D. A. P. Bundy, "Hookworm-related anaemia among pregnant women: a systematic review," *PLoS Neglected Tropical Diseases*, vol. 2, no. 9, article e291, 2008.

[51] UNICEF, UNU, and WHO, *Iron Deficiency Anemia: Assessment, Prevention, and Control*, WHO, Geneva, Switzerland, 2001.

2

Validation of the WHO Hemoglobin Color Scale Method

Leeniyagala Gamaralalage Thamal Darshana and Deepthi Inoka Uluwaduge

Medical Laboratory Sciences Unit, Department of Allied Health Sciences, Faculty of Medical Sciences, University of Sri Jayewardenepura, Gangodawila, Nugegoda 10250, Sri Lanka

Correspondence should be addressed to Leeniyagala Gamaralalage Thamal Darshana; darshana0031@gmail.com

Academic Editor: Eitan Fibach

This study was carried out to evaluate the diagnostic accuracy of WHO color scale in screening anemia during blood donor selection in Sri Lanka. A comparative cross-sectional study was conducted by the Medical Laboratory Sciences Unit of University of Sri Jayewardenepura in collaboration with National Blood Transfusion Centre, Sri Lanka. A total of 100 subjects participated in this study. Hemoglobin value of each participant was analyzed by both WHO color scale method and cyanmethemoglobin method. Bland-Altman plot was used to determine the agreement between the two methods. Sensitivity, specificity, predictive values, false positive, and negative rates were calculated. The sensitivity of the WHO color scale was very low. The highest sensitivity observed was 55.55% in hemoglobin concentrations >13.1 g/dL and the lowest was 28.57% in hemoglobin concentrations between 7.1 and 9.0 g/dL. The mean difference between the WHO color scale and the cyanmethemoglobin method was 0.2 g/dL (95% confidence interval; 3.2 g/dL above and 2.8 g/dL below). Even though the WHO color scale is an inexpensive and portable method for field studies, from the overall results in this study it is concluded that WHO color scale is an inaccurate method to screen anemia during blood donations.

1. Introduction

Anemia is a public health problem that affects both developed and developing countries. Pregnant women and young children are the most affected groups by its overwhelming effects. Hemoglobin concentration is considered as the most reliable indicator of anemia than the clinical findings [1]. The World Health Organization (WHO) color scale method is an inexpensive method for estimating hemoglobin concentration from a drop of blood by means of a color scale [2]. The color scale comprises a small card with six shades of red that represent hemoglobin levels at 4, 6, 8, 10, 12, and 14 g/dL, respectively [3]. Although many absorbent papers were tested, it was concluded that the Whatman 31 ET paper gave the best results with regular round stain of a limited spread. The color standards are printed in a continuous row without any separation and are mounted on a rigid white polyvinyl chloride or polypropylene sheet or thick card with a neutral pale-grey matt background. Estimation of the hemoglobin is done by matching the blood sample with the color standards through circular apertures which are placed in the center of each color standard [4]. The WHO color scale was primarily designed for anemia screening in obstetrical management, pediatric clinics, malaria and hookworm control programs, blood transfusion donor selection, and epidemiological surveys [2, 5, 6].

WHO color scale is a semiqualitative method and over the years it has been a useful tool in identifying anemia in field studies. Efficiency in terms of cost, accuracy, and time makes it an important resource in primary health care settings in developing countries. At present WHO color scale is the most widely used method for detecting anemia in settings where there is no laboratory. It performs better than clinical diagnosis alone in detecting mild to moderate anemia. However color scale's detecting ability is reduced as anemia becomes more severe [7].

Sensitivity and specificity of WHO color scale were very high in laboratory based studies but reduced considerably in field studies [7]. A comparative cross-sectional study done in Ethiopia showed a very low sensitivity in detecting anemia among pregnant mothers [5]. Sensitivity for the hemoglobin values <9 g/dL was 42.9% and for values <10 g/dL was 33.3%

whereas sensitivity for the hemoglobin values <11 g/dL was 43.5%. However specificity remained relatively high in all three categories [5]. Underestimation of the high hemoglobin levels is also reported by Montresor et al. in a field study conducted to detect the anemia among preschool children in Zanzibar [6]. High number of false positives is another problem associated with the WHO color scale. Barduagni et al. have reported very low positive predictive value (PPV) for the color scale (26.7%) in a study which assessed the prevalence of anemia among school children in Northern Egypt suggesting that high number of healthy individuals can be labeled as anemic [8]. Similar results were reported by van den Broek et al. in a study assessing the potential of WHO color scale in anemia screening of pregnant mothers. Positive predictive values were very low for hemoglobin concentrations of ≤8 g/dL and ≤6 g/dL (11.1% and 15.8%, resp.) giving large amounts of false positives as anemic [9].

The predonation assessment of the blood donor hemoglobin is the best approach to determine the iron-status of the donor. Hemoglobin screening prior to blood donation is essential to safeguard anemic individuals from blood donating and protects returning donors from donation-induced iron deficiency [10]. WHO color scale is a common tool that is used to screen anemia during blood donation because of its simplicity [1]. However, some issues have been raised regarding its screening accuracy. Shahshahani and Amiri have reported relatively low sensitivity for the WHO color scale (54.5%) in a study which screened individuals prior to blood donation in Iran. Hemoglobin levels measured by color scale were significantly lower (0.32 ± 0.65 g/dL; $P < 0.001$) than the levels measured by the standard method [11]. In Sri Lanka too WHO color scale is the mostly used tool to screen anemia prior to blood donation. The present study was undertaken to evaluate the diagnostic accuracy of WHO color scale in screening anemia during blood donor selection in Sri Lanka.

2. Materials and Methods

A comparative cross-sectional study was conducted by the Medical Laboratory Sciences Unit of University of Sri Jayewardenepura in collaboration with National Blood Transfusion Centre, Sri Lanka. Study subjects were chosen from the donors who were attending above center and the data was collected between January and April 2010. Informed written consents were obtained from each and every participant prior to the inclusion. Ethical clearances were obtained in written statements form Ethical Review Committee of University of Sri Jayewardenepura and National Blood Transfusion Centre, Sri Lanka. A total of 100 subjects were selected as the participants for the study.

Finger pricked blood was used to measure the color scale hemoglobin value. A blood drop was placed on the test strip provided with the color scale and after waiting for 30 seconds the color of the blood spot was immediately matched against the given color standards (4, 6, 8, 10, 12, and 14 g/dL) and the corresponding value was recorded. Venous blood (2 mL) was collected from each subject into

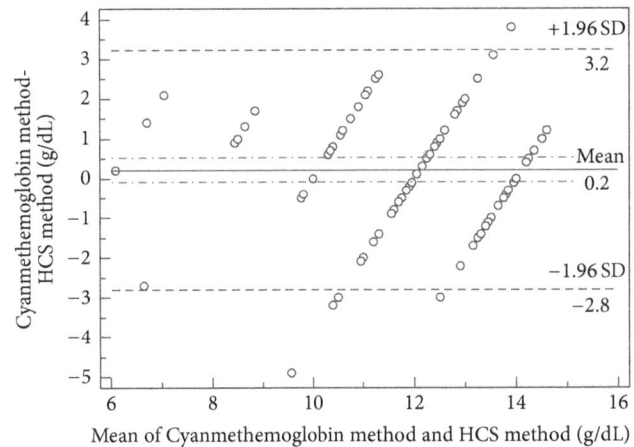

FIGURE 1: Bland-Altman plot for the haemoglobin colour scale compared with the reference method (cyanmethemoglobin method).

EDTA (ethylenediamine tetraacetic acid) containers for the laboratory assessments. Internationally recommended (gold standard) cyanmethemoglobin method was used to determine the reference hemoglobin concentrations of the blood samples [12]. Anticoagulated venous blood (20 μL) was mixed with Drabkin's diluting fluid (5 mL) and after 5 minutes absorbance was taken at 540 nm by using a Labomed UV-VIS AUTO-UV-2602 spectrophotometer. Hemoglobin concentration was measured from a previously prepared standard curve with a hemoglobin standard (concentration of 660 mg/L to 250 times diluted blood of 16.5 g/dL). All the laboratory procedures including preparation of dilutions, absorbance reading, and measuring of hemoglobin concentration from the standard curve were done by single qualified laboratory technician to avoid the operator bias. Laboratory reference hemoglobin value was recorded in g/dL to one single decimal point and WHO color scale results were compared with the laboratory reference readings. Sensitivity, specificity, positive predictive value, and negative predictive values were measured. Bland-Altman plot and proximities of the color scale value to the reference value were obtained (Figure 1). All the statistical analyses were done by using Microsoft Office Excel 2007 and SPSS software version 12.0.

3. Results

Subjects were divided into five categories depending on their reference hemoglobin concentrations (Table 1). Sensitivity and the specificity of the WHO color scale remained low in all five categories; however, the sensitivity showed tendency to increase slightly when the hemoglobin concentration is increasing. Positive predictive value was very low in severe-moderate anemic regions (2.08%, in 5–7 g/dL; 4.44%, in 7.1–9 g/dL) indicating high rate of false positives at very low hemoglobin concentrations. Contrastingly, negative predictive value of the color scale remained relatively high in severe to mild anemic regions.

WHO color scale readings of 53 subjects out of 100 were within the range of the reference hemoglobin value ±1.0.

TABLE 1: Reliability of WHO color scale with the reference method (cyanmethemoglobin method).

Hemoglobin concentration (g/dL)	5–7	7.1–9	9.1–11	11.1–13	>13.1
Specificity %	52.04	53.76	52.94	49.01	50.68
Sensitivity %	50	28.57	46.66	55.10	55.55
Positive prediction %	2.08	4.44	14.89	50.94	29.41
Negative prediction %	98.08	90.9	84.90	53.19	75.51

TABLE 2: Proximity of the test results to the reference method (cyanmethemoglobin method).

	Proximity to reference hemoglobin (g/dL)			
	±1.0	±1.1–2.0	±2.1–3.0	± >3.0
Number of subjects	53	30	12	05

Color scale results of the other 47 subjects were deviated from the reference value ±1.0. Seventeen subjects (17) had their hemoglobin values deviated from reference value ±2.0 (Table 2).

The mean difference value for the two methods (WHO color scale and cyanmethemoglobin method) was 0.2 g/dL. The limits of agreements for the two methods given by Bland-Altman plot were shown as the mean difference ±1.96 standard deviation. The limits of agreements for the WHO color scale were 2.8 g/dL below and 3.2 g/dL above.

4. Discussion

Sensitivity and specificity are two of the very important parameters required by a screening test to be validated. Diagnostic ability of a test method highly depends on these parameters. In the present study we observed low sensitivity and specificity values for all five hemoglobin concentrations (Table 1). Although slight increase in the sensitivity was observed when the hemoglobin concentration is increasing, that too was relatively low (55.55%) being the maximum sensitivity observed. The lowest sensitivity (28.57%) was observed in moderate anemic region (7.1–9 g/dL) and this result is somewhat similar to Gies et al. who have reported the lowest sensitivity (33.3%) of color scale for hemoglobin concentration <10 g/dL region indicating the poor accuracy of color scale in low hemoglobin concentrations [5].

In the present study, we observed low positive predictive values for the color scale. Lowest positive predictive value (2.08%) was observed in severe anemic (hemoglobin 5–7 g/dL) category. This implies high number of healthy nonanemic individuals can be diagnosed as anemic individuals. Our positive predictive value (4.44% for hemoglobin 7.1–9 g/dL) is even lower than van den Broek et al. who have reported positive predictive value (11.1%) for a similar hemoglobin range (≤8 g/dL) [9].

WHO color scale, at best, can measure hemoglobin value ±1 g/dL of reference hemoglobin value. Any value given by color scale outside this range would be inaccurate. In the present study only 53% of the data procured the appropriate range. Almost half of the values (47%) given by color scale

being different from more than ±1 g/dL of reference value imply the poor performance of the color scale in field studies.

When examining the diagnostic accuracy of a test method (in this case WHO color scale) examining the agreement between test method and the gold standard method is vital. Bland-Altman plot was designed to measure the agreement and establish a limit of agreement of two test methods [13]. Therefore we used Bland-Altman plot to compare the agreement between the color scale and the reference instead of correlation coefficient or regression analysis. According to the results obtained from Bland-Altman plot the limits of agreement (the scattering area in which 95% of data are distributed) were 2.8 g/dL below and 3.2 g/dL above demonstrating a wide range of agreement (6 g/dL) for the color scale which is poor and unacceptable. The agreement would have been acceptable if it were 2 g/dL as ±1 g/dL change in color scale result to the reference value can be acceptable. Similar results were reported in a study done in England in which the limits of agreement for the WHO color scale were 3.50 g/dL below and 3.11 g/dL above and the range of agreement was slightly higher (6.61 g/dL) than the present study [14].

In the present study overall performance of the WHO color scale is not satisfactory. Interobserver variation could be a factor for the poor accuracy of the color scale. In this study color scale readings were taken by 3 public health inspectors who were working at the National Blood Transfusion Centre. Reading of the color scale under faded light or under weak light and the discoloration could be the factors interfering with the reading of color scale. Although it was made with Whatman 31 ET special chromatographic paper, there is a tendency to discoloration of the paper as it becomes older. This could substantially affect the reading of the color scale.

5. Conclusion

The WHO color scale is an inexpensive, portable, and easy method to screen anemia. Although its accuracy remains high in laboratory based studies, when it comes to field studies the accuracy becomes questionable. It was developed to be an alternative of the clinical evaluation of anemia and not of a spectrophotometer, but whenever a spectrophotometer is available that method should be preferred to the WHO color scale method in measuring the hemoglobin level. For the areas where spectrophotometers are not available clinical evaluation could be better than the WHO color scale. In future studies large sample numbers are recommended to obtain better results.

Conflict of Interests

The authors declare that there is no conflict of interests regarding the publication of this paper.

Acknowledgments

The authors gratefully acknowledge the support given by the director and the staff of National Blood Transfusion

Centre, Sri Lanka, and the staff of Medical Laboratory Sciences Unit, Faculty of Medical Sciences of University of Sri Jayewardenepura.

References

[1] World Health Organization, *Worldwide Prevalence of Anaemia 1993–2005, WHO Global Database on Anaemia*, WHO, Geneva, Switzerland, 2008.

[2] S. M. Lewis, G. J. Stott, and K. J. Wynn, "An inexpensive and reliable new haemoglobin colour scale for assessing anaemia," *Journal of Clinical Pathology*, vol. 51, no. 1, pp. 21–24, 1998.

[3] World Health Organization, *Haemoglobin Colour Scale: Practical Answer to a vital Need*, Department of Blood Safety and Clinical Technology, WHO, Geneva, Switzerland, 2001.

[4] G. J. Stott and S. M. Lewis, "A simple and reliable method for estimating haemoglobin," *Bulletin of the World Health Organization*, vol. 73, no. 3, pp. 369–373, 1995.

[5] S. Gies, B. J. Brabin, M. A. Yassin, and L. E. Cuevas, "Comparison of screening methods for anaemia in pregnant women in Awassa, Ethiopia," *Tropical Medicine and International Health*, vol. 8, no. 4, pp. 301–309, 2003.

[6] A. Montresor, M. Albonico, N. Khalfan et al., "Field trial of a haemoglobin colour scale: an effective tool to detect anaemia in preschool children," *Tropical Medicine and International Health*, vol. 5, no. 2, pp. 129–133, 2000.

[7] J. Critchley and I. Bates, "Haemoglobin colour scale for anaemia diagnosis where there is no laboratory: a systematic review," *International Journal of Epidemiology*, vol. 34, no. 6, pp. 1425–1434, 2005.

[8] P. Barduagni, A. S. Ahmed, F. Curtale, M. Raafat, and L. Soliman, "Performance of Sahli and colour scale methods in diagnosing anaemia among school children in low prevalence areas," *Tropical Medicine and International Health*, vol. 8, no. 7, pp. 615–618, 2003.

[9] N. R. van den Broek, C. Ntonya, E. Mhango, and S. A. White, "Diagnosing anaemia in pregnancy in rural clinics: assessing the potential of the haemoglobin colour scale," *Bulletin of the World Health Organization*, vol. 77, no. 1, pp. 15–21, 1999.

[10] World Health Organization, *Blood Donor Selection: Guidelines on Assessing Donor Suitability for Blood Donation*, WHO, Geneva, Switzerland, 2012.

[11] H. J. Shahshahani and F. Amiri, "Validity of hemoglobin color scale in blood donor screening based on Standard Operating Procedures of Iranian Blood Transfusion Organization," *Sci J Blood Transfus Organ*, vol. 5, no. 4, pp. 281–286, 2009.

[12] B. J. Bain, I. Bates, and S. M. Lewis, *Dacie and Lewis Practical Haematology*, Churchill Livingstone, Philadelphia, Pa, USA, 11th edition, 2011.

[13] J. M. Bland and D. G. Altman, "Statistical methods for assessing agreement between two methods of clinical measurement," *The Lancet*, vol. 1, no. 8476, pp. 307–310, 1986.

[14] J. J. Paddle, "Evaluation of the Haemoglobin colour scale and comparison with the HemoCue haemoglobin assay," *Bulletin of the World Health Organization*, vol. 80, no. 10, pp. 813–816, 2002.

3

Diagnosis of Fanconi Anemia: Chromosomal Breakage Analysis

Anneke B. Oostra, Aggie W. M. Nieuwint, Hans Joenje, and Johan P. de Winter

Department of Clinical Genetics, VU University Medical Center, Van der Boechorststraat 7, 1081 BT Amsterdam, The Netherlands

Correspondence should be addressed to Johan P. de Winter, j.dewinter@vumc.nl

Academic Editor: Stefan Meyer

Fanconi anemia (FA) is a rare inherited syndrome with diverse clinical symptoms including developmental defects, short stature, bone marrow failure, and a high risk of malignancies. Fifteen genetic subtypes have been distinguished so far. The mode of inheritance for all subtypes is autosomal recessive, except for FA-B, which is X-linked. Cells derived from FA patients are—by definition—hypersensitive to DNA cross-linking agents, such as mitomycin C, diepoxybutane, or cisplatinum, which becomes manifest as excessive growth inhibition, cell cycle arrest, and chromosomal breakage upon cellular exposure to these drugs. Here we provide a detailed laboratory protocol for the accurate assessment of the FA diagnosis as based on mitomycin C-induced chromosomal breakage analysis in whole-blood cultures. The method also enables a quantitative estimate of the degree of mosaicism in the lymphocyte compartment of the patient.

1. Introduction

Fanconi anemia (FA) is a cancer-prone chromosomal instability disorder with diverse clinical symptoms (Table 1) [1]. Because of its rarity and variable presentation FA may be heavily underdiagnosed [2, 3]. Clinical suspicion of FA is mostly based on growth retardation and congenital defects in combination with life-threatening bone marrow failure (thrombocytopenia and later pancytopenia), which usually starts between 5 and 10 years of age. However, the clinical manifestations are highly variable, while some of the symptoms may overlap with those observed in other syndromes, making a reliable diagnosis on the basis of clinical features virtually impossible (Table 1). Even patients presenting with a number of "typical" FA symptoms may not be suffering from FA. Cells derived from true FA patients must exhibit a hypersensitivity to chromosomal breakage induced by DNA cross-linking agents such as mitomycin C (MMC), diepoxybutane (DEB), or cisplatinum.

Indications to test for FA are typical congenital abnormalities with/without thrombocytopenia and/or marrow failure. However, congenital abnormalities may be absent, while isolated thrombocytopenia may be the only presenting symptom. In all children with aplastic anemia FA should

be tested as the possible underlying disease. In children and adults with cancer and an unusual response to DNA-damaging agents such as chemotherapy or radiotherapy (severe skin reactions or mucositis, longlasting aplasia), FA should also be tested for. Similarly, in adults with carcinomas (typically located in the mouth/esophagus or anogenital region) at relatively young age, FA should be considered. Cancer or leukemia may be the first symptom of FA, while congenital abnormalities and marrow failure may be absent altogether, the latter especially in cases with hematopoietic mosaicism [4–6].

The cellular phenotype typical for FA is ascertained using phytohaemagglutinin-stimulated whole-blood (T lymphocyte) cultures. Although it has been considered the gold standard for diagnosing FA, the test is not 100% specific. A few cases of Nijmegen breakage syndrome have been reported to give a false positive result [7–9], which can be excluded by screening the *NBS1* gene for mutations. In addition, patients suffering from the cohesinopathies Roberts syndrome (mutated in *ESCO2*) and Warsaw breakage syndrome (mutated in *DDX11*) may score positive in the test [10]. Additional "atypical FA" or "FA-like" patients have been reported as case reports [11, 12]. Somewhat controversially, the "FA-like" patient found to be mutated in

TABLE 1: General features and symptoms associated with Fanconi anemia.

Birth prevalence	$0.5–2.5$ per 10^5 newborns; varies with ethnic background.
Mode of inheritance	Autosomal recessive ($>98\%$) and X-linked (~ 1-2%).
Carrier frequency	Traditional overall estimate: "1/300 worldwide." Needs reassessment according to subtype and ethnic background.
Congenital abnormalities*	Radial ray abnormalities (aplastic or hypoplastic radii and absent or extra thumbs) and other skeletal abnormalities; small head circumference; abnormal shape of the ears; **microphthalmia**; ectopic or horse-shoe kidney; **hypogonadism**; heart abnormalities; intestinal or anal atresia.
Other somatic abnormalities*	**Short stature/retarded growth; reduced fertility; skin pigmentation abnormalities (hyperpigmentation, café-au-lait spots)**; deafness. Endocrinopathy affecting the pancreas (diabetes mellitus), growth hormone deficiency, and hypothyroidism; early menopause.
Hematological symptoms	Bone marrow failure or aplastic anemia typically starting at 5–10 years with thrombocytopenia. Exception: D1 and N patients may die before that age from AML or other childhood solid tumors (such as medullo- or nephroblastoma).
Cancer risk	800-fold increased risk of AML, mostly occurring at age 5–15 years, typically after the onset of marrow failure. At older ages there is a similarly increased risk of solid tumors, mainly carcinomas of the head and neck or oesophagus, as well as, in females, the vulva and vagina. D1 and N patients typically develop malignancies during early childhood (<5 years).
Overlapping syndromes**	*Inherited bone marrow failure syndromes*: Dyskeratosis congenita, Diamond-Blackfan anemia, Shwachman-Diamond syndrome, severe congenital neutropenia, thrombocytopenia absent radii (TAR) syndrome, amegakaryocytic thrombocytopenia. *Other overlapping syndromes*: Baller-Gerold syndrome, *Nijmegen breakage syndrome*, Rothmund-Thomson syndrome, *Roberts syndrome*, *Warsaw Breakage syndrome*, DK-phocomelia, VACTERL hydrocephalus syndrome, Wiskott-Aldrich syndrome.

*Many symptoms show highly variable penetrance. In a sizable proportion of patients (ca. 30%), congenital abnormalities may be absent altogether. Features in bold are most consistently associated with the FA phenotype.
**For an overview of the overlapping inherited bone marrow failure syndromes, see [5, 25]. For the other overlapping syndromes, the reader is referred to the OMIM database. Three overlapping syndromes may score positive in a chromosomal breakage test (italic): Nijmegen breakage syndrome [7–9], Roberts syndrome, and Warsaw Breakage Syndrome [10].

RAD51C has been assigned to a distinct genetic FA subtype (FA-O) [13].

Approximately 80% of the patients referred for FA diagnostic testing because of bone marrow failure score negative in the chromosomal breakage test. These "true negatives" have other causes of marrow failure and most often represent cases with acquired aplastic anemia.

Lymphocyte mosaicism occurs in a sizable proportion of FA patients (estimated at 10–30%) and is caused by spontaneous genetic reversion at the disease locus in hematopoietic progenitor cells; the reverted cells may (partially) correct the bone marrow failure [14–18]. In most of these cases FA can still be diagnosed by testing peripheral blood, since a portion of the cells will still show hypersensitivity to crosslinking agents. Occasionally, the percentage of reverted cells has reached such a high level as to produce a false negative diagnosis. In such cases cross-linker sensitivity may be tested in skin fibroblasts, which are not known to be affected by mosaicism. After a positive breakage test result has been obtained, screening for mutations in the known FA genes is warranted.

Laboratory studies have revealed as many as 15 distinct "complementation groups" or genetic subtypes: FA-A, -B,
-C, -D1, -D2, -E, -F, -G, -I, -J, -L, -M, -N, -O, and -P [13, 19–21]. For all subtypes known to date the disease genes have been identified. Global relative prevalences are difficult to estimate, as the values may differ considerably depending on the ethnic background, due to founder effects. All FA genes are localized on autosomes, except *FANCB*, which is X-linked and subject to X inactivation in female carriers [22]. These two different modes of inheritance have important consequences for the counseling of FA families.

Recognition of FA as a chromosomal instability disorder was originally based on chromatid-type aberrations spontaneously occurring in standard cytogenetic preparations. However, this phenomenon was later found to be highly variable and considered not reliable for diagnostic purposes. After the discovery of an extreme sensitivity of FA cells to the chromosome-breaking effect of the cross-linking agents mitomycin C (MMC) [23] and diepoxybutane (DEB) [24], this feature has become routinely utilized to diagnose FA by a "chromosomal breakage test." In this test, T lymphocytes in a peripheral blood sample are cultured in the presence of a cross-linking agent, after which chromosomal aberrations are quantified in metaphase spreads. Numerous variations of the test are used in the various cytogenetic laboratories, with significant differences in exposure times and drug concentrations. Also, the ways in which data are evaluated are diverse. We have encountered opposite conclusions from different laboratories based on the very same primary data set, due to a lack of experience in performing the test and evaluating the resulting data. Evidently, there is a great need for a clearly described reliable protocol for the accurate diagnosis of FA patients.

2. Methods and Results

Here we describe a laboratory protocol that has evolved during 30 years of experience and which we can recommend for the unambiguous diagnosis of the vast majority of FA patients, including patients with hematopoietic mosaicism. The test is based on the 72 hour whole-blood cultures as routinely applied in cytogenetics laboratories to make chromosomal preparations for karyotypic analysis. Metaphase spreads are Giemsa-stained (not banded) and analyzed for microscopically visible chromatid-type aberrations. For technical details the reader is referred to the appendices. Laboratories that are not set up to do this type of assay or have no experience with diagnosing FA on a regular basis should be advised to refer to a laboratory where the test is applied on a routine basis, rather than attempting to carry out a "similar" test that is considered a plausible alternative. The test might be omitted if a proband belongs to an ethnic population with a high carrier frequency for a specific FA gene mutation. Demonstrating this mutation in the proband would be diagnostic for FA, although the result may not provide information about possible mosaicism.

3. Discussion

It should be pointed out that, even though we have chosen to use MMC as the cross-linking agent, DEB is used in a widely accepted alternative protocol [1, 26–28]. Pros and cons for using the various cross-linking agents are further discussed in the appendices.

Cell cycle analysis via flow cytometry has been used as an alternative way to diagnose FA in skin fibroblasts [29], amniocytes [30], and peripheral blood mononuclear cells [31–34]. This test is based on the fact that cells from FA patients are hypersensitive towards DNA cross-linking agents and tend to be delayed and arrested with a 4c DNA content in the late S/early G2 phase of the cell cycle [35–38]. With the exception of overt leukemia and complete lymphocyte mosaicism, the cell cycle test reliably differentiates between FA and non-FA blood samples, including non-FA patients with aplastic anemia, Nijmegen breakage syndrome, Roberts syndrome, Baller-Gerold syndrome, VACTERL, and other thrombo- and erythropenia syndromes, as these conditions lack elevated G2-phase cell fractions [39]. For details of the cell cycle assay, readers are referred to the published protocols [39, 40].

FANCD2 western blotting is another alternative procedure to diagnose FA [40]. With this method stimulated T lymphocytes are tested for the occurrence of the ubiquitinated isoform of FANCD2, which readily reveals FA in cases where this isoform is lacking (subtypes A, B, C, D2, E, F, G, I, L, and M). This is a convenient alternative for diagnosing >90% of all FA patients. A disadvantage is that the subtypes with a defect downstream of FANCD2 ubiquitination (D1, J, M, N, O, P and possibly new subtypes) are not diagnosed as FA. In addition, true FA cases with significant lymphocyte mosaicism may also be missed by FANCD2 western blotting.

Why would a relatively laborious breakage test still be relevant now that next-generation sequencing (NGS) is available to determine mutations in FA genes? Two types of result from NGS would require assessment of the cross-linker sensitive cellular phenotype. First, unclassified sequence variations may be identified, whose pathogenic status remains uncertain until functionally tested. Second, if all known FA genes were found to be unaffected by mutations, a putative new FA gene may be found mutated. Proof of identity as a new FA gene requires the demonstration of cellular hypersensitivity to cross-linking agents and some form of functional test where introduction of a wild-type allele should correct the phenotype.

Appendices

A. Laboratory Protocol for Testing MMC-Induced Chromosomal Breakage

A.1. Materials

(1) Heparinized venous blood (≥ 2 mL; preferably freshly drawn, or kept at room temperature for no longer than 48 h) from the patient to be tested and from a healthy control.

(2) RPMI or Ham's F10 culture medium, including 15% fetal bovine serum, streptomycin, penicillin, and phytohemagglutinin, as utilized in standard cytogenetic whole-blood cultures.

(3) Mitomycin C (MMC, mol. wt. 334.33, Kyowa Hakko Kogyo Co., Ltd., Tokyo, Japan, clinical grade), available in vials of 2 mg with 48 mg NaCl, to be stored at 4°C.

(4) Materials for the preparation of metaphase spreads.

A.2. Culturing and Cytogenetics Methods

(1) Prepare a stock solution of MMC at 1.5 mM (0.5 mg/mL) by adding 4 mL sterile water per vial; this solution is stable for 3 months at 4°C. It is mandatory "not" to freeze the MMC stock solution, since—upon thawing—an unknown quantity of MMC appears as crystals that do not readily redissolve.

(2) Prepare whole-blood cultures from the patient and the healthy control, as usual for a standard cytogenetic analysis [25]. You need 4 cultures for the patient and 4 for the healthy control, who should *not* be

a brother or sister of the patient. Initiate the cultures by adding 0.5 mL blood to 4.5 mL complete medium.

(3) Add, at the time of culture initiation, to each set of 4 cultures: 0, 50, 150, and 300 nM MMC, as indicated below.

    (i) Dilute 1 part stock solution plus 9 parts H_2O → *solution A* (150 μM).

    (ii) Dilute 1 part solution A plus 4 parts H_2O → *solution B* (30 μM).

    (iii) Add to the 4 cultures from each individual:

        (a) 50 μL saline → final concentration: 0 nM,

        (b) 8.3 μL solution B → final concentration: 50 nM (optional),

        (c) 25 μL solution B → final concentration: 150 nM,

        (d) 50 μL solution B → final concentration: 300 nM.
        N.B. If insufficient blood should be available, the 50 nM cultures may be omitted.

(4) Harvest at 72 h, after colcemid treatment during the last 40 min (Sigma, demecolcine final concentration 200 ng/mL). Prepare at least 4 microscope slides for every culture; make more slides if mitotic activity is low, to end up with at least several hundreds of metaphases, accounting for the possibility that a large proportion will later be judged unacceptable for microscopic analysis. Stain with Giemsa only. Do not apply any banding technique. Store remaining suspension at –20°C, for future use, if necessary.

A.3. Scoring the Aberrations. It is important to realize that quantification of chromosomal aberrations shows significant differences between laboratories. From a comparative study it appeared that the most important source of disagreement was about whether particular aberrations really existed or not, and about the definition and scoring of gaps [41]. It is therefore mandatory to score metaphases from coded slides ("blind"), that is, without knowing the identity of the preparation you are scoring. Do not score more than 25 cells per slide. This is to reduce the possibility of biased scoring, which would result from inspecting too many metaphases from the same slide. To obtain sufficient statistical power of the breakage data, attempt to find and score at least 50 scorable metaphases per culture (to be scored from at least two slides).

A.3.1. Coding and Organizing the Slides before Scoring. After staining, divide the slides into two equal sets per culture, each set containing 2, 3, or more slides (depending on metaphase yield) to allow the analysis of 25 scorable metaphases per set (see also Appendix A.2, point 4). Cover the unique identifier information on the slide with a piece of nontransparent tape. Write a random code on each set of slides and distinguish multiple slides within a set by adding A, B, C, and so forth.

Example 1. for every culture, you end up with 4 slides or more (depending on the mitotic index), coded as follows:

[random code-1]A, [random code-1]B, and so forth; *[random code-2]A, [random code-2]B,* and so forth.

The scoring of metaphases (see below) starts with slide *[random code-1]A* until 25 metaphases have been examined. If fewer metaphases were found on the slide, proceed with slide *[random code-1]B,* and so forth, until the desired number of metaphases (in our case: 25) have been scored. Follow the same procedure for *[random code-2]A, -B, -C,* and so forth. After finishing the scoring of all preparations, the codes are uncovered and the two data sets from the various cultures are combined to provide results per 50 metaphases.

A.3.2. How to Score Chromosomal Aberrations. Systematically select the metaphases to be analysed: search, at 400x magnification, for metaphases judged suitable for evaluation of chromosomal integrity. To avoid a bias for relatively undamaged metaphases, do not at this stage select on the basis of "quality," since "nice-" looking metaphases tend to have fewer aberrations. Rather, every next metaphase encountered should—in principle—be scored, unless it must be rejected because it fails to meet the observer's criteria for adequate spreading, state of condensation of the chromosomes (not too long or too short), adequate staining and morphology (clearly recognizable chromosomes with clearly visible centromeres), and adequate ploidy. When a metaphase meets these criteria, that metaphase *must* be scored, at 1000x magnification, even if "difficult" aberrations are subsequently encountered. However, be sure to score only the *really convincing* aberrations while ignoring the unconvincing ones. Distinguish the following types of aberration:

(1) chromatid gap, an interruption in the staining of a chromatid 1-2 times the width of that chromatid (Figure 1(a));

(2) chromatid break, where the interruption is more than 2 times the width or where the broken piece of chromatid appears dislocated, as in Figure 1(b);

(3) triradial chromosome, an interchange figure presumably having resulted from the misrepair of two breaks in two distinct chromosomes (Figure 1(c));

(4) quadriradial chromosome, an interchange figure resulting from the misrepair of two broken chromatids in different chromosomes (Figure 1(d));

(5) Other chromatid interchange figures, such as illustrated in Figure 1(e).

Chromosome-type changes, such as dicentrics, acentric fragments, and ring chromosomes, may be recorded, but these aberrations, which are extremely rare with the protocol used, should not be included in the final analysis.

A.3.3. How to Record the Aberrations. The aberrations observed should be recorded with the coordinates of the metaphase, so that aberrant metaphases can be retrieved whenever considered necessary. This can be achieved manually, or with the help of an automated metaphase finder

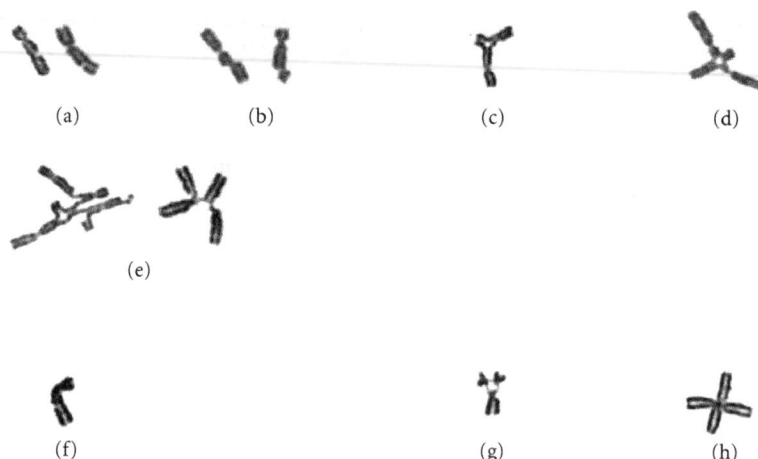

FIGURE 1: Examples of chromosomal aberrations typically observed in a MMC-induced chromosomal breakage assay to diagnose FA. (a) Chromatid gap (broken piece in place); (b) chromatid break (broken piece dislocated); (c) chromatid interchange figure ("triradial"); (d) chromatid interchange figure ("quadriradial"); (e) other chromatid interchange figures. In the eventual analysis, (a) and (b) are counted as one, (c) and (d) as two break events. The left figure in (e) is counted as 8 break events (5 centromeres plus 3 open breaks); the right figure is equivalent to a quadriradial as in (d) (2 break events), in which two break points remained disconnected. (f), (g), and (h), are examples of nonconvincing "aberrations" that should be ignored in the analysis. (f) A gap that is not 100% convincing and should be ignored. (g) An association of 3 acrocentric chromosomes showing "satellite association", not to be confused with a triradial, as in (c). (h) Two overlapping chromosomes, not to be confused with a true quadriradial, as in (d).

equipped with a customisable scoring sheet for the evaluation of chromosomal aberrations, such as developed by Metasystems, Altlussheim, Germany. A sheet developed for manual evaluation may be obtained from the authors, upon request.

A.4. Analyzing the Results

A.4.1. Converting Aberrations into Break Events. The ratio between gaps/breaks ("open breaks") and interchange-type aberrations ("wrongly repaired breaks") may vary considerably. Therefore, for the final evaluation, all aberrations are converted into "break events", which represent the primary type of aberration in an FA cell.

Chromatid gaps or breaks are counted as single break events, tri- and quadriradials as two break events each. Other interchange figures are converted into the minimum number of breaks required for their theoretical reconstruction; in practice, this means that the number of centromeres in an interchange figure is added up to the number of open breaks/gaps, see Figure 1. To avoid spending too much time on reconstructing complex interchange figures, cells showing more than 10 break events are not further quantified and are included in a common category "≥10 breaks/cell". Evaluate the data from a histogram, in which the percentage of cells is plotted against the number of break events/cell, as illustrated in Figure 2.

A.4.2. Evaluating the Results: "FA", "Non-FA", or "Mosaic FA". In cultures from a typical full-fledged FA patient a substantial proportion of the cells should show chromosomal breakage already at 50 nM MMC (Figure 2). At 150 nM MMC, the majority of cells should be aberrant, while at 300 nM no undamaged cells should be left and most cells should be in the category "≥10 breaks/cell". In contrast, cultures from the healthy control should hardly or not be affected, except at 300 nM, where typically 30% of the cells may show 1 to ≤5 break events/cell.

In cultures from FA patients with lymphocyte mosaicism, two cell populations are distinguished at 300 nM MMC, one behaving like typical FA cells, that is, showing ≥10 breaks/cell, and one behaving like healthy controls, that is, largely represented by the categories 0-, 1-, and 2-breaks/cell.

In the event of a positive result (FA or mosaic FA), all asymptomatic sibs of the patient should be tested as well, which is particularly important if the sibs are considered as potential stem cell donors. A positive result indicative of FA should immediately be evident from the histogram (Figure 2). If statistical analysis is considered necessary to "prove" a dubious diagnosis, the diagnosis "FA" is likely to be wrong.

If the result indicates "non-FA", an important question is whether the MMC concentration was correct. This is another reason why the highest concentration (300 nM) is included, since at this concentration the healthy control should show significantly elevated breakage. The difference between treated and untreated control cultures may be tested by comparing the percentages of aberrant metaphases, using a 2-sample Chi-square test. If the healthy control should fail to show a clear response to the MMC at 300 nM, the result "non-FA" is inconclusive and the test should be repeated.

B. Technical Notes and Comments

B.1. Breaks and Gaps. In the 1980s the distinction between chromatid gaps and breaks has been the subject of much

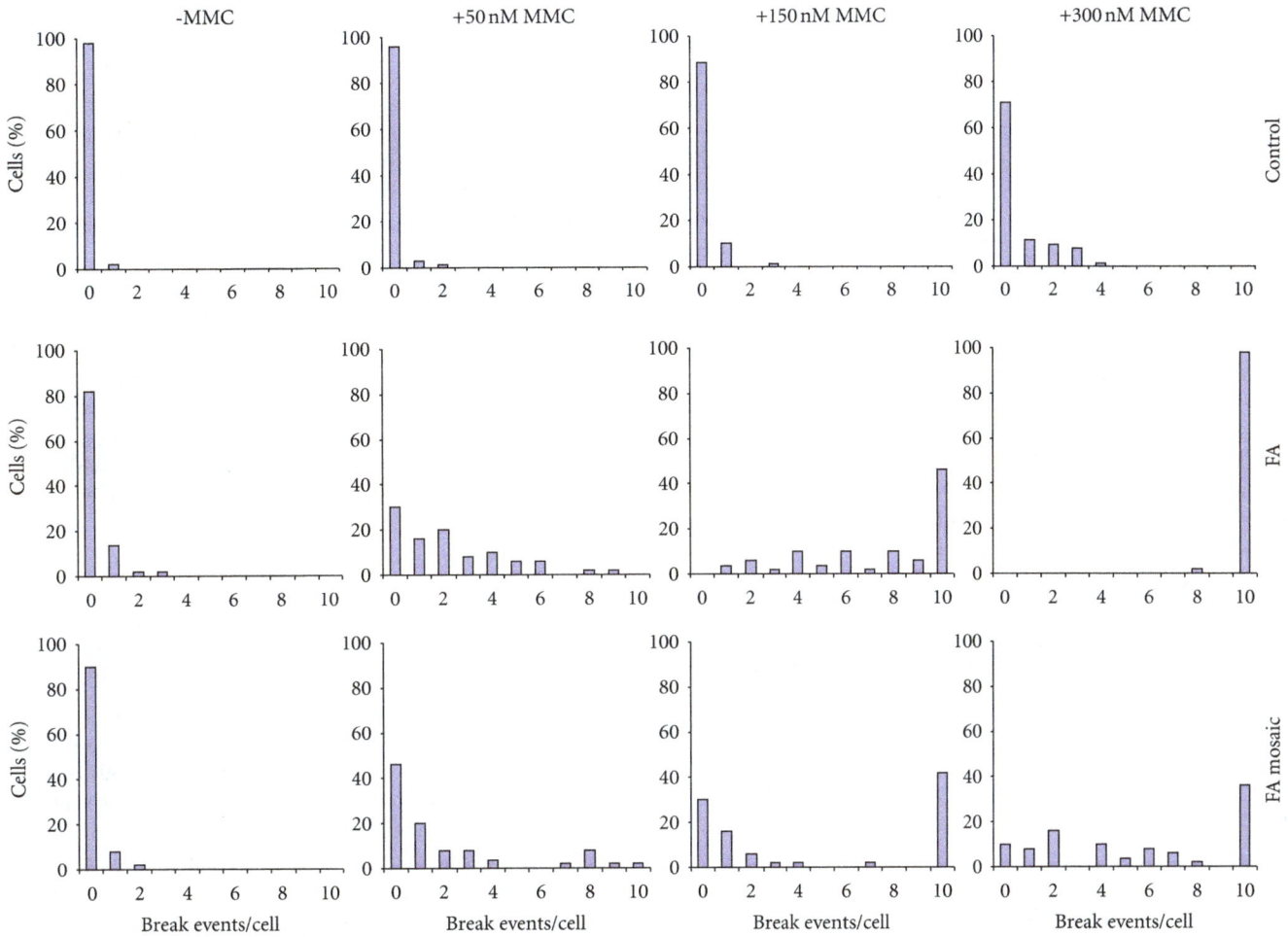

FIGURE 2: Evaluation of MMC-induced chromosomal breakage in stimulated T lymphocyte cultures. Upper row: healthy control; middle row: FA patient; lower row: mosaic FA patient. The healthy control shows breakage only at 300 nM, where the FA patient shows massive breakage (no normal cells present). Mosaicism is evident from the two highest concentrations of MMC, where there are still normal cells present next to cells showing an FA-like breakage rate (>10 breaks/cell). A crude estimate of the proportion of reverted T cells in this mosaic patient would be ~40%.

discussion, the issue being whether a gap represented a true double-stranded break in the DNA of a chromatid. A problem during the evaluation of aberrations is to decide which gap-like feature should be scored as a true aberration. A consensus was reached by accepting an aberration as a gap if the discontinuity in the staining of a chromatid is at least as wide as the width of the chromatid. If wider than twice the width of the chromatid, the aberration may be scored as a break [42]. If the "broken" piece appears dislocated the aberration is always scored as a break. If the interruption is considered doubtful, it should be ignored (Figure 1); this holds for all other aberrations that appear not entirely convincing.

The main reason to distinguish between chromatid gaps and breaks is that their biological impact may be different; conclusions based on significant differences in the frequency of gaps only, should be viewed with caution.

B.2. Saving Time on the Breakage Test

B.2.1. Finding Metaphases.
In cases of low mitotic activity considerable time may be gained by utilizing a metaphase finding apparatus, which can perform unattended metaphase searches on multiple slides. Such apparatus may also be equipped with software for chromosomal aberration scoring, see for example, http://www.metasystems-international.com/

B.2.2. Scoring Aberrations.
To save time, the scoring process may be divided into phases. Score first the cultures exposed to 0 and 300 nM MMC, which may already give you an unambiguous answer.

(1) The diagnosis "FA" is warranted if all cells from the proband contain multiple aberrations, whereas the majority of the control cells is normal.

(2) A result *excluding* FA should be based on a modest but significantly elevated breakage level at 300 nM MMC, both in the proband and in the healthy control.

If there are too few evaluable metaphases, or if there is an indication of mosaicism, score the samples exposed to 150 nM, and—with again too few metaphases present—the 50 nM samples as well. If, however, the 300 or 150 nM cultures have provided a conclusive answer, the 50 nM cultures may be skipped.

Some laboratories score only chromatid interchanges (often referred to as "radials") as aberrations, while ignoring chromatid breaks and gaps. Even though this is a considerable time saver, there are several disadvantages. First, with full-fledged (nonmosaic) FA patients "normal" cells (i.e., cells without interchange aberrations) are still observed at the higher MMC concentrations, leading to a false impression of mosaicism. Second, at the highest MMC concentration the aberration rate in the control does not reach statistical significance, which eliminates the internal check for drug activity. Third, chromatid interchanges are generated from chromatid breaks by an unknown joining mechanism, the precise nature of which is unclear, while variations in this process will affect the ratio between breaks and interchanges. As this ratio may vary from patient to patient, some FA patients might go unrecognised when scoring chromatid interchanges only.

B.2.3. High-Level Mosaicism. With the protocol described, most patients with mosaicism will be correctly diagnosed as FA, because even a minor proportion of FA-like lymphocytes will show up in the ≥ 10 breaks/cell category. When no FA cells can be detected in a patient with a "compelling" clinical phenotype, fibroblasts can be used to establish the diagnosis. We have encountered several FA patients whose T lymphocytes' response was indistinguishable from that in the healthy control, but whose skin fibroblasts' response clearly revealed the cellular FA phenotype (see, e.g., [6, 15]).

Breakage Test Using Fibroblasts. Add MMC (50 nM) or saline to either of two 80 cm^2 tissue culture flasks containing 1-2 $\times$ 10^6 freshly trypsinized fibroblasts (preferably fewer than 8 *in vitro* passages) from the following individuals: (1) the patient to be tested, (2) a healthy control, and (3) a known FA patient (positive control). After 48 h at 37°C, harvest the cultures by trypsinization, following colcemid treatment for 45 min, and prepare chromosome slides. Code the slides and score for aberrations (50 cells per culture). Typical results are as follows.

"*Control (non-FA) fibroblasts*", untreated: 3% aberrant cells (0.03 breaks/cell); *MMC-treated*: 13% aberrant cells (0.2 breaks/cell).

"*FA fibroblasts*", untreated: 7% aberrant cells (0.07 breaks/cell); *MMC-treated*: 95% aberrant cells (7 breaks/cell).

B.2.4. Alternative Cross-Linking Agents. Several other DNA cross-linking agents, besides MMC, have been used to demonstrate the hypersensitive phenotype of FA cells, for example, diepoxybutane (DEB), and cis-diamminedichloroplatinum(II) (cisplatin). DEB is on the Special Health Hazard Substance List because it is a (volatile) carcinogen that should be handled with great caution. DEB is hygroscopic and—upon contact with water—slowly loses activity, with a half-life of approximately 4 days, because it hydrolyzes into 1,2,3,4-tetrahydroxybutane, a compound with no cross-linking activity. DEB is commercially available from Sigma/Aldrich. Since different batches may vary in activity, comparative testing is required, since relatively small differences may lead to incorrect conclusions regarding mosaicism in a patient (compare the standard concentration of 0.1 μg/mL with 0.15 μg/mL in [14]). MMC, which—as a clinically approved chemotherapeutic agent produced by Kyowa Hakko Kogyo (not by Sigma)—is under rigorous quality control and is stable when stored in the vials provided by the manufacturer. A similar argument would favour the use of cisplatin, which is also clinically approved, over DEB as the diagnostic reagent for FA. On the other hand, provided the reagents are properly handled, DEB, MMC, and cisplatin are similarly effective in establishing the FA diagnosis in a chromosomal breakage assay. According to a single comparative study, MMC appeared slightly more suitable for the assessment of lymphocyte mosaicism [14]. It should be pointed out that, unlike DEB and cisplatin, MMC requires metabolic activation in order to become active as a cross-linking agent. If metabolic activation were a variable parameter, this may be considered a disadvantage for MMC and an argument in favour of choosing cisplatin as the diagnostic cross-linker.

B.2.5. Conversion of Interchanges into Break Events. Although the idea of two breaks underlying each interchange between two chromosomes (often referred to as "radial") has been considered commonplace in the genetic toxicology literature, this hypothesis is challenged by the observations of Godthelp et al. [43], who found the frequency of interchanges to increase linearly with drug dosage (rather than exponentially), implying single-hit rather than two-hit kinetics. If the single-hit principle were to be accepted, this would change the conversion factor for the quantification of interchange aberrations into break events from 2 to 1; however, adopting a conversion factor of 1 would not affect the general principle of the FA diagnosis, as described here.

Acknowledgments

The authors thank B. P. Alter, A. D. Auerbach, P. P. van Buul, H. Hoehn, D. Schindler, J. Surrallés, R. M. L. Vervenne, and M. Z. Zdzienicka, for valuable comments on an earlier version of the paper, and the Fanconi Anemia Research Fund, Inc., Eugene, OR, The Netherlands Organization for Health and Development, and the Dutch Cancer Society, for financial support.

References

[1] A. D. Auerbach, "Fanconi anemia and its diagnosis," *Mutation Research*, vol. 668, no. 1-2, pp. 4–10, 2009.

[2] P. F. Giampietro, B. Adler-Brecher, P. C. Verlander, S. G. Pavlakis, J. G. Davis, and A. D. Auerbach, "The need for more accurate and timely diagnosis in Fanconi anemia: a report from the International Fanconi Anemia Registry," *Pediatrics*, vol. 91, no. 6, pp. 1116–1120, 1993.

[3] P. F. Giampietro, P. C. Verlander, J. G. Davis, and A. D. Auerbach, "Diagnosis of Fanconi anemia in patients without congenital malformations: an International Fanconi Anemia Registry Study," *American Journal of Medical Genetics*, vol. 68, no. 1, pp. 58–61, 1997.

[4] B. P. Alter, "Cancer in Fanconi anemia, 1927–2001," *Cancer*, vol. 97, no. 2, pp. 425–440, 2003.

[5] B. P. Alter, "Bone marrow failure: a child is not just a small adult (but an adult can have a childhood disease)," *Hematology*, pp. 96–103, 2005.

[6] B. P. Alter, H. Joenje, A. B. Oostra, and G. Pals, "Fanconi anemia: adult head and neck cancer and hematopoietic mosaicism," *Archives of Otolaryngology*, vol. 131, no. 7, pp. 635–639, 2005.

[7] K. Nakanishi, T. Taniguchi, V. Ranganathan et al., "Interaction of FANCD2 and NBS1 in the DNA damage response," *Nature Cell Biology*, vol. 4, no. 12, pp. 913–920, 2002.

[8] A. R. Gennery, M. A. Slatter, A. Bhattacharya et al., "The clinical and biological overlap between Nijmegen Breakage Syndrome and Fanconi anemia," *Clinical Immunology*, vol. 113, no. 2, pp. 214–219, 2004.

[9] H. V. New, C. M. Cale, M. Tischkowitz et al., "Nijmegen breakage syndrome diagnosed as fanconi anaemia," *Pediatric Blood and Cancer*, vol. 44, no. 5, pp. 494–499, 2005.

[10] P. van der Lelij, A. B. Oostra, M. A. Rooimans, H. Joenje, and J. P. de Winter, "Diagnostic overlap between Fanconi anemia and the cohesinopathies: roberts syndrome and Warsaw Breakage Syndrome," *Anemia*, vol. 2010, Article ID 565268, 7 pages, 2010.

[11] S. Bakhshi, H. Joenje, D. Schindler et al., "A case report of a patient with microcephaly, facial dysmorphism, mitomycin-c-sensitive lymphocytes, and susceptibility to lymphoma," *Cancer Genetics and Cytogenetics*, vol. 164, no. 2, pp. 168–171, 2006.

[12] M. L. Kwee, J. M. van der Kleij, A. J. van Essen et al., "An atypical case of Fanconi anemia in elderly sibs," *American Journal of Medical Genetics*, vol. 68, no. 3, pp. 362–366, 1997.

[13] F. Vaz, H. Hanenberg, B. Schuster et al., "Mutation of the RAD51C gene in a Fanconi anemia-like disorder," *Nature Genetics*, vol. 42, no. 5, pp. 406–409, 2010.

[14] M. L. Kwee, E. H. A. Poll, J. J. P. van de Kamp, H. de Koning, A. W. Eriksson, and H. Joenje, "Unusual response to bifunctional alkylating agents in a case of Fanconi anaemia," *Human Genetics*, vol. 64, no. 4, pp. 384–387, 1983.

[15] J. R. Lo Ten Foe, M. L. Kwee, M. A. Rooimans et al., "Somatic mosaicism in Fanconi anemia: molecular basis and clinical significance," *European Journal of Human Genetics*, vol. 5, no. 3, pp. 137–148, 1997.

[16] Q. Waisfisz, N. V. Morgan, M. Savino et al., "Spontaneous functional correction of homozygous Fanconi anaemia alleles reveals novel mechanistic basis for reverse mosaicism," *Nature Genetics*, vol. 22, no. 4, pp. 379–383, 1999.

[17] J. J. Gregory, J. E. Wagner, P. C. Verlander et al., "Somatic mosaicism in Fanconi anemia: evidence of genotypic reversion in lymphohematopoietic stem cells," *Proceedings of the National Academy of Sciences of the United States of America*, vol. 98, no. 5, pp. 2532–2537, 2001.

[18] M. Gross, H. Hanenberg, S. Lobitz et al., "Reverse mosaicism in Fanconi anemia: natural gene therapy via molecular self-correction," *Cytogenetic and Genome Research*, vol. 98, no. 2-3, pp. 126–135, 2002.

[19] J. P. de Winter and H. Joenje, "The genetic and molecular basis of Fanconi anemia," *Mutation Research*, vol. 668, no. 1-2, pp. 11–19, 2009.

[20] C. Stoepker, K. Hain, B. Schuster et al., "SLX4, a coordinator of structure-specific endonucleases, is mutated in a new Fanconi anemia subtype," *Nature Genetics*, vol. 43, no. 2, pp. 138–141, 2011.

[21] Y. Kim, F. P. Lach, R. Desetty, H. Hanenberg, A. D. Auerbach, and A. Smogorzewska, "Mutations of the SLX4 gene in Fanconi anemia," *Nature Genetics*, vol. 43, no. 2, pp. 142–146, 2011.

[22] A. R. Meetei, M. Levitus, Y. Xue et al., "X-linked inheritance of Fanconi anemia complementation group B," *Nature Genetics*, vol. 36, no. 11, pp. 1219–1224, 2004.

[23] M. S. Sasaki and A. Tonomura, "A high susceptibility of Fanconi's anemia to chromosome breakage by DNA cross linking agents," *Cancer Research*, vol. 33, no. 8, pp. 1829–1836, 1973.

[24] A. D. Auerbach and S. R. Wolman, "Susceptibility of Fanconi's anaemia fibroblasts to chromosome damage by carcinogens," *Nature*, vol. 261, no. 5560, pp. 494–496, 1976.

[25] P. S. Moorhead, P. C. Nowell, W. J. Mellman, D. M. Battips, and D. A. Hungerford, "Chromosome preparations of leukocytes cultured from human peripheral blood," *Experimental Cell Research*, vol. 20, no. 3, pp. 613–616, 1960.

[26] A. D. Auerbach, "Fanconi anemia diagnosis and the diepoxybutane (DEB) test," *Experimental Hematology*, vol. 21, no. 6, pp. 731–733, 1993.

[27] A. D. Auerbach, "Diagnosis of Fanconi anemia by Diepoxybutane Analysis," in *Current Protocols in Human Genetics*, N. C. Dracopoli, J. L. Haines, B. R. Korf et al., Eds., pp. 8.7.1–8.7.15, John Wiley & Sons, Hoboken, NJ, USA, 2003.

[28] M. Castella, R. Pujol, E. Callén et al., "Chromosome fragility in patients with Fanconi anaemia: diagnostic implications and clinical impact," *Journal of Medical Genetics*, vol. 48, no. 4, pp. 242–250, 2011.

[29] T. N. Kaiser, A. Lojewski, and C. Dougherty, "Flow cytometric characterization of the response of Fanconi's anemia cells to mitomycin C treatment," *Cytometry*, vol. 2, no. 5, pp. 291–297, 1982.

[30] A. Bechtold, R. Friedl, R. Kalb et al., "Prenatal exclusion/confirmation of fanconi anemia via flow cytometry: a pilot study," *Fetal Diagnosis and Therapy*, vol. 21, no. 1, pp. 118–124, 2006.

[31] D. Schindler, M. Kubbies, and H. Hoehn, "Confirmation of Fanconi's anemia and detection of a chromosomal aberration (1Q12-32 triplication) via BRDU/Hoechst flow cytometry," *American Journal of Pediatric Hematology/Oncology*, vol. 9, no. 2, pp. 172–177, 1987.

[32] R. Miglierina, M. Le Coniat, M. Gendron, and R. Berger, "Diagnosis of Fanconi's anemia by flow cytometry," *Nouvelle Revue Francaise d'Hematologie*, vol. 32, no. 6, pp. 391–393, 1990.

[33] H. Seyschab, R. Friedl, Y. Sun et al., "Comparative evaluation of diepoxybutane sensitivity and cell cycle blockage in the diagnosis of fanconi anemia," *Blood*, vol. 85, no. 8, pp. 2233–2237, 1995.

[34] F. Timeus, N. Crescenzio, P. Saracco, L. Leone, G. Ponzio, and U. Ramenghi, "Cell cycle analysis in the diagnosis of Fanconi's anemia," *Haematologica*, vol. 85, no. 4, pp. 431–432, 2000.

[35] B. Dutrillaux, A. Aurias, and A. M. Dutrillaux, "The cell cycle of lymphocytes in Fanconi anemia," *Human Genetics*, vol. 62, no. 4, pp. 327–332, 1982.

[36] M. Kubbies, D. Schindler, and H. Hoehn, "Endogenous blockage and delay of the chromosome cycle despite normal recruitment and growth phase explain poor proliferation and frequent endomitosis in Fanconi anemia cells," *American Journal of Human Genetics*, vol. 37, no. 5, pp. 1022–1030, 1985.

[37] H. Seyschab, Y. Sun, R. Friedl, D. Schindler, and H. Hoehn, "G2 phase cell cycle disturbance as a manifestation of genetic cell damage," *Human Genetics*, vol. 92, no. 1, pp. 61–68, 1993.

[38] Y. M. N. Akkari, R. L. Bateman, C. A. Reifsteck, A. D. D'Andrea, S. B. Olson, and M. Grompe, "The 4N cell cycle delay in Fanconi anemia reflects growth arrest in late S phase," *Molecular Genetics and Metabolism*, vol. 74, no. 4, pp. 403–412, 2001.

[39] D. Schindler and H. Hoehn, "Flow cytometric testing for syndromes with chromosomal instability, aplastic anemia and related hematological disorders," in *Diagnostic Cytogenetics*, R. D. Wegner, Ed., pp. 269–281, Springer, Heidelberg, Germany, 1999.

[40] R. Miglierina, M. Le Coniat, and R. Berger, "A simple diagnostic test for Fanconi anemia by flow cytometry," *Analytical Cellular Pathology*, vol. 3, no. 2, pp. 111–118, 1991.

[41] A. Brøgger, R. Norum, I. L. Hansteen et al., "Comparison between five Nordic laboratories on scoring of human lymphocyte chromosome aberrations," *Hereditas*, vol. 100, no. 2, pp. 209–218, 1984.

[42] A. Brogger, "The chromatid gap—a useful parameter in genotoxicology?" *Cytogenetics and Cell Genetics*, vol. 33, no. 1-2, pp. 14–19, 1982.

[43] B. C. Godthelp, P. P. W. van Buul, N. G. J. Jaspers et al., "Cellular characterization of cells from the Fanconi anemia complementation group, FA-D1/BRCA2," *Mutation Research*, vol. 601, no. 1-2, pp. 191–201, 2006.

4

Anemia in Patients with Type 2 Diabetes Mellitus

Jéssica Barbieri,[1] Paula Caitano Fontela,[2] Eliane Roseli Winkelmann,[3,4]
Carine Eloise Prestes Zimmermann,[5,6] Yana Picinin Sandri,[4,6]
Emanelle Kerber Viera Mallet,[6] and Matias Nunes Frizzo[3,6]

[1]Regional University of Northwestern Rio Grande do Sul (UNIJUÍ), Ijuí, RS, Brazil
[2]Program in Respiratory Sciences, the Federal University of Rio Grande do Sul (UFRGS), Porto Alegre, RS, Brazil
[3]Department of Life Sciences, the Regional University of Northwestern Rio Grande do Sul (UNIJUÍ),
Rua do Comércio No. 3000, Bairro Universitário, 98700 000 Ijuí, RS, Brazil
[4]Program in Integral Attention to Health (PPGAIS-UNIJUI/UNICRUZ), Ijuí, RS, Brazil
[5]Program in Pharmacology of the Health Sciences Center, The Federal University of Santa Maria (UFSM), RS, Brazil
[6]Cenecista Institute for Higher Education, Rua Dr. João Augusto Rodrigues 471, 98801 015 Santo Ângelo, RS, Brazil

Correspondence should be addressed to Carine Eloise Prestes Zimmermann; carine_zimmermann@yahoo.com.br
and Matias Nunes Frizzo; matias.frizzo@gmail.com

Academic Editor: Eitan Fibach

The objective of this study was to evaluate the prevalence of anemia in DM2 patients and its correlation with demographic and lifestyle and laboratory variables. This is a descriptive and analytical study of the type of case studies in the urban area of the Ijuí city, registered in programs of the Family Health Strategy, with a total sample of 146 patients with DM2. A semistructured questionnaire with sociodemographic and clinical variables and performed biochemical test was applied. Of the DM2 patients studied, 50 patients had anemia, and it was found that the body mass items and hypertension and hematological variables are significantly associated with anemia of chronic disease. So, the prevalence of anemia is high in patients with DM2. The set of observed changes characterizes the anemia of chronic disease, which affects quality of life of diabetic patients and is associated with disease progression, development, and comorbidities that contribute significantly to increasing the risk of cardiovascular diseases.

1. Introduction

Diabetes mellitus (DM) is a metabolic disorder of great impact worldwide. Epidemiological data showed that in 2010 there were 285 million people affected with the disease in the world, and it is estimated that in the year of 2030 we will have about 440 million diabetics [1]. Its worldwide prevalence is increasing fast among developing countries. The type 2 diabetes affects about 7% of the population [2].

The increasing prevalence of type 2 diabetes mellitus (DM2) has become a major public health concern. The diabetic patients' number has been increasing due to population and urbanization growth, increase in the prevalence of obesity and sedentary lifestyle, and the longer survival of patients with DM [3]. Diabetes is a highly disabling disease, which can cause blindness, amputations, kidney disease,

anemia, and cardiovascular and brain complications, among others, impairing the functional capacity and autonomy and individual quality of life [4].

The disease can be classified into two predominant types, as type 1 DM (DM1), defined by the destruction of pancreatic β-cells and the absence of endogenous insulin, and as DM2, insulin resistance characterized by a frame, generally associated with obesity. Both types are featured by hyperglycemia above. Insulin resistance reduces glucose tolerance especially in muscle cells and adipocytes, where glucose uptake is insulin dependent. This causes glucose accumulation in the circulation and consequently a hyperglycemic state, generating homeostatic and systemic imbalance [5].

Diabetes is considered a major cause of premature death, because of the increased risk for developing cardiovascular diseases, which contribute to 50% to 80% of patients deaths due to increased levels of serum cholesterol and triglycerides. Cardiovascular diseases include diseases of the circulatory system, comprising a wide range of clinical syndromes, the main cause of atherosclerosis, which also increases the risk of acute coronary syndromes. The incidence of cardiovascular diseases reaches 20% in diabetics after a period of about 7 years [6].

Hyperglycemia has a direct relationship with the development of an inflammatory condition showed by the increased expression of proinflammatory cytokines such as IL-6, TNF-α, and NFκB. Thus, diabetes, as well as hyperglycemia due to its nature, is also an inflammatory disease character. Studies show that the longer the duration of the disease and/or loss of glycemic control, the higher the inflammatory process [7, 8].

The elevation of proinflammatory cytokines plays an essential role in insulin resistance and induces the appearance of cardiovascular complications diabetic micro- and macrovascular, kidney disease and anemia. By increasing especially IL-6, antierythropoietic effect occurs, since this cytokine changes the sensitivity of progenitors to erythropoietin (erythroid growth factor) and also promotes apoptosis of immature erythrocytes causing a decrease, further, in the number of circulating erythrocytes and consequently causing a reduction of circulating hemoglobin [7, 9].

It should also be noted that, due to the development of diabetes mellitus, the nephropathy may arise, which further undermines the renal production of erythropoietin, positively contributing to an increased anemic framework [9, 10]. According to Escorcio et al. [11] approximately 40% of diabetic patients are affected by kidney diseases. The decreased renal function and proinflammatory cytokines are the most important factors in determining reduction of hemoglobin levels in those patients. The inflammatory situation created by kidney disease also interferes with intestinal iron absorption and mobilization of inventories [12]. Therefore, diabetic patients with kidney disease have the highest risk for developing anemia [11].

The National Kidney Foundation defines anemia in chronic kidney disease as Hb level < 13,5 g/dL in men and 12,0 g/dL in women [13]. Anemia represents an emerging global health problem that negatively impacts quality of life and requires an ever-greater allocation of healthcare resources [14]. The anemic framework promotes reduced exercise capacity, fatigue, anorexia, depression, cognitive dysfunction, decreased libido, and other factors, which increase cardiac risk patients and depress the quality and life expectancy of the same [15]. Under these circumstances, anemia in patients with diabetes must be treated once diagnosed, since it may contribute to the pathogenesis and progression of cardiovascular disease and serious diabetic nephropathy and retinopathy. The regular screening for anemia, along with other complications associated with diabetes, can help slow the progression of vascular complications in these patients [16].

Anemia in diabetic person has a significant adverse effect on quality of life and is associated with disease progression and the development of comorbidities [7], as obesity and dyslipidemia that are strongly associated with diabetic framework and significantly contribute to increasing the risk of cardiovascular diseases [8]. Thus, the present study is to evaluate the prevalence of anemia in a sample of patients with type 2 diabetes who are living in a city in the northwest of the Rio Grande do Sul state, registered in the Family Health Strategies, and check its correlation with demographic, lifestyle, and laboratory variables of patients.

2. Methods

This is a descriptive and analytical study of the type of case studies in patients with DM2 and ages less than 75 years living in the urban area in the city of Ijuí RS, registered in programs of the Family Health Strategy (FHS) in this city. The study was conducted from January 2010 to January 2013, after agreement by the Research Ethics Committee of the Regional University of Rio Grande do Sul State Northwest (UNIJUÍ) (Opinion number 091/2010). All participants signed the informed consent in this research.

The sample size was calculated by StatCalc application EpiInfo 3.5.3, considering the prevalence of nonspecific outcome of 50%, 5% error, and 95% level of reliability, which resulted in a sample of 269 patients. Foreseeing possible losings a percentage of 5% of this number was added, a total sample of 283 patients with DM2.

The study excluded those patients who had difficulties to understand the proposed procedures, those who were bedridden, and those who had difficulty walking.

The invitation to participate in the study was made to patients during home visits, with the monitoring of community health workers when possible. At the moment of visit, the research objectives were explained for the patient and the dates of the interviews were fixed with those who agreed to participate, in addition to scheduling the clinical and laboratory reviews, held, respectively, in Physiotherapy Clinic and the Laboratory of Clinical Analysis of UNIJUÍ (UNILAB).

The interviews and tests were conducted by trained health professionals. Data collection was performed by applying a semistructured instrument. The presence of anemia was considered as the dependent variable; the patient was considered anemic, according to the World Health Organization reference values [17]. Thus, the patient was considered anemic patient when the blood count hemoglobin < 12 g/dL and <14 g/dL for females and males, respectively. The independent variables analyzed were as follows:

(a) Sociodemographic characteristics:

   (i) age (in years);

   (ii) sex (female/male).

(b) Health condition:

   (i) time of diagnosis of type 2 diabetes (in years);

   (ii) advanced age (over 60 years).

(c) Comorbidities:

   (i) presence of hypertension (yes/no);

(ii) cardiac and/or respiratory (yes or no), analyzed according to the patient's report when asked about the presence of these diseases;

(iii) dyslipidemia (yes/no), diagnosed by biochemical tests;

(iv) obesity (yes/no), when the value of body mass index was $\geq 30,0 \, kg/m^2$ for patients up to 59 years old and $\geq 27,0 \, kg/m^2$ for patients aged 60–75 [18].

(d) Lifestyle:

(i) smoking (yes/no);

(ii) alcohol consumption (yes/no);

(iii) physical inactivity (yes/no);

(iv) stress (yes/no).

(e) Eating habits, investigated through questioning a high salt diet (yes/no).

Every patient who declared himself a smoker at the moment of evaluation is considered smoker, regardless of the amount of cigarettes consumed; and alcoholic is the person who reported excessive consumption of alcohol during the study period, at any frequency. Excessive salt intake was measured by the question: Do you put much salt in your food? Stress was assessed by the question: Do you consider yourself a stressed person? There were classified physically inactive patients who reported not performing any type of regular exercise with the lowest frequency of three times a week.

The evaluation of anthropometric data, including the measurement of body weight (in kilograms) on digital scale, was performed (Toledo); height (in meters) in stadiometer (Toledo) and waist circumference (WC) were measured at the midpoint between the last rib and the iliac crest using flexible standard tape and nonextensible, defining measure of 0,1 cm, according to techniques recommended [19]. The body mass index (BMI) was calculated by dividing body weight and the square of height: kg/m^2.

At the end of the clinical evaluation, an appointment was made with the date and the time of collection of blood from each patient. Patients personally received clarification on the procedures of collection and were instructed to fast for at least eight hours prior to the blood collection, in addition to writing instructions and containers for the collection of the first urine in the morning. Among the laboratory tests that were performed are the creatinine dosage and blood glucose by enzymatic Trinder method [20]. In addition, the collection and enforcement of the blood count were performed to evaluate the presence of hematological disorders in patients with DM2. The blood sample, was also used the serum of patients after venipuncture and centrifugation of whole blood for biochemical measurements, as well as whole blood anticoagulant containing standard for hematologic examinations.

The patient who presented two or more of the following criteria proposed by the National Cholesterol Education Program was classified as having metabolic syndrome: [21] increased waist circumference (>88 cm women and >102 cm men); elevated serum triglycerides ($\geq 150 \, mg/dL$) or

decreased HDL cholesterol (<40 mg/dL men and <50 mg/dL women); and hypertension (diagnosed or identified through the use of antihypertensive medication).

Renal function was assessed by the value of serum creatinine, obtained by biochemical tests. The glomerular filtration rate is estimated by the Cockcroft-Gault calculated using the formula available on the websites of the Brazilian Society of Nephrology (SBN) of the National Kidney Foundation [22]. We considered impaired renal function the values above 1,2 mg/dL in the serum creatinine [23] and the GFR less than $60 \, mL/min/1,73 \, m^2$ estimated by the Cockcroft-Gault equation [24] representing a decrease of about 50% of normal renal function and, below this level, increasing the prevalence of complications of chronic kidney disease [25]. For the use of the Cockcroft-Gault equation, the ideal weight of the patient was computed using the Lorenz formula, which puts the ideal body weight for the subjects height in cm function [26].

For processing the data, we used the Statistical Package for Social Science (SPSS) (version 18.0, one Chicago, IL, USA). In the statistical analysis, all variables were tested for normality using the Kolmogorov-Smirnov (KS) test. The qualitative variables are presented as frequencies and percentages and quantitative variables as average and standard deviation (average $\pm$ SD) ormedian (minimumand maximum). Mann-Whitney tests were used to compare two independent groups with abnormal distribution, Student's t-test was used for normally distributed variables, and the Chi-square test and Fisher's exact Pearson were used to compare categorical variables in order to verify differences of variables between patients with and without anemia. The Spearman correlation coefficient was used to evaluate the correlation between clinical and biochemical parameters with the hemoglobin level. $p < 0,05$ was considered statistically significant. All tests were applied with a Confidence Interval (CI) of 95%.

3. Results

283 patients with DM2 were suitable to the study inclusion criteria and were selected for home visits and invitation to participate in the study, according to data collected from health professionals in FHS or the medical records of the patients belonging to nine FHS in the city of Ijuí, RS. Of these, 64 patients were not included in the study for the following reasons: contact absence; refusal to participate; and not identifying the address informed and 73 individuals were not included due to insufficient data to evaluate the hematologic changes, since they did not undergo blood tests for hemoglobin count, a total sample of 146 type 2 diabetic patients in this study, of which 50 had anemia, corresponding to 34,2%.

The study population had an average age of 60,9 $\pm$ 8,9 years, body mass index of 31,2 $\pm$ 5,8 kg/m^2, and a median of disease diagnosis time of 5,0 years (0,5–40,0 years).

We analyzed the dependent variable "anemia" according to some characteristics of patients with DM2. For time of diagnosis of the disease, old age, metabolic syndrome, renal dysfunction by creatinine, and the Cockcroft-Gault equation, there was no difference between the presence and absence

TABLE 1: Characteristics of patients with diabetes mellitus type 2 according to the presence of anemia.

Variables	Anemia		
	Yes ($n = 50$)	No ($n = 96$)	p value
Gender			$0,059^{£}$
Male	23 (46,0)	29 (30,2)	
Female	27 (54,0)	67 (69,8)	
Age (in years)	$61,8 \pm 9,5$	$60,5 \pm 8,7$	$0,274^{\mu}$
Body mass (kg)	$83,6 \pm 16,8$	$77,5 \pm 13,5$	$0,019^{¥*}$
Height (m)	$1,61 \pm 0,08$	$1,59 \pm 0,09$	$0,287^{¥}$
BMI (kg/m^2)	$32,2 \pm 6,0$	$30,6 \pm 5,7$	$0,126^{¥}$
Waist circumference (cm)	$105,9 \pm 15,9$	$104,7 \pm 11,5$	$0,626^{¥}$
Time of diagnosis of DM2 (in years)	6 (0,5–40,0)	5 (0,6–40,0)	$0,148^{\mu}$
Advanced age	30 (60,0)	55 (57,3)	$0,753^{£}$
Hypertension	42 (84,0)	65 (67,7)	$0,035^{£*}$
Dyslipidemia	23 (46,0)	48 (50,0)	$0,646^{£}$
Obesity	38 (76,0)	65 (67,7)	$0,297^{£}$
Metabolic syndrome	35 (70,0)	56 (58,3)	$0,167^{£}$
Heart disease	10 (20,0)	18 (18,8)	$0,856^{£}$
Respiratory disease	6 (12,0)	15 (15,6)	$0,627^{€}$
Smoking	8 (18,0)	14 (14,6)	$0,179^{£}$
Alcoholism	4 (8,0)	6 (6,3)	$0,924^{€}$
Physical inactivity	23 (46,0)	50 (52,1)	$0,485^{£}$
Stress	23 (46,0)	53 (55,2)	$0,291^{£}$
Hypersodic diet	6 (12,0)	19 (19,8)	$0,259^{€}$
Alteration of renal function by creatinine	9 (18,0)	18 (18,8)	$0,912^{£}$
Alteration of renal function by Cockcroft-Gault equation	12 (24,0)	25 (26,0)	$0,788^{£}$

DM2: diabetes mellitus type 2; ¥ indicates p value according to Student's t-test; μ indicates p value according to test of Mann-Whitney; £ indicates p value according to test of Chi-square of Pearson; € indicates p value according to the exact test of Fischer; results presented on average ± standard deviation or median (minimal and maximal value) and number (percentage); * was considered statistically significant.

TABLE 2: Biochemical and hematological variables in patients with DM2 according to the presence of anemia.

Variables	Anemia		
	Yes ($n = 50$)	No ($n = 96$)	p value
Hemoglobin (g/dL)	$11,68 \pm 0,81$	$13,32 \pm 0,85$	$<0,0001^{¥*}$
Hematocrit (%)	$35,08 \pm 5,23$	$40,45 \pm 2,88$	$<0,0001^{\mu*}$
Red cells (millions/mm^3)	$4,23 \pm 0,37$	$4,68 \pm 0,34$	$<0,0001^{¥*}$
Glycemia (mg/dL)	$109,4 \pm 40,5$	$133,6 \pm 55,2$	$0,005^{\mu*}$
Creatinine (mg/dL)	$1,05 \pm 0,39$	$1,03 \pm 0,27$	$0,944^{\mu}$
Glomerular filtration rate (mL/min)	$91,7 \pm 41,9$	$79,9 \pm 27,2$	$0,277^{**}$

¥ indicates p value according to Student's t-test; μ indicates p value according to test of Mann-Whitney; * was considered statistically significant; results presented in average ± standard deviation or median (minimal and maximal value). ** indicates mean glomerular filtration rate by Cockcroft-Gault equation.

TABLE 3: Coefficients of correlation between clinical and biochemical parameters with the hemoglobin in patients with diabetes mellitus type 2.

Variables	Hemoglobin	
	p	R
Age (in years)	0,492	−0,057
BMI (kg/m^2)	0,051	−0,155
Time of diagnosis of DM2	0,466	−0,061
Glycemia (mg/dL)	$0,004^*$	0,235
Creatinine (mg/dL)	0,209	0,105
Glomerular filtration rate by the Cockcroft-Gault equation (mL/min./1,73 m^2)	0,526	0,053

Spearman rank correlation test; * was considered statistically significant.

of anemia ($p > 0,05$). However, variables, body mass, and hypertension showed significance to the outcome studied ($p < 0,05$). These data are presented in Table 1.

We observed statistically significant difference in hematological variables between groups with and without anemia ($p < 0,05$). The same is observed with respect to glucose,

however, with higher values in the group without anemia. There was no statistically significant difference in creatinine variable ($p > 0,05$). These data are presented in Table 2.

Table 3 shows the correlations between the clinical and biochemical parameters with hemoglobin. It is observed that there are positive and weak correlation between glucose and hemoglobin and negative and weak correlation between BMI and hemoglobin.

4. Discussion

Often, chronic diseases, such as DM, are accompanied by mild-to-moderate anemia, often called anemia of inflammation or infection or anemia of chronic disease [27]. Andrews and Arredondo [28] determined the presence of anemia in type 2 diabetic patients as well as evaluating the expression of genes related to inflammation and immune response. The results found by the authors demonstrate that diabetic patients with anemia exhibit increased expression of proinflammatory cytokines as compared to diabetic patients only. In anemic patient increase in IL-6 production, as well as B cell activity, was confirmed which reinforces the association between IL-6 and antierythropoietic action. Moreover, the diabetic and anemic patients had high levels of C-reactive protein and ferritin ultrasensible; however, these diabetic and anemic patients had low iron contents, showing that ferritin increases were associated with chronic inflammatory process present in diabetes [28].

In this study, there was a higher prevalence of obesity and higher mean BMI and waist circumference in anemic patients when compared to nonanemic ones; however, there was a statistically significant difference between the groups only for body mass variable. Anemia in diabetic patients is also related to obesity, BMI, and high waist circumference. The obesity or accumulation of circulating fatty acids is associated with the development of an inflammatory state that predisposes the development of insulin resistance. Insulin resistance reduces glucose tolerance especially in adipocytes and muscle cells, in which glucose uptake is insulin. This causes glucose accumulation in the circulation and consequently a hyperglycemic state [29].

Adipose tissue has more recently been recognized as a metabolically active organ system linking the endocrine and immune systems; furthermore it is the source of a variety of cytokines. Higher baseline BMI remained a predictor of additional adjustments for blood pressure level and the presence or absence of diabetes mellitus. Similar to TNF-alpha, IL-6 is a proinflammatory adipokine that correlates with body weight and insulin resistance [30].

The increased inflammatory activity in adipose tissue of obese patients favors the production of hepcidin that in anemia of chronic disease is increased during infection and inflammation, causing a decrease in serum iron level through a mechanism that limits the availability of iron. The association of higher iron stores with diabetes and insulin resistance has been repeatedly confirmed by many investigators. Ferritin levels were found to predict a higher rate of diabetes in prospective studies and case-control cohorts. Furthermore, serum ferritin was positively associated with body mass index (BMI), visceral fat mass, serum glucose levels, insulin sensitivity, and cholesterol levels [31–33].

In addition, it was found in this study that the prevalence of hypertension in diabetic patients that were anemic was significantly higher when compared to nonanemic ones. This association is of concern considering that hypertension in diabetic increases the risk of cardiovascular complications such as heart failure, stroke, tissue inflammation, and atherosclerosis [4].

According to Ximenes et al. [34] anemia is a prevalent comorbidity in patients with hypertension and when present, patients have more severe symptoms and worse functional capacity as well as increased mortality. The knowledge that anemia worsens the symptoms of hypertension is not new, but, in recent years, the magnitude of the anemia associated with this disease has become more evident. The main causes that contribute to anemia in patients with hypertension are nutritional deficiencies especially iron deficiency and chronic inflammation [34].

It was observed in the present study that there are decreased values of hemoglobin, hematocrit, and red blood cells in anemic patients, which can be associated with a normocytic normochromic anemia, characteristic of an anemia of chronic disease (ACD). ACD is a light-to-moderate anemia shortening the survival of red blood cells (about 80 days instead of 120 days normal). This phenomenon is attributed to hyperactivity state mononuclear phagocyte system, triggered by infectious, inflammatory, or neoplastic process, leading to early removal of circulating red blood cells. Inadequate bone marrow response observed is due basically to inappropriately low Secretion of Erythropoietin (EPO), decreased bone marrow response to EPO, and decreased erythropoiesis consequent to lower supply of iron to the bone marrow [35].

One explanation for this bone marrow response is directly related to the activation of macrophages and the release of inflammatory cytokines, particularly IL-1, IL-6, tumor necrosis factor (TNF a), and interferon gamma (INF g) which act by inhibiting the proliferation of erythroid precursors and therefore inhibit erythropoiesis. Furthermore, the suppressive action of these cytokines on erythropoiesis stimulating overcomes the action of EPO resulting in decreased bone marrow response to EPO and erythropoiesis [36].

Also it should be noted that there was no hemoglobin correlation with creatinine or statistical differences in creatinine values and glomerular filtration rate estimated between groups, indicating once again that anemia by chronic disease was inflammation triggered and the reduction renal function affects the production of EPO.

The limitations in this study refer to the fact that the assessment of glycemic control in diabetic patients was performed by means of fasting glucose that is a momentary biochemical analysis, does not represent the average glucose of patients, and may also occur interfering in the examination, as the effect of hypoglycemic agents, promoting a reduction in glucose levels. In this sense, the gold standard for assessing glycemic control would be the achievement of HbA1c (glycated hemoglobin), which is one of the most important tools to assess glycemic control of patients with diabetes, as they express the average amount of glucose in the last three months, and this can infer the diabetes control efficiency and suggest the need for adjustments.

Therefore, it is suggested that further studies should be conducted using test glycated hemoglobin, which currently is already considered an essential parameter in the DM control evaluation, in order to relate hyperglycemia, inflammation, and anemia.

5. Conclusion

Patients with DM2 and anemia were those with high body mass, hypertension, increased waist circumference, and longer time of the disease. This set of changes characterizes the anemia as chronic disease, which has a significant adverse effect on quality of life of diabetic patients and is associated with the progression of the disease; the development of comorbidities significantly contributes to the increased risk of cardiovascular disease. However, against what was expected, the results of blood glucose were higher in nonanemic patients, which is contradictory due to the anemia of these patients being associated with an inflammatory condition, for being characterized as normocytic normochromic anemia. Deepening the study of the issues raised throughout this work provides knowledge for the establishment of new strategies for glycemic control, which can increase the research and correlate some analytical parameters, such as HbA1c, Il-6, VHS, and PCR.

Conflict of Interests

The authors declare that there is no conflict of interests.

References

[1] J. E. Shaw, R. A. Sicree, and P. Z. Zimmet, "Global estimates of the prevalence of diabetes for 2010 and 2030," *Diabetes Research and Clinical Practice*, vol. 87, no. 1, pp. 4–14, 2010.

[2] P. F. Pereira, R. D. C. G. Alfenas, and R. M. A. Araújo, "Does breastfeeding influence the risk of developing diabetes mellitus in children? A review of current evidence," *Jornal de Pediatria*, vol. 90, no. 1, pp. 7–15, 2014.

[3] Brasil Ministério da Saúde, *Diretrizes da Sociedade Brasileira de Diabetes 2013-2014*, AC Farmacêutica, 2014.

[4] P. M. S. B. Francisco, A. P. Belon, M. B. A. Barros, L. Carandina, M. C. G. P. Alves, and C. L. G. Cesar, "Self-reported diabetes in the elderly: prevalence, associated factors, and control practices," *Cadernos de Saúde Pública*, vol. 26, no. 1, pp. 175–184, 2010.

[5] X. Zhang, X. Cui, F. Li et al., "Association between diabetes mellitus with metabolic syndrome and diabetic microangiopathy," *Experimental and Therapeutic Medicine*, vol. 8, no. 6, pp. 1867–1873, 2014.

[6] T. R. Silva, J. Zanuzzi, C. D. M. Silva, X. S. Passos, and B. M. F. Costa, "Prevalence of cardiovascular diseases in diabetic and nutritional status of patientes," *Journal of the Health Sciences Institute*, vol. 30, no. 3, pp. 266–270, 2012.

[7] A. Angelousi and E. Larger, "Anaemia, a common but often unrecognized risk in diabetic patients: a review," *Diabetes & Metabolism*, vol. 41, no. 1, pp. 18–27, 2015.

[8] B. Martínez-Pérez, I. De La Torre-Díez, and M. López-Coronado, "Mobile health applications for the most prevalent conditions by the World Health Organization: review and analysis," *Journal of Medical Internet Research*, vol. 15, no. 6, article e120, 2013.

[9] S. Fava, J. Azzopardi, S. Ellard, and A. T. Hattersley, "ACE gene polymorphism as a prognostic indicator in patients with type 2 diabetes and established renal disease," *Diabetes Care*, vol. 24, no. 12, pp. 2115–2120, 2001.

[10] V. Jha, G. Garcia-Garcia, K. Iseki et al., "Chronic kidney disease: global dimension and perspectives," *The Lancet*, vol. 382, no. 9888, pp. 260–272, 2013.

[11] C. S. M. Escorcio, H. F. Silva, G. B. S. Junior, M. P. Monteiro, and R. P. Gonçalves, "Evaluation of anemia treatment with EPO and oral and iv iron in patients with chronic kidney disease under hemodialysis," *RBSA*, vol. 42, no. 2, pp. 87–90, 2010.

[12] G. Weiss and L. T. Goodnough, "Anemia of chronic disease," *The New England Journal of Medicine*, vol. 352, no. 10, pp. 1011–1059, 2005.

[13] I. C. Macdougall, K.-U. Eckardt, and F. Locatelli, "Latest US KDOQI Anaemia Guidelines update—what are the implications for Europe?" *Nephrology Dialysis Transplantation*, vol. 22, no. 10, pp. 2738–2742, 2007.

[14] A. Macciò and C. Madeddu, "Management of anemia of inflammation in the elderly," *Anemia*, vol. 2012, Article ID 563251, 20 pages, 2012.

[15] T. D. Moreira and M. A. Mascarenhas, *Avaliação da prevalência de anemia em grupos diabéticos e não diabéticos e sua relação com insuficiência renal crônica*, 62nd edition, 2004.

[16] D. K. Singh, P. Winocour, and K. Farrington, "Erythropoietic stress and anemia in diabetes mellitus," *Nature Reviews Endocrinology*, vol. 5, no. 4, pp. 204–210, 2009.

[17] WHO, *Anaemia*, World Health Organization, 2012.

[18] D. A. Lipschitz, "Screening for nutritional status in the elderly," *Primary Care*, vol. 21, no. 1, pp. 55–67, 1994.

[19] V. H. Hevward and L. M. Stolarczyc, *Avaliação da composição corporal aplicada*, Manole, São Paulo, Brazil, 2000.

[20] J. B. Henry, *Diagnósticos Clínicos e Tratamento por Métodos Laboratoriais*, São Paulo, Brazil, Manole, 2008.

[21] Expert Panel on Detection, Evaluation, and Treatment of High Blood Cholesterol in Adults, "Executive summary of the third report of the National Cholesterol Education Program (NCEP) Expert Panel on Detection, Evaluation, and Treatment of High Blood Cholesterol in Adults (Adult Treatment Panel III)," *Journal of the American Medical Association*, vol. 285, no. 19, pp. 2486–2497, 2001.

[22] National Kidney Foundation, "K/DOQI clinical practice guidelines for chronic kidney disease: evaluation, classification and stratification," *American Journal of Kidney Diseases*, vol. 39, no. 2, supplement 1, pp. S1–S266, 2002.

[23] F. M. Di Napoli, J. E. Burmeister, D. R. Miltersteiner, B. M. Campos, and M. G. Costa, "Estimation of renal function by the cockcroft and gault formula in overweighted or obese patients," *Jornal Brasileiro de Nefrologia*, vol. 30, pp. 185–191, 2008.

[24] E. J. C. Magacho, A. C. Pereira, H. N. Mansur, and M. G. Bastos, "Nomogram for estimation of glomerular filtration rate based on the CKD-EPI formula," *Jornal Brasileiro de Nefrologia*, vol. 34, no. 3, pp. 313–315, 2012.

[25] M. G. Bastos, R. Bregman, and G. M. Kirsztajn, "Chronic kidney diseases: common and harmful, but also preventable and treatable," *Revista da Associacao Medica Brasileira*, vol. 56, no. 2, pp. 248–253, 2010.

[26] T. P. Sanso, "Neurofisiologia dela alimentación: su incidencia en la obesidade común," *Estudios de Psicologia*, vol. 14, pp. 126–138, 1983.

[27] M. C. Carvalho, E. C. E. Baracat, and V. C. Sgarbieri, "Anemia ferropriva e anemia de doença crônica: distúrbios do metabolismo de ferro," *Revista Segurança Alimentar e Nutricional*, vol. 13, no. 2, pp. 54–63, 2006.

[28] M. Andrews and M. Arredondo, "Ferritin levels and hepcidin mRNA expression in peripheral mononuclear cells from anemic type 2 diabetic patients," *Biological Trace Element Research*, vol. 149, no. 1, pp. 1–4, 2012.

[29] P. L. Hooper and P. L. Hooper, "Inflammation, heat shock proteins, and type 2 diabetes," *Cell Stress and Chaperones*, vol. 14, no. 2, pp. 113–115, 2009.

[30] C. Rüster and G. Wolf, "Adipokines promote chronic kidney disease," *Nephrology Dialysis Transplantation*, vol. 28, supplement 4, pp. iv8–iv14, 2013.

[31] T. Iwasaki, A. Nakajima, M. Yoneda et al., "Serum ferritin is associated with visceral fat area and subcutaneous fat area," *Diabetes Care*, vol. 28, no. 10, pp. 2486–2491, 2005.

[32] C. E. Wrede, R. Buettner, L. C. Bollheimer, J. Schölmerich, K.-D. Palitzsch, and C. Hellerbrand, "Association between serum ferritin and the insulin resistance syndrome in a representative population," *European Journal of Endocrinology*, vol. 154, no. 2, pp. 333–340, 2006.

[33] P. Galan, N. Noisette, C. Estaquio et al., "Serum ferritin, cardiovascular risk factors and ischaemic heart diseases: a prospective analysis in the SU.VI.MAX (SUpplementation en VItamines et Minéraux AntioXydants) cohort," *Public Health Nutrition*, vol. 9, no. 1, pp. 70–74, 2006.

[34] R. M. O. Ximenes, A. C. P. Barretto, and E. P. Silva, "Anemia in heart failure patients: development risk factors," *Revista Brasileira de Cardiologia*, vol. 27, no. 3, pp. 189–194, 2014.

[35] R. D. Cançado, "Multiple myeloma and anemias," *Revista Brasileira de Hematologia e Hemoterapia*, vol. 29, no. 1, pp. 67–76, 2007.

[36] L. F. Amador-Medina, "Anemia in chronic kidney disease," *Revista Médica del Instituto Mexicano del Seguro Social*, vol. 52, no. 6, pp. 660–665, 2014.

5

FK228 Analogues Induce Fetal Hemoglobin in Human Erythroid Progenitors

Levi Makala,[1] Salvatore Di Maro,[2, 3] Tzu-Fang Lou,[4] Sharanya Sivanand,[5] Jung-Mo Ahn,[2] and Betty S. Pace[1]

[1] Department of Pediatrics, Georgia Health Sciences University, Augusta, GA 30912, USA
[2] Department of Chemistry, University of Texas at Dallas, Richardson, TX 75083, USA
[3] Department of Pharmacological and Toxicological Chemistry, University of Naples Federico II, 80100 Naples, Italy
[4] Department of Molecular and Cell Biology, University of Texas at Dallas, TX 75080, USA
[5] Department of Developmental Biology, University of Texas Southwestern Medical Center, Dallas, TX 75390, USA

Correspondence should be addressed to Betty S. Pace, bpace@georgiahealth.edu

Academic Editor: Solomon F. Ofori-Acquah

Fetal hemoglobin (HbF) improves the clinical severity of sickle cell disease (SCD), therefore, research to identify HbF-inducing agents for treatment purposes is desirable. The focus of our study is to investigate the ability of FK228 analogues to induce HbF using a novel KU812 dual-luciferase reporter system. Molecular modeling studies showed that the structure of twenty FK228 analogues with isosteric substitutions did not disturb the global structure of the molecule. Using the dual-luciferase system, a subgroup of FK228 analogues was shown to be inducers of HbF at nanomolar concentrations. To determine the physiological relevance of these compounds, studies in primary erythroid progenitors confirmed that JMA26 and JMA33 activated HbF synthesis at levels comparable to FK228 with low cellular toxicity. These data support our lead compounds as potential therapeutic agents for further development in the treatment of SCD.

1. Introduction

Several classes of pharmacological compounds that reactivate γ-globin gene transcription have been identified. They include cytotoxic agents, DNA methyl transferase, and histone deacetylase (HDAC) inhibitors. Cytotoxic compounds terminate actively cycling progenitors and perturb cellular growth to trigger rapid erythroid regeneration and γ-globin gene activation. S-stage cytotoxic drugs, such as cytosine arabinoside [1], myleran [2], vinblastine [3], and hydroxyurea [4, 5], induce HbF production in primates and humans [4, 6, 7]. The Multicenter Study of Hydroxyurea established this agent as the first FDA-approved treatment for SCD [7]. Hydroxyurea was shown to reduce vaso-occlusive episodes in the majority of sickle-cell patients treated. However, limitations to using hydroxyurea such as bone marrow suppression

[8], concerns over long-term carcinogenic complications, and a 30% non-response rate [7, 9], make the development of alternative therapies desirable.

The HDAC inhibitors have also been shown to be potent HbF inducers. These agents target HDACs, which play a dynamic role in regulating cell cycle progression and chromatin conformation by changes in histone acetylation status. Aberrant transcriptional repression mediated by Class I and II HDACs has been demonstrated in many cancers [10]. Thus, HDAC inhibitors have been developed as promising anticancer therapeutics [11]. Structurally diverse classes of natural and synthetic HDAC inhibitors bind target HDACs to block histone deacetylation [12] and produce an open chromatin confirmation and gene activation [13].

There has been great interest in HDAC inhibitors as HbF inducers to treat SCD. They include (1) short-chain fatty acids such as sodium butyrate (NaB), the first HDAC inhibitor reported [14, 15]; (2) the benzamides (i.e., MS-275); (3) non cyclic and cyclic hydroxamates, like SAHA (suberoylanilide hydroxamic acid) and TSA (Trichostatin A); (4) cyclic peptides including FK228 (depsipeptide). NaB induces differentiation in mouse erythroleukemia cells via Stat5 phosphorylation and HbF synthesis through p38 mitogen-activated protein kinase signaling [16–18]. Other fatty acids including phenylacetate and propionate [19–21], induce HbF in erythroid progenitors, however, these agents are rapidly metabolized and oral preparations are not available. These published studies serve as the basis for research efforts to develop HDAC inhibitors as therapeutic agents for SCD.

Of the hydroxamic acid derivatives, the prototype TSA is a potent HDAC inhibitor [22, 23]. It interacts with a divalent zinc-binding motif in the binding pocket of Class I and II HDACs [24]. Other HDAC inhibitors in the hydroxamic acid class include the second-generation analogues of TSA, identified from a library screen of 600 synthesized compounds [25]. The most widely studied TSA analogues are SAHA and Scriptaid. SAHA targets HDAC1, 3, and 4 and inhibits prostate cancer cell growth *in vitro* and *in vivo* [26, 27]. Recently, it was demonstrated by Pace and colleagues that SAHA and Scriptaid induce HbF synthesis comparable to NaB and TSA in erythroid cells and β-YAC transgenic mice respectively [28]. However, limitations to the further development of these agents included toxicity in primary cells.

Another potent HDAC inhibitor is FK228, also known as depsipeptide, isolated from *Chromobacterium violaceum* [29]. This compound has a unique bicyclic structure and is a stable pro-drug activated by the reduction of the disulfide bond by glutathione to produce an active form (redFK) after uptake into cells [30]. The reduced sulfhydryl group interacts strongly with the zinc ion at the active site of the enzyme and has been shown to inhibit tumor proliferation *in vitro* and *in vivo* at nanomolar concentrations [27, 31, 32]. Recently, FK228 was tested in the $\mu LCR\beta_{pr}R_{luc}{}^A\gamma_{pr}F_{luc}$ GM979 stable cell line and erythroid progenitors grown in methylcellulose colonies produced from peripheral blood mononuclear cells [33]. FK228 was shown to induce HbF in both systems. The level of γ-globin and β-globin promoter activity was quantified indirectly using firefly (γ) and renilla (β) luciferase activity.

Drug-mediated HbF induction remains the best approach to ameliorate the symptoms and complications of SCD. Among many compounds, FK228 showed efficacy in inducing γ-globin transcription at low concentrations, however, cell toxicity was observed and the drug is difficult to synthesize. It is a bicyclic depsipeptide almost exclusively comprised of unnatural amino acids, D-valine, D-cysteine and, (Z)-dehydrobutyrine (Dhb) as well as a (3S, 4E)-3-hydroxy-7-mercapto-4-heptenoic acid, which is a key component to form the highly constrained bicyclic structure. The high content of the unnatural amino acids and the constrained bicyclic structure make it extremely stable in physiological condition. Simon and coworkers first reported its total synthesis in 1996 [34], and suggested a laborious

synthetic route with moderate yield (18% overall yield with over 16 steps).

Despite its exceptionally high *in vitro* and *in vivo* activity, FK228 has not been explored due to its non-trivial and challenging synthesis, which hampered its production and the design of analogues. The latter would aide our understanding of the molecular mechanism of FK228 and to achieve higher potency and selectivity for HbF induction. In fact, only a few FK228 analogues have been created to date even after intensive synthetic efforts were made [34–36]. To circumvent this problem, we used *in silico* structure analysis and molecular modeling to design twenty FK228 structural analogues that can be easily synthesized [37]. Furthermore, two isosteric substitutions were made without altering its global conformation.

The objective of our study was to investigate the ability of the newly synthesized FK228 analogues to induce γ-globin gene transcription using a dual luciferase-based assay system. We identified two lead compounds, JMA26 and JMA33, which induce HbF expression in primary erythroid progenitors. The potential of HDAC enzymes as druggable targets in the treatment of SCD is discussed.

2. Materials and Methods

2.1. Synthesis of FK228 Analogues. The synthesis of all FK228 analogues described in this study was accomplished by following the previously reported solid-phase synthetic procedure outlined in Scheme 1 [37]. Briefly, S-trityl cysteamine was loaded on aminomethylated polystyrene (AM-PS) resin that was previously functionalized with a backbone amide linker (BAL) [38]. The resulting secondary amine 1 was then coupled with the first amino acid, Fmoc-L-Asp(OAl) to give the aspartylcysteamine 2 with high yield (98%). Thus, the aspartylcysteamine moiety designed to replace the heptenoic acid in the native FK228, was constructed in a single reaction step. The remaining four amino acids were introduced sequentially using the standard N-Fmoc/^{t}Bu solid-phase peptide synthesis strategy to build the linear pentapeptides 6a-f. After the allyl and N-Fmoc protecting groups were removed, the macrolactams 7a-f were formed with HBTU (O-benzotriazole-N,N,N′,N′-tetramethyluronium hexafluorophosphate) as a coupling reagent with high yields and purity (>95%). S-Trityl protecting groups were removed with dilute 1% trifluoroacetic acid and the resulting free thiols were oxidized with iodine to produce the bicyclic FK228 analogues. The analogues were cleaved from the resin with TFA (>95%) and characterized by reverse phase—high performance liquid chromatography and electrospray ionization mass spectrometry.

2.2. Cell Culture. Human KU812 leukemia cells were grown in Iscove's Modified Dulbecco's medium (IMDM) (Invitrogen, Carlsbad, CA) with 10% fetal bovine serum (Atlanta Biologicals, Atlanta, GA), penicillin (100 U/mL), and streptomycin (0.1 mg/mL). The cells were incubated at 37°C with 5% CO_2. Cell count and viability were determined using a hemocytometer and 2% Trypan blue exclusion. Inductions

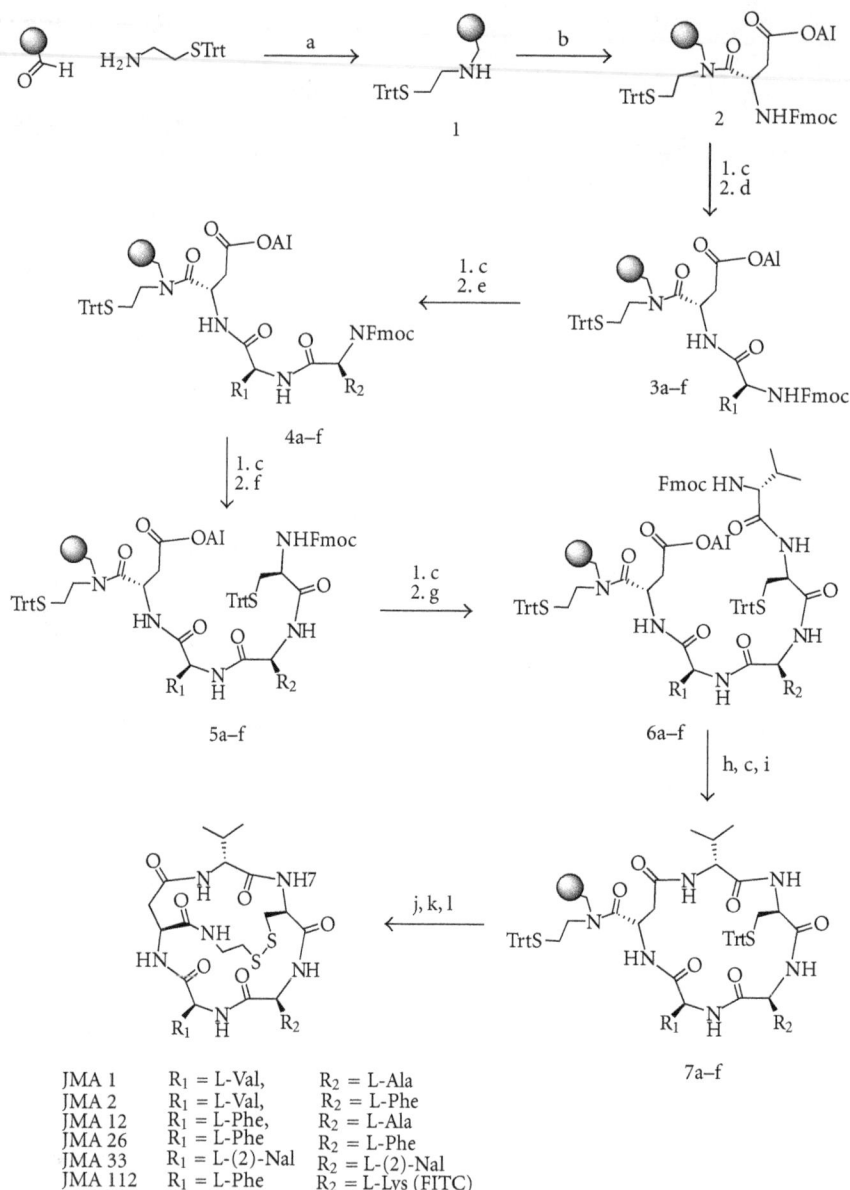

SCHEME 1: Synthesis of FK228 analogues. Shown in the schematic are the steps, reagents, and conditions used for FK228 analogue synthesis. Compounds 1–7 are the intermediates during the synthesis. For steps 7a–f, the different R_1 and R_2 group substitutions were made to generate the various JMA analogues shown. Symbols: (a) NaBH$_3$CN; (b) Fmoc-Asp(OAl), DIC; (c) Piperidine; (d) Fmoc-AA$_1$, HBTU; (e) Fmoc-AA$_2$, HBTU; (f) Fmoc-D-Cys(Trt), HBTU; (g) Fmoc-D-Val, HBTU; (h) Pd(PPh$_3$)$_4$, DMBA; (i) HBTU; (j) 1% TFA; (k) I$_2$; (l) TFA (>95%).

were performed with one million cells treated for 48 hr with the following drugs purchased from Sigma (St Louis, MO): 50 μM Hem (hemin), 2 mM NaB (sodium buytrate), 0.5 μM TSA, 10 mM Cys (cysteine), 1.5 nM FK228, and 100 μM HU (hydroxyurea). We also tested 5 μM SAHA, a gift from Merck & Co. Inc. (Whitehouse Station, NJ).

2.3. KU812 Stable Lines. KU812 stable cell lines were created by co-transfecting wild-type KU812 cells with p*EGFP-NI* (G418 selectable marker) *and the* μLCRβ_{pr}R$_{luc}$$^A\gamma_{pr}F_{luc}$ dual-reporter a kind gifts from Dr. George Stamatoyannopoulos

(University of Washington). Briefly, the 315-bp human β-globin gene promoter sequence was inserted upstream of the Renilla along with a polyadenylation signal downstream to create Pβ_{pr}R$_{luc}$. Likewise, 1.4 kb of human Aγ-globin promoter was inserted upstream of firefly luciferase to create $^A\gamma_{pr}$F$_{luc}$. The μLCR (locus control region), Pβ_{pr}R$_{luc}$, and $^A\gamma_{pr}$F$_{luc}$ fragments were subsequently cloned into the mammalian vector, pRL-null [39].

The dual-luciferase reporter lines were produced using 10 μg each of linearized μLCRβ_{pr}R$_{luc}$$^A\gamma_{pr}F_{luc}$ and p*EGFP-NI* plasmids co-transfected into KU812 cells by electroporation

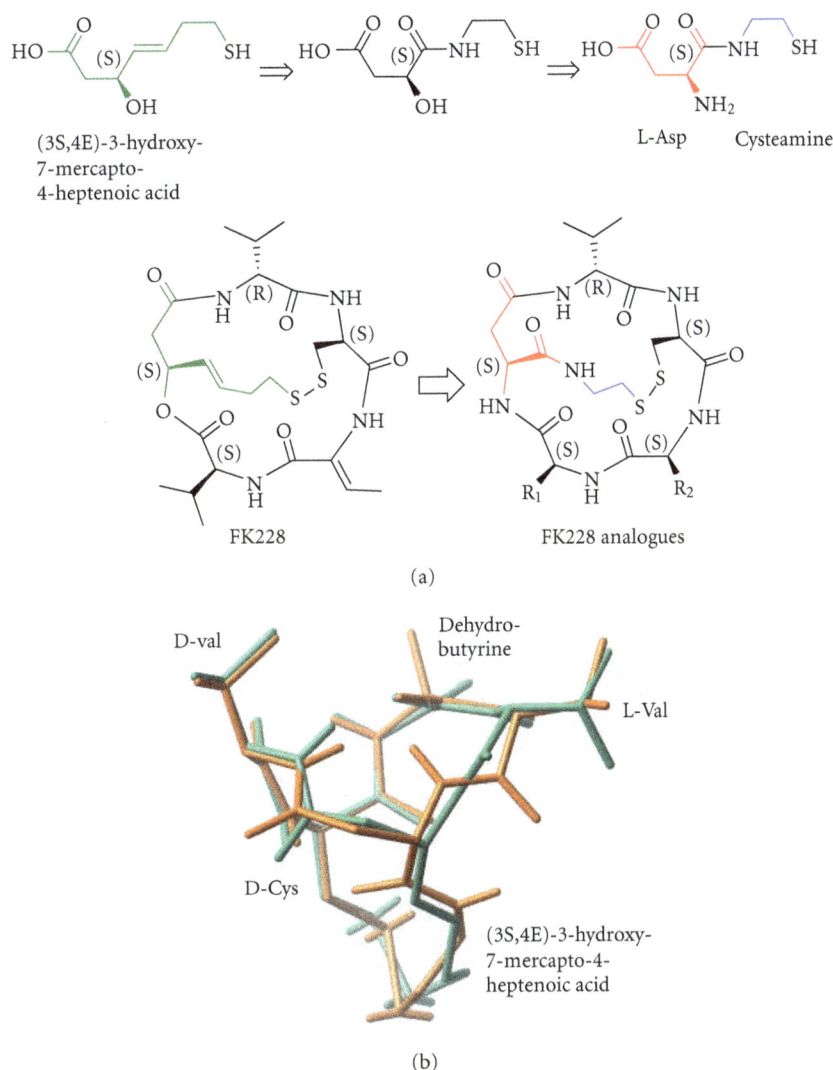

FIGURE 1: Structures of FK228 analogues. (a) The parent compound FK228 was transformed into novel structural analogues by two isosteric substitutions. The modification of the trans-double bond and ester linkage in the native FK228 with two isosteric amide functional groups allows facile synthesis of analogues as well as retention of the same backbone structure. Various amino acids such as Val, Ala, Phe, 2-Nal, and Lys were introduced to investigate potency of the analogues. (b) Superimposed structures of FK228 (green) and a modified FK228 analogue (orange).

at 260 V, 975 μF (Bio-Rad, Hercules CA). After 72 hr, G418 was added at a concentration of 900 μg/μl for 3 days then maintained under selection pressure indefinitely at a concentration of 400 μg/μl. KU812 stable lines were treated with the various drugs at the same concentrations described above. FK228 and analogues were screened at concentrations between 1–1000 nM for 48 hr and cell toxicity was monitored by 2% Trypan blue exclusion. The effect of drug treatments on γ-globin and β-globin promoter activity was monitored by luciferase assay.

2.4. Dual Luciferase Assay. Luciferase activity was monitored under the different experimental conditions using the Dual Luciferase Assay Reporter System (Promega, Madison, WI). The activity of firefly luciferase represents γ-globin promoter activity (γF), while the renilla luciferase is the read-out for β-globin promoter activity (βR). The β-globin promoter was strategically cloned between the LCR and γ-globin promoter to increase β expression, while simultaneously increasing the sensitivity of detection of γ-globin gene inducers [40].

After drug treatments, KU812 stable cells were washed with 1X phosphate buffered saline and lysed in 1X Passive Lysis Buffer for 15 min, then protein extracts were added to the Luciferase Assay Reagent II and firefly luciferase activity quantified in a Turner Designs TD-20/20 luminometer (Sunnyvale, CA). To measure βR activity, Stop & Glo Reagents was added to measure the renilla luciferase activity. Total protein was determined by Bradford assay on a Beckman DU 640 spectrophotometer (Chaska, MN) and luciferase activity was corrected for total protein.

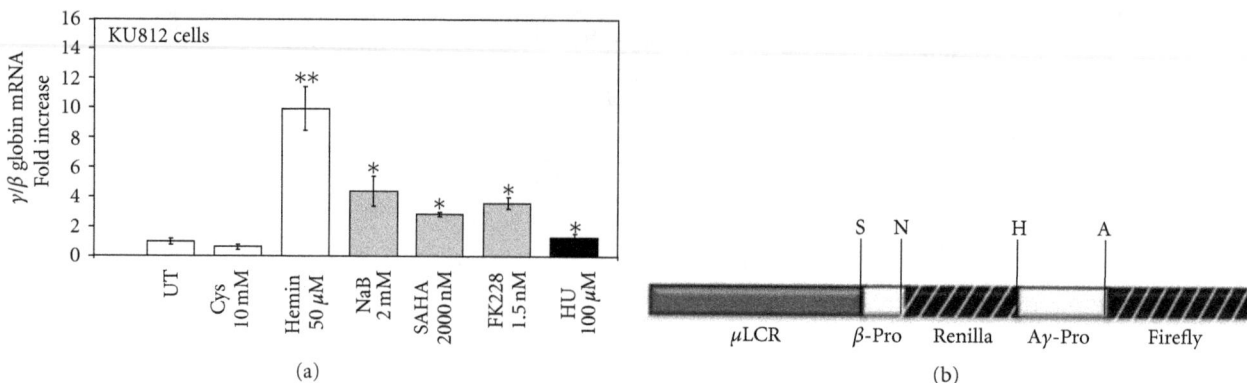

FIGURE 2: Known HbF inducers activate γ-globin expression in KU812 cells. (a) Induction of γ-globin transcription by known HbF inducers. Cells were treated for 48 hr with the different drug inducers and γ-globin and β-globin gene transcription were measured by RT-qPCR (see Section 2). The relative mRNA levels were plotted as fold increase. Untreated cells (UT) were used as a control and normalized to one. Data were calculated as the means $\pm$ standard error of the mean (SEM); $*P < 0.05$ and $**P < 0.01$. (b) Shown is a schematic of the dual luciferase reporter construct $\mu LCR\beta_{pr}R_{luc}\gamma_{pr}F_{luc}$ which contains a 3.1-kb μLCR cassette linked to a 315-bp human β-globin gene promoter driving the renilla luciferase gene and a 1.4-kb Aγ promoter driving the firefly luciferase gene [33, 39].

2.5. Two-Phase Erythroid Liquid Culture System.

The two-phase liquid culture system was established as previously published by Fibach et al. [41] using buffy coat mononuclear cells, purchased from Carter Blood Care (Fort Worth, TX) in accordance with the guidelines of the Institutional Review Board at the University of Texas at Dallas. During phase 1, cells were grown in IMDM medium with 30% fetal bovine serum and 50 ng/mL each of the granulocyte-monocyte colony-stimulating factor, Interleukin-3, and stem cell factor. Subsequently, phase 2 was initiated on day 7 with the addition of erythropoietin (2 U/mL) and stem cell factor (50 ng/mL). The cells were treated on Day 11 with the different test compounds and harvested on Day 14 (72 hr incubation).

2.6. Reverse Transcription—Quantitative PCR (RT-qPCR) Analysis.

Total RNA was isolated from samples using RNA Stat-60 (TEL-TEST "B" Inc., Friendswood, TX) and used for RT-qPCR analysis as previously published [42]. Briefly, cDNA was prepared using the Improm-II reverse transcriptase system and oligo (dT)$_{15}$ primers (Promega). qPCR was performed on an iCycler iQ machine (Bio-Rad) using a master mix containing Sybergreen iQ Supermix (BioRad) and 100 pM of each gene-specific primer pairs for γ-globin, β-globin and the internal control GAPDH. Standard curves were generated using serial 10-fold dilutions of Topo7 base plasmids carrying a γ-globin cDNA sequence (Topo7-γ-globin), Topo7-β-globin, and Topo7-GAPDH. The globin mRNA levels were calculated as a ratio of GAPDH (γ/GAPDH, β/GAPDH), and the γ/β-globin mRNA ratio was calculated by dividing γ/GAPDH by β/GAPDH.

2.7. Immunohistochemistry.

Primary erythroid progenitor cytospin cell preparations were fixed with 4% paraformaldehyde in phosphate buffered saline for 15 min, washed, and then permeabilized with 0.3% Trition-100 solution for 10 min. Cells were then blocked in a 5% bovine serum albumin solution and immunostaining performed at 4°C overnight with anti-HbF fluorescein isothiocyanate (FITC) conjugated antibody (Bethyl Laboratories Inc., TX). Cell nuclei were stained with mounting medium containing 4′,6-diamidino-2-phenylindole (DAPI; Santa Cruz Biotechnology, CA). Primary cells were photographed with an Olympus BX 51 phase contrast epifluorescent microscope equipped with Hoffman Modulation optics. Phase-contrast images were recorded with a CCD camera (1/100 sec exposure) and fluorescence images were photographed through 485/520 nm emission filter. The percent of HbF positive cells was calculated by dividing the number of FITC positive cells by total cells (DAPI positive).

2.8. Enzyme-Linked Immunosorbent Assay (ELISA).

Total hemoglobin was quantified using 20 μL of protein extract from one million KU812 cells mixed with 5 mL of Drabkin's reagent (Sigma); then cyanmethemoglobin was measured at the 540 nm wavelength. HbF levels were quantified using the human Hemoglobin F ELISA Quantitation Kit (Bethyl Laboratory, Montgomery, TX). Briefly, 96-well plates were coated with sheep anti-human HbF antibody (1 mg/mL). After blocking with 1% bovine serum albumin, horse radish peroxidase-conjugated secondary antibody (1 mg/mL) was added. Raw data were analyzed using GraphPad PRISM (GraphPad Software, Inc., La Jolla, CA) and HbF levels were calculated as a ratio of total hemoglobin corrected for total protein (HbF/total Hb/total protein).

2.9. HDAC Inhibition Assay.

The HDAC Fluorescent Activity Assay (Enzo Life Science, Farmingdale, NY) was used to measure HDAC inhibition in HeLa cells in a 96-well format using Trichostatin A as the positive control per the manufacturer's protocol. This assay is based on the Fluor de Lys (Fluorogenic Histone Deacetylase Lysyl (FDL)) Substrate/ Developer. The procedure was as follows: the test compounds FK228, JMA26, and JMA33 were added to HeLa cells along

(a)

(b)

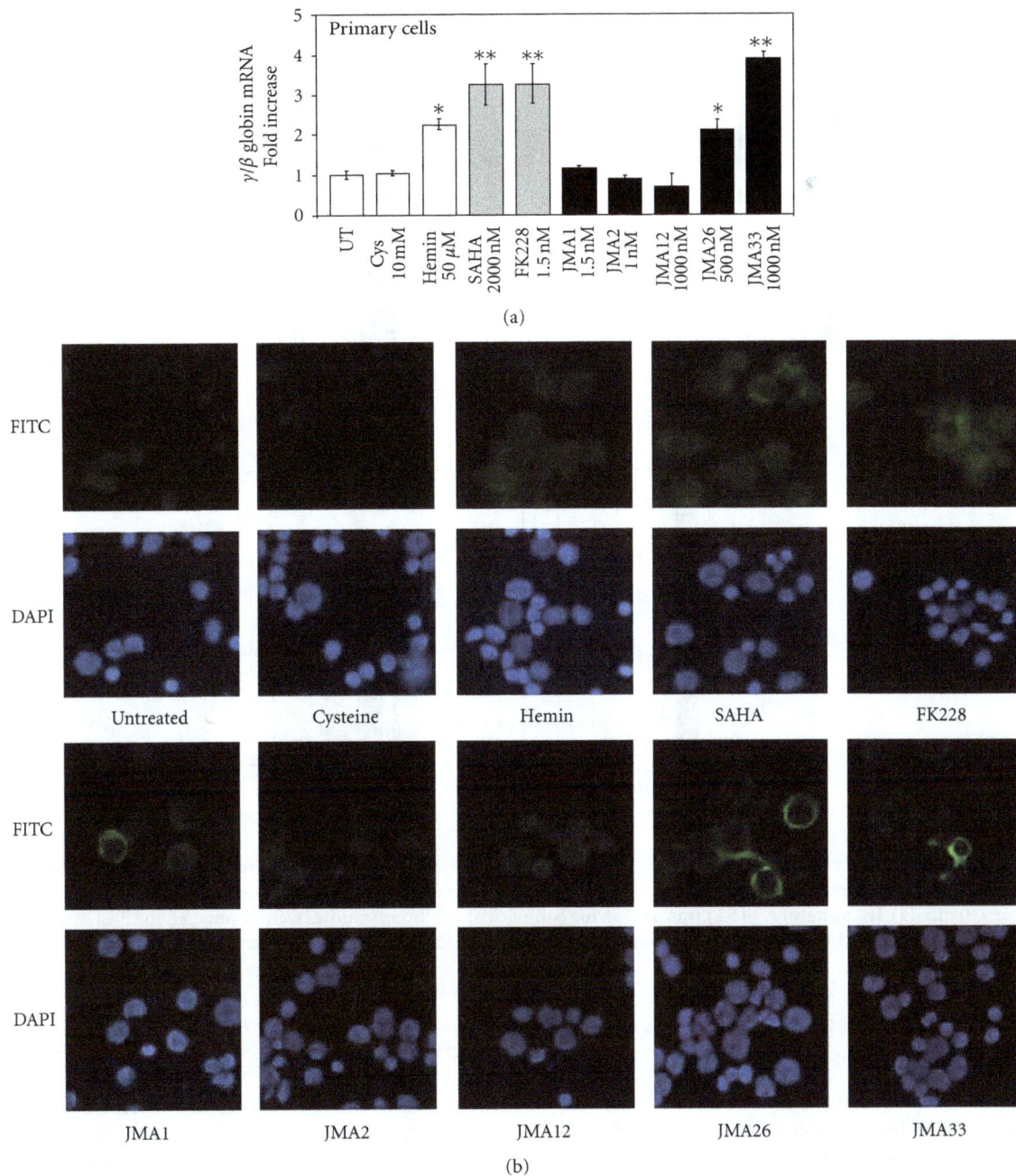

FIGURE 3: JMA33 and JMA26 induce HbF in primary erythroid cells. (a) Day 11 erythroid progenitors were treated for 48 hr with the controls agents and the FK228 analogues shown and then analyzed by RT-qPCR. Untreated cells (UT) were used as a control and normalized to one. Data were calculated as the means ± SEM. (b) Progenitors were stained with anti-γ-globin FITC conjugated antibody overnight and HbF positive cells for were visualized. DAPI staining was performed to identify cell nuclei and to determine cell counts. Images were photographed at 40X power. The images generated were used to count 500 DAPI positive cells and the %FITC positive cells were calculated accordingly.

with the FDL substrate to allow intracellular drug activation then fluorescence levels were read on the fluorometer at 440 nm (CytoFluor II, PerSeptive Biosystems, Farmingdale, NY). The drug concentrations tested were based on the amount required for HbF induction in primary cells. Data was reported as the mean ± standard deviation (SD) for at least five replicates.

2.10. Statistical Analysis. The data are reported as the mean ± standard error of the mean (SEM) from at least five data points generated from independent drug treatments. Data were analyzed by a two-tailed student's t-test, and values of $P < 0.05$ were considered statistically significant. Statistical analyses were performed using Microsoft Excel (Redmond, WA, USA).

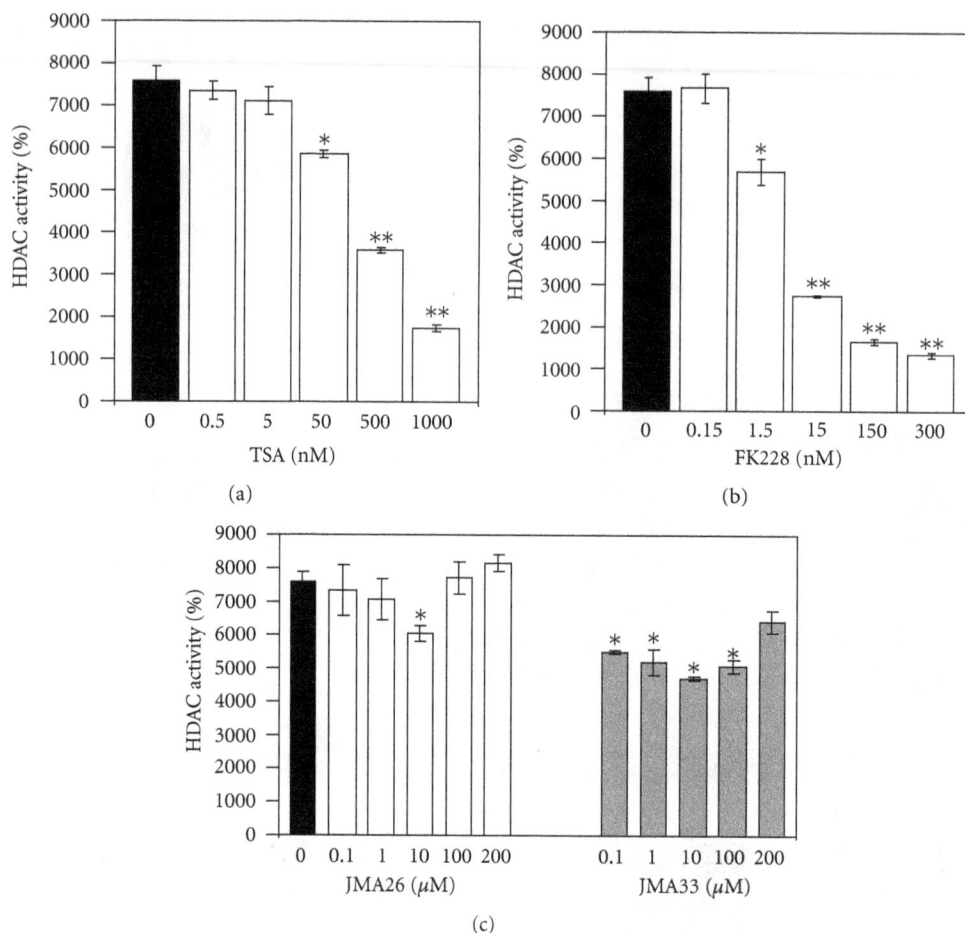

FIGURE 4: HDAC inhibition assay. The HDAC Fluorescent Activity Assay was used to measure HDAC inhibition in HeLa cells (See Section 2). Compounds and FDL substrate were added to HeLa cells to allow drug activation *in vivo* then fluorescence levels were quantified on the fluorometer at 440 nm. (a) Trichostatin A (TSA) was used as the control. (b) Inhibition studies were conducted for FK228 showing maximal HDAC inhibition at the 300 nm concentration. (c) Similar studies were performed for JMA33 and JMA26. The data are reported as the means ± SEM.

3. Results

3.1. Isosteric Substitutions Do Not Alter the Global Structure of FK228. For the facile synthesis of FK228 analogues, the most synthetically challenging moiety, hydroxy-mercapto-heptenoic acid was modified to a structure that can be easily constructed but has the capability of retaining the structure required for biological activity. We used *in silico* structure analysis and molecular modeling to design structural analogues of FK228 that met these requirements and could be easily synthesized [37]. The design of a novel FK228 analogue is summarized in Figure 1. These compounds were synthesized by modifying the most synthetically challenging unit, (3*S*,4*E*)-3-hydroxy-7-mercaptoheptenoic acid, with two isosteric substitutions without altering its global conformation compared to native FK228. First, the trans-double bond in the heptenoic acid was replaced by an isosteric amide bond. Second, the ester bond required to form the depsipeptide was replaced by another amide bond for facile ring closure that provided higher synthetic yield and increased *in vivo* stability. As shown in Figure 1(b), the

structure of the FK228 analogue was found to be almost identical in structure (RMSD = 0.20 Å), indicating that the two isosteric changes neither disturbed the global structure nor altered the backbone structure compared to FK228. However, these changes enabled facile and rapid synthesis using readily available starting materials and high-yielding reactions. While retaining the original stereochemical configurations, the functional groups R_1 and R_2 (Figure 1(b)) were substituted with a variety of amino acids such as Ala, Leu, Phe, 2-Nal, Thr, Asp, and Lys (Scheme 1) to examine the side chain consisting of small, large, aromatic, hydrophilic, and charged alterations.

Twenty FK228 analogues were prepared with high overall yield (75–90%) and purity (80–94%) using the solid-phase synthetic strategy. To further characterize the compounds, selected FK228 analogues were examined by 2D-NMR spectroscopy in (dimethyl sulfoxide) DMSOd$_6$ using Double-quantum filtered, total correlation, and rotating frame Overhauser effect spectroscopy to confirm structures and stereochemistry (data not shown). The FK228 analogues were shown to have outstanding solubility (10 mM) in the

TABLE 1: γ-globin induction in KU812-γF/βR stable lines by FK228 derivatives[1].

Line 1	Drug concentration	$\gamma/\gamma + 2\beta$ Mean	SEM	P value	Fold change
Untreated	none	0.0402	0.0091	n/a	1
Cys	10 mM	0.0388	0.0092	0.8528	0.950
Hemin	50 μM	0.1732	0.0399	0.0050	4.325
SAHA	2000 nM	0.2157	0.0142	0.0001	5.400
FK228	1.5 nM	0.1197	0.0325	0.0150	2.975
1127Ox	1000 nM	0.0363	0.0022	0.8167	0.900
JMA1	1.5 nM	0.0473	0.0149	0.6720	1.175
JMA2	1.0 nM	0.0157	0.0003	0.1629	0.400
JMA12	1000 nM	0.0187	0.0009	0.2156	0.475
JMA26	500 nM	0.1460	0.0234	0.0004	3.650
JMA33	1000 nM	0.1373	0.0117	0.0002	3.425
JMA112	100 nM	0.0187	0.0007	0.2156	2.453
Line 2	Drug concentration	$\gamma/\gamma + 2\beta$ Mean	SEM	P value	Fold change
Untreated	none	0.1573	0.0150	n/a	1
Cys	10 mM	0.1200	0.0056	0.1977	0.764
Hemin	50 μM	0.6593	0.0839	0.0001	4.261
SAHA	2000 nM	0.6500	0.0208	0.0001	4.140
FK228	1.5 nM	0.6167	0.0338	0.0001	3.929
1127Ox	1000 nM	0.6133	0.0371	0.0001	3.904
JMA1	1.5 nM	0.1260	0.0152	0.2896	0.803
JMA2	1.0 nM	0.1183	0.0071	0.1814	0.752
JMA12	1000 nM	0.1470	0.0027	0.7093	0.936
JMA26	500 nM	0.2487	0.0308	0.0153	1.579
JMA33	1000 nM	0.3313	0.0256	0.0002	2.108
JMA112	100 nM	0.1070	0.0076	0.0938	0.682
Line 3	Drug concentration	$\gamma/\gamma + 2\beta$ Mean	SEM	P value	Fold change
Untreated	none	0.0721	0.0052	n/a	1
Cys	10 mM	0.0860	0.0050	0.1814	1.194
Hemin	50 μM	0.2508	0.0153	0.0001	3.486
SAHA	2000 nM	0.2520	0.0066	0.0001	3.500
FK228	1.5 nM	0.1583	0.0198	0.0007	2.194
1127Ox	1000 nM	0.0370	0.0095	0.0076	0.514
JMA1	1.5 nM	0.0770	0.0036	0.6179	1.069
JMA2	1.0 nM	0.0740	0.0036	0.8463	1.027
JMA12	1000 nM	0.0537	0.0023	0.0779	0.750
JMA26	500 nM	0.2560	0.0192	0.0001	3.555
JMA33	1000 nM	0.5120	0.1765	0.0007	7.111
JMA112	100 nM	0.0467	0.0019	0.0216	0.653

[1] Using three independent KU812-γF/βR stable cell lines, the FK228 analogues were examined for their ability to induce γ-globin. After 48 hr drug treatments, cells were harvested and dual luciferase assay performed. Untreated cells were used as a control and normalized to one. Data were calculated as the means ± standard error of the mean (SEM).

organic solvents ethanol and DMSO and were stable for over one year.

3.2. FK228 Analogues Are Potent Inducers of γ-Globin Expression. We first performed drug induction studies in wild type KU812 cells to determine the ability of analogues to induce endogenous γ-globin gene transcription. KU812 cells have been classified as a multipotential leukemia cell line with the ability to differentiate down the basophilic [43, 44], eosinophilic [45] and erythroid/megakaryocytic lineages [46]. Previous studies from our laboratory demonstrated that KU812 cells express γ-globin, β-globin and the erythroid markers CD36, and erythropoietin receptor [47]. Therefore, we used these cells to perform initial drug screens to determine the suitability of KU812 cells for our dual luciferase reporter stable lines. We observed a 1.5- to 10-fold increase in the γ/β-globin mRNA levels after Hem (50 μM), NaB (2 mM), SAHA (2 μM)), and FK228 (1.5 nM) treatment (Figure 2(a)). In the untreated and negative controls, cysteine-treated cells, γ-globin gene expression was not induced. These data demonstrated that the intracellular environment in KU812 is conducive to identifying γ-globin gene activators in our FK228 analogue drug screen.

Subsequently, three independent dual-luciferase reporter KU812 stable cell lines were established to analyze the ability FK228 analogues to induce γ-globin promoter activity without an effect on β-globin transcription. The stable cell lines were created with the μLCRβ_{pr}R$_{luc}\gamma_{pr}$F$_{luc}$ construct (Figure 2(b)) containing a 3.1-kb μLCR cassette linked to a 315-bp human β-globin promoter driving the renilla (R) and a 1.4-kb Aγ-globin promoter driving the firefly (F) luciferase genes [33, 39]. Since the firefly luciferase gene (γF) has approximately 50% greater luminescence than the renilla gene (βR), the renilla activity was multiplied by two to adjust for the difference in luminescence [33] yielding the $\gamma/\gamma+2\beta$ final measurement. The FK228 analogues were examined at concentrations ranging from 1–1000 nM in the three stable lines. After 48-hour treatments, cells were harvested and protein isolated for luciferase activity using the Dual Luciferase Reporter Assay. Of the twenty compounds tested, five induced γ-promoter activity. The remaining agents were either toxic at the concentrations tested or did not induce γ-globin (data not shown). Table 1 summarizes the γ-promoter activity for FK228 analogues that were tested further in primary erythroid cells. Cell viability by Trypan blue exclusion remained at 90–95% for the concentrations shown. Of note are the FK228 analogues, JMA26 and JMA33 (Table 2) containing aromatic side chains in the functional R$_1$ and R$_2$ groups which produced statistically significant γ-promoter activation comparable to FK228. Additional analogues can be designed based on these observations to increase potency, while sparing toxicity.

3.3. FK228 Analogues Activate HbF Synthesis in Primary Erythroid Progenitors. Next, we examined the ability of the lead FK228 analogues to induce HbF expression in primary erythroid progenitors grown from peripheral blood mononuclear cells in the two-phase liquid culture system. As shown in Figure 3(a), JMA26 and JMA33 induced γ-globin transcription at the mRNA level 2.1-fold and 3.9-fold, respectively, compared to a maximal 3.2-fold, induction by SAHA and FK228. However, FK228 derivatives induce γ-promoter activity at significantly lower drug concentrations compared to SAHA and Hem. At the concentrations tested, greater than 90% cell viability was observed in primary cells at all concentrations tested for the synthesized compounds. The similarity of these results to those acquired with the KU812 dual-luciferase reporter cell lines also validates the system for drug screening.

TABLE 2: FK228 structural analogues.

FK228 analogues	R$_1$	R$_2$
JMA1	Val	Ala
JMA2	Val	Phe
JMA12	Phe	Ala
JMA26	Phe	Phe
JMA33	2Nal	2Nal
JMA112	Phe	Lys(FITC)

Val: valine; Phe: phenylalanini; Ala: alanine; 2Nal: 2-naphthylmethyl; Lys: lysine; FITC: fluorescein isothiocyanate.

The next set of studies was performed to determine the ability of JMA26 and JMA33 to induce HbF in primary erythroid progenitors. Using anti-HbF fluorescein isothiocyanate (FITC) antibody, we observed 15.5% HbF-positive progenitors at baseline in untreated cells (Figure 3(b)). Treatment with JMA26 and JMA33 produced 3.0-fold, and 2.5-fold increase in HbF-positive cells, respectively. A similar increase in HbF-positive cells, were produced by hemin, SAHA and FK228 (3.0-fold, 3.2-fold and 3.5-fold). Complementary ELISA data (Table 3) showed a 1.9-fold and 2.5-fold increase in HbF levels produced by JMA26 and JMA33, respectively, compared to a 2.4-fold HbF induction by FK228. We concluded that these lead compounds have the capability to induce HbF in physiologically normal primary erythroid progenitors.

3.4. JMA26 and JMA33 Exhibit HDAC Inhibition Activity. To ascertain the mechanism of HbF induction by the lead compounds, we performed an *in vivo* assay to investigate the ability of JMA26 and JMA33 to act as HDAC inhibitors. The HDAC Fluorescent Activity Assay designed to measure HDAC activity in HeLa cells was completed in a 96-well format. The assay is based on the fact that the Fluor de Lys substrate is deacetylated by HDACs to generate a fluorescent readout. TSA (0.5 to 1000 nM) was used to establish the assay in HeLa cells, showing about 80% HDAC inhibition in our system (Figure 4(a)). By contrast, FK228 produced about 85% inhibition at the 300 nM concentration, which produces marked cell toxicity (Figure 4(b)). Similar studies performed for JMA26 and JMA33 showed 20% and 37% HDAC inhibition, respectively (Figure 4(c)), suggesting HbF induction in erythroid cells occurs by other mechanisms.

4. Discussion

Drug-mediated HbF induction remains the best treatment approach to ameliorate the symptoms and complications of SCD due to its ability to inhibit hemoglobin S polymerization. In addition, HbF provides an effective treatment for β-thalassemia by correcting globin chain imbalance [48]. Other therapies aimed at the underlying molecular causes of the β-hemoglobinopathies include hematopoietic stem cell transplantation [49] and gene therapy involving the transfer of normal γ- or β-globin genes into hematopoietic stem cells. Despite promising results and ongoing research, the option for stem cell transplantation is limited by the lack of suitable

TABLE 3: Fetal hemoglobin quantification in primary erythroid cells.

	Drug concentration	Mean	SEM	P value	Fold change
Untreated	none	0.683	0.0291	n/a	1
Cys	10 mM	0.737	0.1201	0.7773	1.079
Hemin	50 μM	1.515	0.0405	0.0001	2.218
SAHA	2000 nM	1.094	0.1049	0.0197	1.602
FK228	1.5 nM	1.676	0.0506	0.0001	2.454
JMA1	1.5 nM	0.7953	0.0849	0.2803	1.164
JMA2	1.0 nM	0.8120	0.0165	0.0183	1.188
JMA26	500 nM	1.3086	0.0535	0.0005	1.916
JMA33	1000 nM	1.7223	0.0725	0.0002	2.521

donors for the majority of SCD patients. On the other hand, gene therapy offers a universal cure but there are concerns about mutagenesis of target genes due to random vector integration and the effects of viral sequences on nearby gene expression [50]. Therefore, pharmacologic HbF induction remains a viable choice for the development of additional therapeutic options for treating SCD.

Hydroxyurea is the only drug approved by the Food and Drug Administration for the treatment of SCD [7, 51], however, it is not effective in all patients [7] and of minimal benefit in β-thalassemia [52]. Moreover, there are concerns about undesirable side effects including long-term carcinogenesis [53]. Clinical trials with other compounds, such as arginine butyrate [54] and decitabine [55] have shown considerable promise, however, orally active preparations need to be developed to make these agents viable treatment alternatives.

For many years, K562 cells have been used to screen pharmacological agents as potential HbF inducers. For example, NaB, decitabine, and hydroxyurea, among others, stimulate erythroid differentiation in K562 cells and induce γ-globin gene transcription [56]. Many HDAC inhibitors including FK228 are also known to induce HbF. However, synthetic difficulties associated with FK228 production have severely deterred structure-activity studies to aid understanding of its mechanism of action and to improve efficacy. Our data shows that JMA26 and JMA33 increased HbF levels by a mechanism independent of HDAC inhibition.

Many published studies have shown that primary erythroid cells remain the best system to confirm HbF-inducing agents and to serve as a predictor of efficacy *in vivo*. Human burst forming units—erythroid cells in clonogenic assays [57] or erythroid progenitors grown in liquid culture [39, 41]—have been used to evaluate putative HbF inducers. However, these assays are not easily adaptable to large-scale drug screening, thus immortalized cell lines have been investigated for this purpose. Previously, FK228 was tested in the $\mu LCR\beta_{pr}R_{luc}{}^A\gamma_{pr}F_{luc}$ GM979 stable line [33] and was shown to induce γ-promoter activity at the 1 nM concentration. We expanded on these studies to establish a dual-luciferase reporter system. Thus, we used KU812 cells derived from an individual with chronic myeloid leukemia

[58] because both γ-globin and β-globin are actively transcribed [47]. Moreover, gene profiling data generated by our laboratory showed that KU812 cells express CD36 and the erythropoietin receptor at levels comparable to day-14 human erythroid progenitors [47].

In this study, when wild-type KU812 cells were treated with Hem, NaB, SAHA, and FK228, we observed a 3- to 10-fold increase in the γ/β-globin ratio. We next tested the FK228 analogues in the KU812 dual-luciferase reporter system created with the $\mu LCR\beta_{pr}R_{luc}{}^A\gamma_{pr}F_{luc}$ construct. Two FK228 analogues identified in the reporter assay, JMA26 and JMA33, showed efficacy as HbF inducer in primary erythroid progenitors suggesting these compounds have the potential for further development.

Our last set of experiments was aimed at understanding the mechanism by which JMA26 and JMA33 induce γ-globin. Histone acetylation is a highly dynamic reversible modification that contributes to gene expression through changes in chromatin conformations. The parent compound FK228 is a class IV cyclic peptide capable of inhibiting Class I HDAC enzymes (HDAC1, 2, 3, and 8) after intracellular reduction of its disulfide bond by glutathione to produce the active reduced form of FK228. The functional sulfhydryl group fits inside the catalytic pocket producing zinc chelation and inhibition of enzymatic activity [59].

The role of HDAC inhibition in HbF induction has been investigated by several laboratories. NaB was the first agent shown to mediate histone H3 and H4 hyperacetylation as a mechanism of HbF induction [60]. Subsequently, many other HDAC inhibitors such as TSA [42], scriptaid [28], SBHA (suberohydroxamic acid), and SAHA (suberoylanilide hydroxamic acid) [59] were shown to be HbF inducers based on the central role of histone hyperacetylation. Subsequently, Perrine and colleagues showed the ability of short-chain fatty acids to induce γ-globin by displacement of an HDAC3-NcoR repressor complex [61]. More recently, there exist chemical genetic screen-identified HDAC1 and HDAC2 as molecular targets facilitating drug-mediated HbF induction [62]. Therefore, to determine the mechanism of action of JMA26 and JMA33, we completed the HDAC inhibition assay.

Using the Fluor de Lys system, FK228 produced strong HDAC inhibition but at a higher concentration (300 nM) than required for HbF induction. Similar studies performed for JMA26 and JMA33 showed 20% and 37% maximal inhibition, respectively. These findings suggest that the alterations in FK228 structure may have uncoupled HDAC inhibition activity as the primary mechanism of HbF induction since higher test drug concentrations did not produce more HDAC inhibition. These data suggests JMA26 and JMA33 may induce γ-globin by mechanisms other than targeting HDACs. Since the FK228 analogues were developed from a structural library designed by molecular modeling, additional compounds can be synthesized with greater HbF inducing potency and selectivity to Class I HDACs. Additional studies will also be conducted to determine other mechanisms by JMA26 and JMA33 that induce HbF such as activation of the p38 mitogen-activated protein kinase or other signaling pathways [17, 63, 64].

5. Conclusions

The current drug treatment options for SCD are limited with hydroxyurea being the only FDA-approved drug. The key finding of this study is the high-efficiency synthesis of FK228 analogues with structural modifications which did not disturb the global chemical structure of the parent compound. The analogues exhibited HbF induction at nanomolar concentrations in primary erythroid progenitors demonstrating physiological relevance. These data support the FK228 analogues as potential therapeutic agents and also validates the KU812 dual-luciferase stable cell lines as an efficacious screening system to identify γ-globin activators. Long-term our goal is to establish a group of HbF inducers that selectively inhibit Class I HDACs to expand our understanding of epigenetic mechanisms of γ-globin gene regulation and to facilitate the development of drug therapy for SCD.

Acknowledgment

This work was supported by a Grant from the National Heart Lung and Blood Institute (R01HL069234; BSP), the Francis J. Tedesco Distinguished Chair in Pediatric Hematology/Oncology (BSP), and the Robert A. Welch Foundation (AT-1595; JMA).

References

[1] T. Papayannopoulou, A. Torrealba De Ron, and R. Veith, "Arabinosylcytosine induces fetal hemoglobin in baboons by perturbing erythroid cell differentiation kinetics," *Science*, vol. 224, no. 4649, pp. 617–619, 1984.

[2] D. P. Liu, C. C. Liang, Z. H. Ao et al., "Treatment of severe β-thalassemia (patients) with myleran," *American Journal of Hematology*, vol. 33, no. 1, pp. 50–55, 1990.

[3] R. Veith, T. Papayannopoulou, S. Kurachi, and G. Stamatoyannopoulos, "Treatment of baboon with vinblastine: insights into the mechanisms of pharmacologic stimulation of hb f in the adult," *Blood*, vol. 66, no. 2, pp. 456–459, 1985.

[4] R. Galanello, G. Stamatoyannopoulos, and Papayannopoulou Th., "Mechanism of hb f stimulation by s-stage compounds. in vitro studies with bone marrow cells exposed to 5-azacytidine, ara-c, or hydroxyurea," *Journal of Clinical Investigation*, vol. 81, no. 4, pp. 1209–1216, 1988.

[5] N. L. Letvin, D. C. Linch, and G. P. Beardsley, "Augmentation of fetal-hemoglobin production in anemic monkeys by hydroxyurea," *New England Journal of Medicine*, vol. 310, no. 14, pp. 869–873, 1984.

[6] M. H. Steinberg, F. Barton, O. Castro et al., "Effect of hydroxyurea on mortality and morbidity in adult sickle cell anemia: risks and benefits up to 9 years of treatment," *Journal of the American Medical Association*, vol. 289, no. 13, pp. 1645–1651, 2003.

[7] S. Charache, M. L. Terrin, R. D. Moore et al., "Effect of hydroxyurea on the frequency of painful crises in sickle cell anemia. Investigators of the Multicenter Study of Hydroxyurea in Sickle Cell Anemia," *The New England Journal of Medicine*, vol. 332, pp. 1317–1322, 1995.

[8] M. H. Steinberg, Z. H. Lu, F. B. Barton, M. L. Terrin, S. Charache, and G. J. Dover, "Fetal hemoglobin in sickle cell anemia: determinants of response to hydroxyurea," *Blood*, vol. 89, no. 3, pp. 1078–1088, 1997.

[9] X. De La Cruz, S. Lois, S. Sánchez-Molina, and M. A. Martínez-Balbás, "Do protein motifs read the histone code?" *Bioessays*, vol. 27, no. 2, pp. 164–175, 2005.

[10] P. A. Marks and X. Jiang, "Histone deacetylase inhibitors in programmed cell death and cancer therapy," *Cell Cycle*, vol. 4, no. 4, pp. 549–551, 2005.

[11] C. Monneret, "Histone deacetylase inhibitors," *European Journal of Medicinal Chemistry*, vol. 40, no. 1, pp. 1–13, 2005.

[12] K. N. Prasad, "Butyric acid: a small fatty acid with diverse biological functions," *Life Sciences*, vol. 27, no. 15, pp. 1351–1358, 1980.

[13] A. E. Smith, P. J. Hurd, A. J. Bannister, T. Kouzarides, and K. G. Ford, "Heritable gene repression through the action of a directed dna methyltransferase at a chromosomal locus," *Journal of Biological Chemistry*, vol. 283, no. 15, pp. 9878–9885, 2008.

[14] S. D. Gore and M. A. Carducci, "Modifying histones to tame cancer: clinical development of sodium phenylbutyrate and other histone deacetylase inhibitors," *Expert Opinion on Investigational Drugs*, vol. 9, no. 12, pp. 2923–2934, 2000.

[15] T. Yamashita, H. Wakao, A. Miyajima, and S. Asano, "Differentiation inducers modulate cytokine signaling pathways in a murine erythroleukemia cell line," *Cancer Research*, vol. 58, no. 3, pp. 556–561, 1998.

[16] O. Witt, K. Sand, and A. Pekrun, "Butyrate-induced erythroid differentiation of human k562 leukemia cells involves inhibition of erk and activation of p38 map kinase pathways," *Blood*, vol. 95, no. 7, pp. 2391–2396, 2000.

[17] B. S. Pace, X. H. Qian, J. Sangerman et al., "P38 map kinase activation mediates γ-globin gene induction in erythroid progenitors," *Experimental Hematology*, vol. 31, no. 11, pp. 1089–1096, 2003.

[18] S. Torkelson, B. White, D. V. Faller, C. Phipps, C. Pantazis, and S. P. Perrine, "Erythroid progenitor proliferation is stimulated by phenoxyacetic and phenylalkyl acids," *Blood Cells, Molecules, and Diseases*, vol. 22, no. 2, pp. 150–158, 1996.

[19] G. J. Dover, S. Brusilow, and S. Charache, "Induction of fetal hemoglobin production in subjects with sickle cell anemia by oral sodium phenylbutyrate," *Blood*, vol. 84, no. 1, pp. 339–343, 1994.

[20] E. Liakopoulou, C. A. Blau, Q. Li et al., "Stimulation of fetal hemoglobin production by short chain fatty acids," *Blood*, vol. 86, no. 8, pp. 3227–3235, 1995.

[21] N. Tsuji, M. Kobayashi, and K. Nagashima, "A new antifungal antibiotic, trichostatin," *Journal of Antibiotics*, vol. 29, no. 1, pp. 1–6, 1976.

[22] M. Yoshida, M. Kijima, M. Akita, and T. Beppu, "Potent and specific inhibition of mammalian histone deacetylase both in vivo and in vitro by trichostatin a," *Journal of Biological Chemistry*, vol. 265, no. 28, pp. 17174–17179, 1990.

[23] M. S. Finnin, J. R. Donigian, A. Cohen et al., "Structures of a histone deacetylase homologue bound to the tsa and saha inhibitors," *Nature*, vol. 401, no. 6749, pp. 188–193, 1999.

[24] V. M. Richon, S. Emiliani, E. Verdin et al., "A class of hybrid polar inducers of transformed cell differentiation inhibits histone deacetylases," *Proceedings of the National Academy of Sciences of the United States of America*, vol. 95, no. 6, pp. 3003–3007, 1998.

[25] L. M. Butler, D. B. Agus, H. I. Scher et al., "Suberoylanilide hydroxamic acid, an inhibitor of histone deacetylase, suppresses the growth of prostate cancer cells in vitro and in vivo," *Cancer Research*, vol. 60, no. 18, pp. 5165–5170, 2000.

[26] P. A. Marks, V. M. Richon, R. Breslow, and R. A. Rifkind, "Histone deacetylase inhibitors as new cancer drugs," *Current Opinion in Oncology*, vol. 13, no. 6, pp. 477–483, 2001.

[27] H. Ueda, H. Nakajima, Y. Hori et al., "Fr901228, a novel antitumor bicyclic depsipeptide produced by chromobacterium violaceum no. 968. i. taxonomy, fermentation, isolation, physico-chemical and biological properties, and antitumor activity," *Journal of Antibiotics*, vol. 47, no. 3, pp. 301–310, 1994.

[28] J. Johnson, R. Hunter, R. McElveen, X. H. Qian, B. S. Baliga, and B. S. Pace, "Fetal hemoglobin induction by the histone deacetylase inhibitor, scriptaid," *Cellular and Molecular Biology*, vol. 51, no. 2, pp. 229–238, 2005.

[29] R. Furumai, A. Matsuyama, N. Kobashi et al., "Fk228 (depsipeptide) as a natural prodrug that inhibits class i histone deacetylases," *Cancer Research*, vol. 62, no. 17, pp. 4916–4921, 2002.

[30] J. J. Xiao, J. Byrd, G. Marcucci, M. Grever, and K. K. Chan, "Identification of thiols and glutathione conjugates of depsipeptide fk228 (fr901228), a novel histone protein deacetylase inhibitor, in the blood," *Rapid Communications in Mass Spectrometry*, vol. 17, no. 8, pp. 757–766, 2003.

[31] H. Kosugi, M. Ito, Y. Yamamoto et al., "In vivo effects of a histone deacetylase inhibitor, fk228, on human acute promyelocytic leukemia in nod/shi-scid/scid mice," *Japanese Journal of Cancer Research*, vol. 92, no. 5, pp. 529–536, 2001.

[32] K. A. Fecteau, M. E. I. Jianxun, and H. C. Wang, "Differential modulation of signaling pathways and apoptosis of ras-transformed 10t1/2 cells by the depsipeptide fr901228," *Journal of Pharmacology and Experimental Therapeutics*, vol. 300, no. 3, pp. 890–899, 2002.

[33] H. Cao and G. Stamatoyannopoulos, "Histone deacetylase inhibitor fk228 is a potent inducer of human fetal hemoglobin," *American Journal of Hematology*, vol. 81, no. 12, pp. 981–983, 2006.

[34] K. W. Li, J. Wu, W. Xing, and J. A. Simon, "Total synthesis of the antitumor depsipeptide fr-901,228," *Journal of the American Chemical Society*, vol. 118, no. 30, pp. 7237–7238, 1996.

[35] T. J. Greshock, D. M. Johns, Y. Noguchi, and R. M. Williams, "Improved total synthesis of the potent hdac inhibitor FK228 (FK-901228)," *Organic Letters*, vol. 10, no. 4, pp. 613–616, 2008.

[36] A. A. Bowers, T. J. Greshook, N. West et al., "Synthesis and conformation-activity relationships of the peptide isosteres of fk228 and largazole," *Journal of the American Chemical Society*, vol. 131, no. 8, pp. 2900–2905, 2009.

[37] S. Di Maro, R. C. Pong, J. T. Hsieh, and J. M. Ahn, "Efficient solid-phase synthesis of fk228 analogues as potent antitumoral agents," *Journal of Medicinal Chemistry*, vol. 51, no. 21, pp. 6639–6641, 2008.

[38] K. J. Jensen, J. Alsina, M. F. Songster, J. Vágner, F. Albericio, and G. Barany, "Backbone amide linker (BAL) strategy for solid-phase synthesis of c-terminal-modified and cyclic peptides," *Journal of the American Chemical Society*, vol. 120, no. 22, pp. 5441–5452, 1998.

[39] E. Skarpidi, G. Vassilopoulos, Q. Li, and G. Stamatoyannopoulos, "Novel in vitro assay for the detection of pharmacologic inducers of fetal hemoglobin," *Blood*, vol. 96, no. 1, pp. 321–326, 2000.

[40] C. Y. Gui and A. Dean, "Acetylation of a specific promoter nucleosome accompanies activation of the ε-globin gene by β-globin locus control region HS2," *Molecular and Cellular Biology*, vol. 21, no. 4, pp. 1155–1163, 2001.

[41] E. Fibach, L. P. Burke, A. N. Schechter, C. T. Noguchi, and G. P. Rodgers, "Hydroxyurea increases fetal hemoglobin in cultured erythroid cells derived from normal individuals and patients with sickle cell anemia or β- thalassemia," *Blood*, vol. 81, no. 6, pp. 1630–1635, 1993.

[42] J. Sangerman, S. L. Moo, X. Yao et al., "Mechanism for fetal hemoglobin induction by histone deacetylase inhibitors involves γ-globin activation by creb1 and atf-2," *Blood*, vol. 108, no. 10, pp. 3590–3599, 2006.

[43] T. Fukuda, K. Kishi, Y. Ohnishi, and A. Shibata, "Bipotential cell differentiation of ku-812: evidence of a hybrid cell line that differentiates into basophils and macrophage-like cells," *Blood*, vol. 70, no. 3, pp. 612–619, 1987.

[44] K. Kishi, "A new leukemia cell line with Philadelphia chromosome characterized as basophil precursors," *Leukemia Research*, vol. 9, no. 3, pp. 381–390, 1985.

[45] M. Yamashita, A. Ichikawa, Y. Katakura et al., "Induction of basophilic and eosinophilic differentiation in the human leukemic cell line ku812," *Cytotechnology*, vol. 36, no. 1–3, pp. 179–186, 2001.

[46] M. Nakazawa, M. T. Mitjavila, N. Debili et al., "Ku 812: a pluripotent human cell line with spontaneous erythroid terminal maturation," *Blood*, vol. 73, no. 7, pp. 2003–2013, 1989.

[47] S. Zein, W. Li, V. Ramakrishnan et al., "Identification of fetal hemoglobin-inducing agents using the human leukemia ku812 cell line," *Experimental Biology and Medicine*, vol. 235, no. 11, pp. 1385–1394, 2010.

[48] D. G. Nathan and R. B. Gunn, "Thalassemia: the consequences of unbalanced hemoglobin synthesis," *the American Journal of Medicine*, vol. 41, no. 5, pp. 815–830, 1966.

[49] M. Bhatia and M. C. Walters, "Hematopoietic cell transplantation for thalassemia and sickle cell disease: past, present and future," *Bone Marrow Transplantation*, vol. 41, no. 2, pp. 109–117, 2008.

[50] C. E. Dunbar, "The yin and yang of stem cell gene therapy: insights into hematopoiesis, leukemogenesis, and gene therapy safety," *Hematology/the Education Program of the American Society of Hematology. American Society of Hematology. Education Program*, pp. 460–465, 2007.

[51] M. H. Steinberg, Z. H. Lu, F. B. Barton, M. L. Terrin, S. Charache, and G. J. Dover, "Fetal hemoglobin in sickle cell anemia: determinants of response to hydroxyurea," *Blood*, vol. 89, no. 3, pp. 1078–1088, 1997.

[52] H. Fathallah, M. Sutton, and G. F. Atweh, "Pharmacological induction of fetal hemoglobin: why haven't we been more successful in thalassemia?" *Annals of the New York Academy of Sciences*, vol. 1054, pp. 228–237, 2005.

[53] S. C. Davies and A. Gilmore, "The role of hydroxyurea in the management of sickle cell disease," *Blood Reviews*, vol. 17, no. 2, pp. 99–109, 2003.

[54] G. F. Atweh, M. Sutton, I. Nassif et al., "Sustained induction of fetal hemoglobin by pulse butyrate therapy in sickle cell disease," *Blood*, vol. 93, no. 6, pp. 1790–1797, 1999.

[55] Y. Saunthararajah, R. Molokie, S. Saraf et al., "Clinical effectiveness of decitabine in severe sickle cell disease," *British Journal of Haematology*, vol. 141, no. 1, pp. 126–129, 2008.

[56] R. Mabaera, R. J. West, S. J. Conine et al., "A cell stress signaling model of fetal hemoglobin induction: what doesn't kill red blood cells may make them stronger," *Experimental Hematology*, vol. 36, no. 9, pp. 1057–1072, 2008.

[57] P. Constantoulakis, G. Knitter, and G. Stamatoyannopoulos, "On the induction of fetal hemoglobin by butyrates: in vivo and in vitro studies with sodium butyrate and comparison of

combination treatments with 5-AZAC and ARAC," *Blood*, vol. 74, no. 6, pp. 1963–1971, 1989.

[58] A. Goga, J. McLaughlin, D. E. H. Afar, D. C. Saffran, and O. N. Witte, "Alternative signals to ras for hematopoietic transformation by the bcr- abl oncogene," *Cell*, vol. 82, no. 6, pp. 981–988, 1995.

[59] R. Furumai, A. Matsuyama, N. Kobashi et al., "FK228 (depsipeptide) as a natural prodrug that inhibits class i histone deacetylases," *Cancer Research*, vol. 62, no. 17, pp. 4916–4921, 2002.

[60] H. Fathallah, R. S. Weinberg, Y. Galperin, M. Sutton, and G. F. Atweh, "Role of epigenetic modifications in normal globin gene regulation and butyrate-mediated induction of fetal hemoglobin," *Blood*, vol. 110, no. 9, pp. 3391–3397, 2007.

[61] R. Mankidy, D. V. Faller, R. Mabaera et al., "Short-chain fatty acids induce γ-globin gene expression by displacement of a hdac3-ncor repressor complex," *Blood*, vol. 108, no. 9, pp. 3179–3186, 2006.

[62] J. E. Bradner, R. Mak, S. K. Tanguturi et al., "Chemical genetic strategy identifies histone deacetylase 1 (HDAC1) and HDAC2 as therapeutic targets in sickle cell disease," *Proceedings of the National Academy of Sciences of the United States of America*, vol. 107, no. 28, pp. 12617–12622, 2010.

[63] O. Witt, K. Sand, and A. Pekrun, "Butyrate-induced erythroid differentiation of human k562 leukemia cells involves inhibition of ERK and activation of p38 map kinase pathways," *Blood*, vol. 95, no. 7, pp. 2391–2396, 2000.

[64] O. Witt, S. Mönkemeyer, K. Kanbach, and A. Pekrun, "Induction of fetal hemoglobin synthesis by valproate: modulation of mapkinase pathways," *American Journal of Hematology*, vol. 71, no. 1, pp. 45–46, 2002.

6

Diagnosis of Fanconi Anemia: Mutation Analysis by Next-Generation Sequencing

Najim Ameziane,[1] Daoud Sie,[2] Stefan Dentro,[1] Yavuz Ariyurek,[3]
Lianne Kerkhoven,[1] Hans Joenje,[1] Josephine C. Dorsman,[1] Bauke Ylstra,[2] Johan J. P. Gille,[1]
Erik A. Sistermans,[1] and Johan P. de Winter[1]

[1] Department of Clinical Genetics, VU University Medical Center, Van der Boechorststraat 7, 1081 BT Amsterdam, The Netherlands
[2] Department of Pathology, VU University Medical Center, De Boelelaan 1117, 1081 HV Amsterdam, The Netherlands
[3] Leiden Genome Technology Center, Center for Human and Clinical Genetics, Leiden University Medical Center, Einthovenweg 20, 2333 ZC Leiden, The Netherlands

Correspondence should be addressed to Najim Ameziane, n.ameziane@vumc.nl

Academic Editor: Stefan Meyer

Fanconi anemia (FA) is a rare genetic instability syndrome characterized by developmental defects, bone marrow failure, and a high cancer risk. Fifteen genetic subtypes have been distinguished. The majority of patients ($\approx$85%) belong to the subtypes A ($\approx$60%), C ($\approx$15%) or G ($\approx$10%), while a minority ($\approx$15%) is distributed over the remaining 12 subtypes. All subtypes seem to fit within the "classical" FA phenotype, except for D1 and N patients, who have more severe clinical symptoms. Since FA patients need special clinical management, the diagnosis should be firmly established, to exclude conditions with overlapping phenotypes. A valid FA diagnosis requires the detection of pathogenic mutations in a FA gene and/or a positive result from a chromosomal breakage test. Identification of the pathogenic mutations is also important for adequate genetic counselling and to facilitate prenatal or preimplantation genetic diagnosis. Here we describe and validate a comprehensive protocol for the molecular diagnosis of FA, based on massively parallel sequencing. We used this approach to identify BRCA2, FANCD2, FANCI and FANCL mutations in novel unclassified FA patients.

1. Introduction

Fanconi anemia (FA) is a recessive chromosomal instability syndrome with diverse clinical symptoms and a high risk for acute myeloid leukemia and squamous cell carcinoma of the head and neck region [1]. Clinical suspicion of FA is mostly based on growth retardation and congenital defects in combination with life-threatening bone marrow failure (thrombocytopenia and later pancytopenia), which usually starts between 5 and 10 years of age. However, the clinical manifestations of FA patients are highly variable, and therefore the FA diagnosis should be confirmed by a positive chromosomal breakage test and/or pathogenic mutations in one of the FA genes. Currently, mutations in 15 different genes are known to cause FA, and their gene products act in a pathway that takes care of specific problems that may arise during the process of DNA replication [2].

The conventional Sanger sequencing-based mutation screening approach for FA is time-consuming, costly, and most importantly may not detect all types of disease-causing aberrations, such as deep intronic mutations, large deletions, and amplifications. Furthermore, the existence of FANCD2 pseudogenes obstructs the identification of pathogenic mutations in this gene when sequencing genomic DNA. Here, we demonstrate a comprehensive mutation detection approach for FA based on massively parallel sequencing (MPS) [3].

2. Methods

We designed an in-solution oligonucleotide hybridization capture kit (SureSelect, Agilent) targeting the open reading frames of all FA genes, except for regions that contain repetitive and low complexity DNA sequences as assessed by RepeatMasker (http://www.repeatmasker.org/). All exons-, 3′-, and 5′-UTR-regions, and exon-intron boundaries were targeted by this approach (the oligonucleotide locations, in a .BED format, are available upon request). In addition, a number of other genes involved in cancer predisposition and routinely screened in our diagnostic lab were included in the enrichment kit. We used the Illumina GAIIx platform for sequencing.

To assess the performance of the custom target kit and the massively parallel sequencing method, we selected FA samples with a spectrum of different types of known variations (Table 1). The pathogenic mutations in these samples have previously been identified either by Sanger sequencing or by multiplex ligation-dependent probe amplification (MLPA) [4]. One of the samples included in the study was from a carrier of a *BRCA1* mutation. Unique barcode sequences were used for 11 DNA libraries to allow distinction between the samples that were run on a single Illumina flow-cell lane. In addition, to evaluate the sensitivity of the approach, two DNA samples were pooled before library preparation to mimic a mosaic condition.

An in-house variation detection pipeline, including a novel tool for large deletion detection, was used to score for relevant mutations.

2.1. Library Preparation. For each sample, 1.5 μg of DNA was resuspended in 75 μL of TE buffer in a Covaris microTube, and subsequently sheared in a Covaris S220 (Covaris, Inc. MS, USA) using the following settings: duty cycle = 10%, Intensity = 5, cycles per burst = 200, time = 360, Set mode = frequency sweeping, and temperature = 4°C. Fragmented DNA containing overhangs is converted into blunt ends using T4 DNA polymerase and Klenow enzyme (New England Biolabs) by incubation for 30 minutes at 20°C. The DNA sample is then purified with QIAquick PCR purification kit (Qiagen) following the manufacturer's instructions and eluted in 32 μL of Qiagen elution buffer. Next, the 3′ ends of the fragmented DNA are adenylated using Klenow exonuclease (New England Biolabs) by incubating for 30 minutes at 37°C. The DNA sample is then purified with MinElute PCR purification kit (Qiagen) following the manufacturer's instructions and eluted in 10 μL of Qiagen elution buffer. Next, Illumina-specific index paired-end adapters (Illumina) are ligated to the 5′ and 3′ ends of DNA fragments by incubation with DNA ligase (New England Biolabs) for 15 minutes at 20°C. The adapter-ligated DNA fragments are purified with MinElute PCR purification kit, and 1 μL is used to assess proper adapter ligation by a control PCR using InPE 1.0, InPE 2.0, and a random index primer with the following PCR conditions: 30 sec at 98°C, 18 cycles of 10 sec at 98°C, 30 sec at 65°C, 30 sec at 72°C, and a final step of 5 minutes at 72°C. The quality and quantity of the library is evaluated with the Agilent 2100 Bioanalyzer on a DNA 1000 chip following the manufacturer's instructions.

For the FA gene enrichment, we used 500 ng of adapter-ligated library following the manufacturer's instructions. Briefly, DNA libraries are incubated with the biotinylated

TABLE 1: Selected FA samples with mutations previously identified by Sanger sequencing and multiplex ligation-dependent probe amplification (MLPA), used for validation of the next-generation sequencing approach.

Sample (affected gene)	Allele 1	Allele 2	Reference
Sam 1 (*BRCA2*)	c.9253dupA	—	BIC DB#
Sam 2 (*FANCA*)	c.3558insG	—	[4]
Sam 3 (*FANCG*)	c.271–272del	c.620delT	[4]
Sam 4a (*FANCA*)	c.1464C>G	c.2632G>C	[4]
Sam 4b (*FANCA*)	Ex 15–23 del	—	[4]
Sam 5 (*BRCA1*)	c.2694dupA	—	BIC DB#
Sam 6 (*FANCC*)	c.376–377del	c.844-1G>C	[4]
Sam 7 (*FANCA*)	Ex 1–20 del	c.893+920 C>A	[5]
Sam 8 (*FANCB*)	c.811insT	absent	[4]
Sam 9 (*FANCE*)	c.91C>T	c.91C>T	[4]
Sam 10 (*PALB2*)	Ex 1–10 del	c.1802T>A	[6]
Sam 11 (*FANCI*)	c.2509G>T	NF*	[4]

#Breast cancer information core database available at http://www.research.nhgri.nih.gov/bic/.
*NF: not found.

RNA custom SureSelect library "baits" for 16 hours at 60°C. Next, DNA library that hybridized to the baits is captured using magnetic beads (Dynabeads, Invitrogen), washed, and eluted in elution buffer. Primers containing unique barcode sequences are used to amplify captured libraries, and equimolar pooling is performed after quantification on a bioanalyzer. The eleven pooled DNA libraries were then sequenced on a single flow cell lane of an Illumina GAIIx using a 72 cycle multiplex paired-end sequence protocol.

3. Results

Sequence data from DNA libraries of eleven carriers of mutations in the FA genes: *FANCA (4)*, *FANCB (1)*, *FANCC (1)*, *FANCD1 (1)*, *FANCE (1)*, *FANCG (1)*, *FANCI (1)*, *FANCN (1)*, and one individual carrying a mutation in *BRCA1*, were generated from an Illumina GAIIx sequencer. An average of 2.8 million unique reads were obtained per library resulting in a median sequence depth of about 100 fold, with an average enrichment efficiency of >75% (Figure 1). Several types of disease-causing genetic aberrations were present in the assayed DNA samples including single nucleotide substitutions, small deletions (1–8 nucleotides), and large deletions (multiple exons). We developed a variation detection pipeline detecting all these types of aberrations.

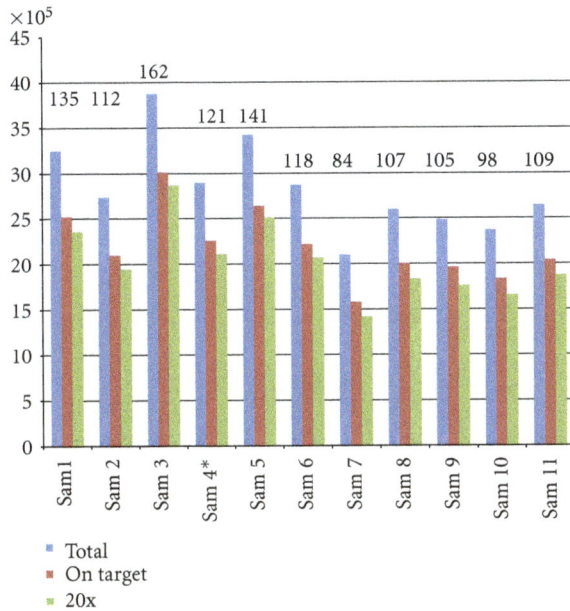

FIGURE 1: Specifications of 11 DNA libraries pooled and sequenced on one flow cell lane of an Illumina GAIIx. Numbers on top of the bars indicate the average sequencing depth obtained for the individual samples. Blue bars indicate total number of unique reads, red bars indicate reads that fall on target of the bait design, green bars indicate reads that fall in target regions covered with at least 20x depth. Sample 4 is a mix of genomic DNA from two individuals 4a and 4b.

3.1. Detection of Single Nucleotide Variations (SNVs) and Small Insertions/Deletions (Indels).

The data analysis pipeline for the detection of SNVs and small indels that was developed is comprised of freely available tools on the web. An initial quality check of the sequence reads is followed by mapping the paired-end reads with the Burrows-Wheeler Aligner (BWA) [14] to the National Center for Biotechnology Information (NCBI) hg19 build reference genome. Subsequently, SNPs and small indels are called using Samtools [15] and Varscan [16]. The resulting list of variations is annotated with Annovar [17] that utilizes information from external databases to generate context around the mutations, such as amino acid change consequence, location to canonical splice site regions, and information about reference to dbSNP and frequencies if available. Finally, a manual filtering step is executed to prioritize relevant mutations. Low-frequency frameshifts and truncating mutations are considered pathogenic. Unreported nonsynonymous amino acid variations are analyzed in silico by the pathogenicity predicting programs, Align-GVGD, Polyphen-2 and SIFT [7–9] to help assess the damaging effect.

The variation detection frequency for all samples was set at a minimum of 31% of the reads covering the aberrations except for sample 4 (pre-library DNA pooling of samples 4a and 4b), for which it was set at 12%. The total number of variations detected in the samples and the subsequent reduction in number of variations through filtering is depicted in Table 2.

Using the variation detection pipeline and filtering procedure 12 SNVs out of the total of 13 were detected. The variation that escaped the initial filtering procedure resided deep in the intronic region; 920 nucleotide upstream of the exon start site. However, the variation was present in the initial variation list.

3.2. Detection of Large Insertions/Deletions.

Large deletions are detected by analyzing local read depth. Firstly, a reference local read depth is established by binning read counts in a preset sliding window using data from all pooled samples. The local read depth is also determined for each sample separately, using the same preset sliding window used for the reference. A Log2 ratio is calculated for each window by dividing the local read depth of the sample by the reference. Normalization is performed through a mean shift to zero. The copy number data is projected on the open reading frame (ORF) of the gene and also projected on an exon scale, where the mean read count is aggregated on a per exon basis.

The large FANCA and PALB2 deletions, previously identified by MLPA (Table 1), were readily detected using the MPS data. The DNA from sample 4b that contained a heterozygous exon 15 to 23 deletion in FANCA was pooled with sample 4a before library preparation. As expected, the read depth Log2 ratio as compared to the reference was approximately −0.5, which corresponds with a loss of one allele in a background of four copies. Interestingly, in sample 11 only one pathogenic nucleotide substitution in FANCI has previously been identified while the other mutation remained undetected. Here we show the deletion of the last exon (exon 38) of the gene as detected by our large indel analysis tool (Figure 2(d)). We confirmed the deletion by PCR and Sanger sequencing by using a SNP in the last unaffected exon 37 and two sets of primers amplifying up- and downstream of the breakpoint (Figure 3).

3.3. Identification of Pathogenic Mutations in Unclassified FA Patients.

To investigate if our next-generation sequencing method also identifies mutations in unclassified FA patients, we investigated five patients that were sent in for FA mutation screening, without prior knowledge about their gene defect. Aberrations in the FANC-A, -C, -E, -F, and -G genes were already excluded in a routine diagnostics analysis by MLPA and Sanger sequencing. In two patients we identified known compound heterozygous pathogenic mutations in BRCA2 and FANCD2. In two other patients, novel homozygous mutations were detected. In one patient (Unc4) a dinucleotide insertion/duplication in exon 9 of FANCL was found, which results in a frameshift and a stop codon in exon 14. The other patient (Unc3) showed a missense mutation in exon 28 of FANCI that changed codon 954 from a cysteine to a tyrosine. The affected amino acid is highly conserved, up to fruit fly, suggesting that it may have an important function. Moreover, in silico analysis by SIFT [9] and Polyphen 2 [8] predicted the amino acid change to be damaging. All the identified variations were confirmed by Sanger sequencing, and the novel variations had a proper segregation within the family.

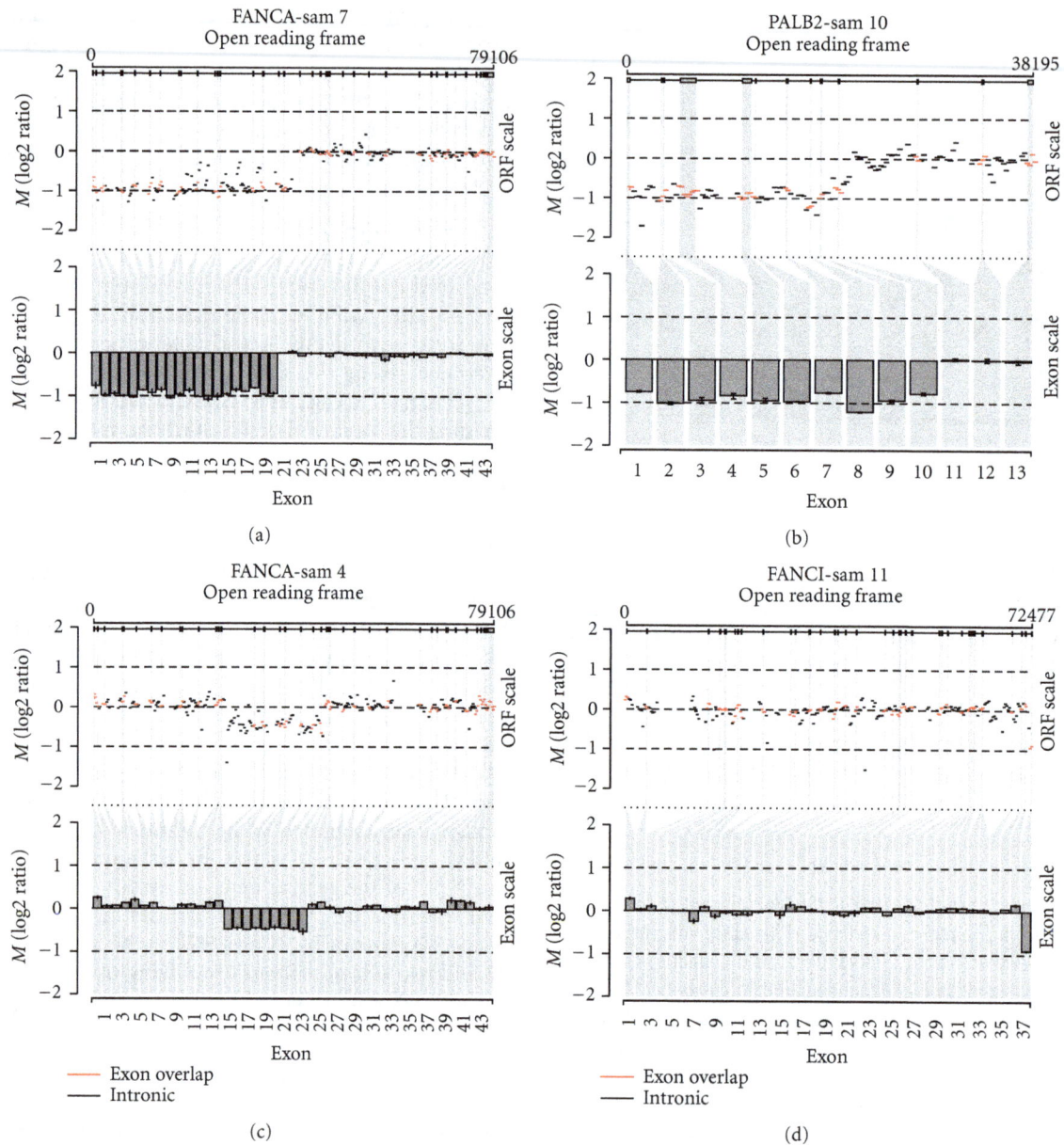

FIGURE 2: Large detection using next-generation sequence data. Copy number data are projected on an open reading frame (ORF) and on an exon scale. The ORF scale (upper panel) shows log2 ratios (M) for all exons and introns. Red segments indicate an overlap with an exon and black segments indicate no overlap with exons. The exon scale (lower panel) only shows the mean log2 ratio per exon with their 25th and 75th percentile. R plots of large deletion analysis. Deletion of exons 1 to 20 of *FANCA* (a), exons 1 to 10 of *FANCN* (b), exons 15 to 23 in *FANCA* (c), and exon 38 in *FANCI* (d).

In one patient no pathogenic variants were detected, although the coding regions of all known FA genes were covered deep enough to call variants. This suggests that the patient has a defect in a new FA gene or is not a true FA patient.

4. Discussion

The mutation detection strategy described here proved to be efficient for the molecular diagnosis of FA although patients with mutations in *FANCF, -J, -M, -O,* and *-P* were not included in our study. All the FA mutations identified by Sanger sequencing were also detected by next-generation sequencing. Moreover, we discovered a novel large deletion in the FA-I patient, for whom only one truncating mutation was previously identified [4]. The exact breakpoint at nucleotide level could be distinguished as also the intronic regions of the FA genes were enriched and sequenced. We confirmed the deletion by PCR and Sanger sequencing, using a SNP in the last unaffected exon and two sets of primers amplifying the regions up- and downstream of the breakpoint (Figure 3). Besides this novel large deletion we

TABLE 2: Pathogenic mutation detection through filtering.

Sample[1]	Variants (total)	Variants (target genes)	NS/SS[2]	Not in dbSNP	FA genes[3]	Pathogenic clue[4]
Sam 1	2535	1579	58	11	4	1
Sam 2	2659	1700	43	6	1	1
Sam 3	2388	1537	40	5	2	2
Sam 5	2490	1570	49	5	4	2
Sam 6	2081	1362	38	5	3	2
Sam 7	2417	1541	34	0	0	0[5]
Sam 8	2267	1416	53	5	3	1
Sam 9	2284	1354	34	4	1	1
Sam 10	2570	1760	51	5	2	1
Sam 11	2277	1491	44	7	2	1

[1] Sample 4 is not included in this table, as it is composed of pooled DNA from sample 4a and 4b. Slightly different analysis parameters were used for that sample.
[2] NS: nonsynonymous, SS: splice site.
[3] Number of variations remaining after filtering for variations in FA genes only.
[4] pathogenic clues are obtained from *in silico* analysis using Align-GVGD, Polyphen-2, and SIFT [7–9].
[5] This patient is a carrier for a large deletion and a deep intronic mutation. The large deletion is detectable by a separate tool, and the intronic variation is filtered out at this stage.

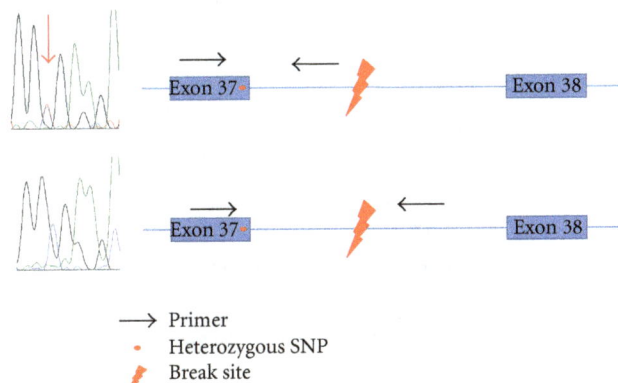

FIGURE 3: Confirmation of the large *FANCI* deletion by Sanger sequencing. A part of exon 37 with a SNP was amplified with primers designed either up- or downstream of the deletion breakpoint. Sequence analyses resulted in the detection of the SNP (red arrow) as heterozygous or hemizygous, respectively.

identified large genomic deletions in *FANCA* (2 samples) and *PALB2* (1 sample). The sensitivity of the method was demonstrated by mixing two DNA samples prior to library preparation and enrichment. A deletion of one allele in a background of four alleles can be detected, suggesting that the method is even applicable for the classification of mosaic FA patients. However, a thorough assessment of the method using serial dilutions with samples harboring large deletions is required to determine the detection limit of the assay. The identification of large deletions is essential for FA molecular diagnostics since about 40% of pathogenic mutations in the major FA complementation group, FA-A, are caused by large deletions in *FANCA*. As large deletions have also been demonstrated for *FANCI* (this study) and *FANCN* [6], it is plausible that these types of aberrations are present in other FA samples, which were previously unclassified by conventional molecular screening methods. Therefore, these types of mutations should be examined in the standard molecular diagnostics of FA.

The presence of *FANCD2* pseudogenes can complicate the identification of pathogenic mutations in this gene, as variations will tend to have a reduced frequency due to the occurrence of multiple highly similar copies. However, this difficulty can be resolved with bioinformatics by flagging variations that tend to have lower frequencies than expected within those regions. In cases where all other FA genes are excluded for mutations, careful inspection is required for flagged variations. Deep intronic mutations represent another type of variation, which are not analyzed with the classical molecular diagnostics approach. Indeed, the hemizygous *FANCA* c.893+920 C>A mutation in sample 7 was only identified after a heterozygous large *FANCA* deletion was detected by MLPA. This suspected the presence of a mutation on the other *FANCA* allele, which was then found after the FANCA cDNA was analyzed [5].

When we applied our novel molecular diagnostics approach on unclassified FA patients, we identified pathogenic mutations in four individuals. All the variations were confirmed with Sanger sequencing and demonstrated proper segregation with the disease. Two patients carried biallelic mutation in *BRCA2* and *FANCD2*, which have been described previously (Table 3). The remaining two patients harbored novel homozygous mutations in *FANCI* and *FANCL*; c.G2861A (p.C954Y) and c.755_756insAT (p.M252fs), respectively. The frameshift mutation in *FANCL* results in a stop codon in the last exon of the gene, which likely produces an mRNA targeted for nonsense mediated decay. The c.2861G>A substitution in *FANCI* affects a highly conserved amino acid and results in a large physiochemical difference, which is predicted to have a damaging effect on the FANCI protein by SIFT and polyphen-2. Nevertheless, functional studies are required to ultimately classify this

Prioritization schema

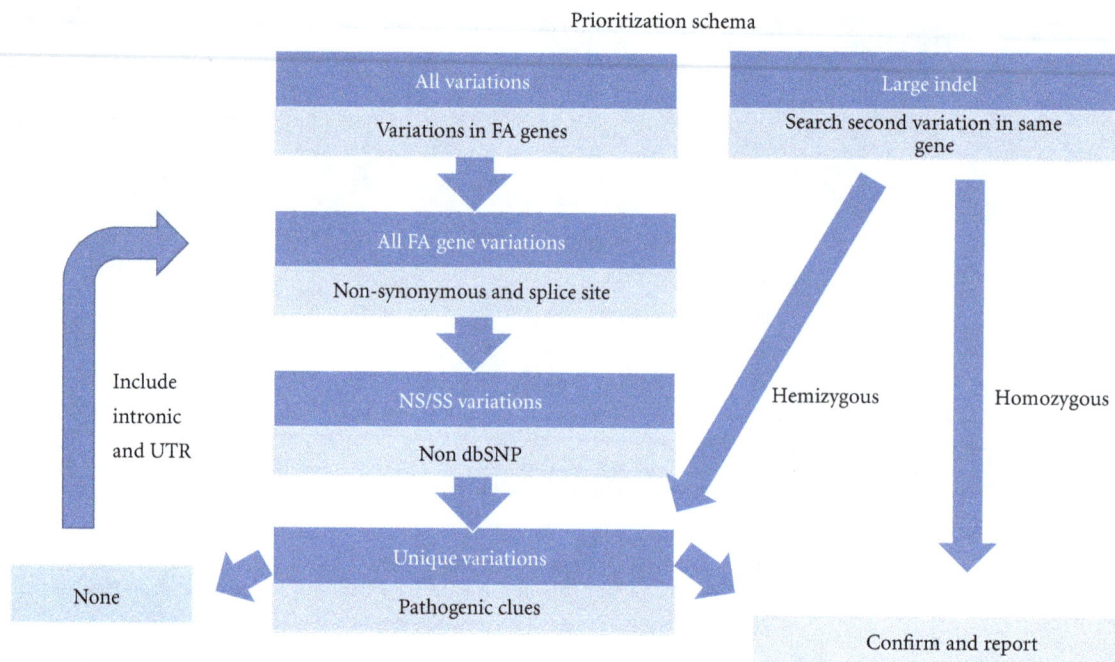

FIGURE 4: Prioritization scheme for the detection of disease-causing mutations by next-generation sequencing.

TABLE 3: Mutation detection in unclassified FA patients.

Sample	Gene	Mut 1	Effect 1	Mut 2	Effect 2	Note
Unc1	BRCA2	c.T8067A	p.C2689X	c.9672_9673insA	p.I3224fs	[10, 11]
Unc2	FANCD2	c.904C>T	p.R302W	c.2715+1G>A	splicing	[12, 13]
Unc3	FANCI	c.G3041A	p.C1014Y	c.G3041A	p.C1014Y	Novel
Unc4	FANCL	c.755_756insAT	p.M252fs	c.755_756insAT	p.M252fs	Novel
Unc5	—	NF*	—	NF*	—	—

Annotations are based on the following transcripts: BRCA2, NM_000059.3; FANCD2, NM_033084.3; FANCI, NM_001113378.1; FANCL, NM_001114636.1.
*NF = not found.

variation as pathogenic. In one FA sample we could not detect the disease causing mutations in any of the known FA genes. This patient might represent a novel FA subtype and whole-exome sequencing might be a useful approach to identify the affected gene.

Altogether, inspection of different variation types and inclusion of intronic regions warrants a comprehensive molecular FA diagnosis. Given the average number of variations of around 2500 per patient, it appears a difficult task to recognize the disease-causing mutation(s). Here we propose a prioritization approach following the recessive mode of inheritance (Figure 4). When no large deletions are identified, an initial filtering for nonsynonymous and canonical splice site variations should be performed. Subsequently, exclusion of variations in dbSNP and an in-house variant database with a frequency above 2%, reduces the number of possible pathogenic variations to less than 4. In cases where only one heterozygous pathogenic mutation is found, close examination of variations in intronic- and UTR regions in the same gene is required. When no pathogenic variations have been detected, assessment of all unique intronic and UTR variations is needed. With an ever expanding variant database of characterized FA patients, the identification of pathogenic mutations will become less complicated. Nevertheless, the necessity for functional tests, such as retroviral complementation or transfection, will remain essential to help assess the pathogenic status of unclassified missense variants.

In conclusion, multiplexed next-generation sequencing based on massively parallel sequencing is an effective molecular diagnostics approach for FA. The procedure, performed on genomic DNA, reduces the turnaround time, number of assays, and costs for a reliable detection of the disease-causing mutation. With the ever decreasing costs of enrichment and sequencing procedures, we expect that in the near future this will be the first test for patients clinically suspected of FA, thus avoiding labor-intensive chromosomal breakage assays and reducing turnaround time for FA diagnosis. To increase the efficiency of the molecular diagnosis, genes involved in other bone marrow failure syndromes (e.g., diamond-Blackfan anaemia and Shwachman-diamond syndrome) can be included, to be able to diagnose these non-FA patients that are often referred for FA diagnosis.

Authors' Contributions

N. Ameziane and D. Sie equally contributed to the work.

References

[1] A. J. Deans and S. C. West, "DNA interstrand crosslink repair and cancer," *Nature Reviews Cancer*, vol. 11, no. 7, pp. 467–480, 2011.

[2] W. Wang, "Emergence of a DNA-damage response network consisting of Fanconi anaemia and BRCA proteins," *Nature Reviews Genetics*, vol. 8, no. 10, pp. 735–748, 2007.

[3] K. V. Voelkerding, S. A. Dames, and J. D. Durtschi, "Next-generation sequencing: from basic research to diagnostics," *Clinical Chemistry*, vol. 55, no. 4, pp. 641–658, 2009.

[4] N. Ameziane, A. Errami, F. Leveille et al., "Genetic subtyping of Fanconi anemia by comprehensive mutation screening," *Human Mutation*, vol. 29, no. 1, pp. 159–166, 2008.

[5] M. Castella, R. Pujol, E. Callen et al., "Origin, functional role, and clinical impact of Fanconi anemia FANCA mutations," *Blood*, vol. 117, pp. 3759–3769, 2011.

[6] B. Xia, J. C. Dorsman, N. Ameziane et al., "Fanconi anemia is associated with a defect in the BRCA2 partner PALB2," *Nature Genetics*, vol. 39, no. 2, pp. 159–161, 2007.

[7] S. V. Tavtigian, A. M. Deffenbaugh, L. Yin et al., "Comprehensive statistical study of 452 BRCA1 missense substitutions with classification of eight recurrent substitutions as neutral," *Journal of Medical Genetics*, vol. 43, no. 4, pp. 295–305, 2006.

[8] I. A. Adzhubei, S. Schmidt, L. Peshkin et al., "A method and server for predicting damaging missense mutations," *Nature Methods*, vol. 7, no. 4, pp. 248–249, 2010.

[9] P. Kumar, S. Henikoff, and P. C. Ng, "Predicting the effects of coding non-synonymous variants on protein function using the SIFT algorithm," *Nature Protocols*, vol. 4, no. 7, pp. 1073–1081, 2009.

[10] T. Peelen, M. van Vliet, A. Bosch et al., "Screening for BRCA2 mutations in 81 Dutch breast-ovarian cancer families," *British Journal of Cancer*, vol. 82, no. 1, pp. 151–156, 2000.

[11] N. G. Howlett, T. Taniguchi, S. Olson et al., "Biallelic inactivation of BRCA2 in Fanconi anemia," *Science*, vol. 297, no. 5581, pp. 606–609, 2002.

[12] C. Timmers, T. Taniguchi, J. Hejna et al., "Positional cloning of a novel Fanconi anemia gene, FANCD2," *Molecular Cell*, vol. 7, no. 2, pp. 241–248, 2001.

[13] R. Kalb, K. Neveling, H. Hoehn et al., "Hypomorphic mutations in the gene encoding a key Fanconi anemia protein, FANCD2, sustain a significant group of FA-D2 patients with severe phenotype," *American Journal of Human Genetics*, vol. 80, no. 5, pp. 895–910, 2007.

[14] H. Li and R. Durbin, "Fast and accurate short read alignment with Burrows-Wheeler transform," *Bioinformatics*, vol. 25, no. 14, pp. 1754–1760, 2009.

[15] H. Li, B. Handsaker, A. Wysoker et al., "The sequence alignment/map format and SAMtools," *Bioinformatics*, vol. 25, no. 16, pp. 2078–2079, 2009.

[16] D. C. Koboldt, K. Chen, T. Wylie et al., "VarScan: variant detection in massively parallel sequencing of individual and pooled samples," *Bioinformatics*, vol. 25, no. 17, pp. 2283–2285, 2009.

[17] K. Wang, M. Li, and H. Hakonarson, "ANNOVAR: functional annotation of genetic variants from high-throughput sequencing data," *Nucleic Acids Research*, vol. 38, no. 16, article e164, Article ID gkq603, 2010.

7

Hematological Indices for Differential Diagnosis of Beta Thalassemia Trait and Iron Deficiency Anemia

Aysel Vehapoglu,[1] **Gamze Ozgurhan,**[2] **Ayşegul Dogan Demir,**[1] **Selcuk Uzuner,**[1] **Mustafa Atilla Nursoy,**[1] **Serdar Turkmen,**[3] **and Arzu Kacan**[4]

[1] *Department of Pediatrics, School of Medicine, Bezmialem Vakif University, 34093 Istanbul, Turkey*
[2] *Department of Pediatrics, Suleymaniye Obstetrics and Gynecology Hospital, 34010 Istanbul, Turkey*
[3] *Department of Biochemistry, Istanbul Training and Research Hospital, 34098 Istanbul, Turkey*
[4] *Department of Pediatrics, Istanbul Training and Research Hospital, Istanbul, Turkey*

Correspondence should be addressed to Aysel Vehapoglu; ayvahap@hotmail.com

Academic Editor: Bruno Annibale

Background. The two most frequent types of microcytic anemia are beta thalassemia trait (β-TT) and iron deficiency anemia (IDA). We retrospectively evaluated the reliability of various indices for differential diagnosis of microcytosis and β-TT in the same patient groups. *Methods.* A total of 290 carefully selected children aged 1.1–16 years were evaluated. We calculated 12 discrimination indices in all patients with hemoglobin (Hb) values of 8.7–11.4 g/dL. None of the subjects had a combined case of IDA and β-TT. All children with IDA received oral iron for 16 weeks, and HbA2 screening was performed after iron therapy. The patient groups were evaluated according to red blood cell (RBC) count; red blood distribution width index; the Mentzer, Shine and Lal, England and Fraser, Srivastava and Bevington, Green and King, Ricerca, Sirdah, and Ehsani indices; mean density of hemoglobin/liter of blood; and mean cell density of hemoglobin. *Results.* The Mentzer index was the most reliable index, as it had the highest sensitivity (98.7%), specificity (82.3%), and Youden's index (81%) for detecting β-TT; this was followed by the Ehsani index (94.8%, 73.5%, and 68.3%, resp.) and RBC count (94.8%, 70.5%, and 65.3%). *Conclusion.* The Mentzer index provided the highest reliabilities for differentiating β-TT from IDA.

1. Introduction

Anemia resulting from lack of sufficient iron to synthesize hemoglobin is the most common hematological disease in infants and children. It has been estimated that 30% of the global population suffers from iron deficiency anemia (IDA), and most of those affected live in the developing countries. Microcytic anemia in a case of thalassemia results from impaired globin chain synthesis and decreased hemoglobin (Hb) synthesis, resulting in microcytosis and hypochromia; 1.5% of the world's population carries genes for β-thalassemia [1]. Individuals with the beta thalassemia trait (β-TT) are usually asymptomatic and may be unaware of their carrier status unless diagnosed by testing. β-TT is the most common type of hemoglobinopathy transmitted by heredity. It is estimated that about 50% of the world's population with β-TT

are in Southeast Asia; it is also common in the Mediterranean region, the Middle East, Southeast Asia, Southwest Europe, and Central Africa [2]. Due to the migration and intermarriage of different ethnic populations, β-TT is found in people with no obvious ethnic connection to the disorder.

A definitive differential diagnosis between β-TT and IDA is based on the result of HbA_2 electrophoresis, serum iron levels, and a ferritin calculation [3]. Electronic cell counters have been used to determine red cell indices as a first indicator of β-TT. The purpose of using indices to discriminate anemia is to detect subjects who have a high probability of requiring appropriate follow-up and to reduce unnecessary investigative costs. Since 1970, a number of complete blood count indices have been proposed as simple and inexpensive tools to determine whether a blood sample is more suggestive of β-TT or IDA [4–12]. Most of these articles include

TABLE 1: Hematological and biochemical date of study groups.

	β-TT (n: 154)		IDA (n: 136)	
	Range	Mean ± SD	Range	Mean ± SD
Hb (g/dL) total	9–11.46	10.39 ± 0.69	8.7–11.42	10.23 ± 0.95
RBC ($\times 10^6$/L)	4.34–6.54	5.56 ± 0.4	3.45–6.33	4.84 ± 0.59
MCV (fL)	52.1–71	60.11 ± 3.49	45.3–79.53	67.49 ± 7.14
MCH (pg)	16.3–23.8	18.9 ± 1.37	13.65–27.7	21.33 ± 3.09
RDW (%)	13.9–24.63	16.76 ± 1.83	12.5–28.66	17.4 ± 3.48
SI (μg/dL)	20–194	76.6 ± 29.2	4.6–31.2	23.74 ± 9.48
SIBC (μg/dL)	257–472	339 ± 40.47	279–495	392 ± 41.74
TS (%)	5.5–55.2	22.88 ± 8.7	0.9–8.7	6.1 ± 2.6
Ferritin (ng/mL)	11.2–96	33.75 ± 22.9	1.1–11.2	7.54 ± 3.2

β-TT: beta thalassemia trait; IDA: iron deficiency anemia; Hb: hemoglobin; RBC: red blood cell; MCV: mean corpuscular volume; MCH: mean corpuscular hemoglobin; RDW: red blood cell distribution width; SI: serum iron; SIBC: serum iron binding capacity; TS: transferrin saturation.

adults but very few data are available on children. An ideal discrimination index has high sensitivity and specificity; that is, it can detect the maximum number of patients with β-TT (high sensitivity) while eliminating patients with IDA (high specificity). In this study, we compared the ability of different 12 indices to distinguish β-TT from IDA by calculating their sensitivity, specificity, and Youden's index values.

2. Material and Methods

We retrospectively analyzed 290 children with microcytic anemia (mean age: 6.2 ± 4.2 years; range: 1.1–16 years). Samples were obtained from 121 boys and 169 girls with no clinical symptoms of acute or chronic inflammation or infectious diseases. None of them had received a transfusion or had an acute bleeding episode in the previous month. The samples were obtained during the course of routine analysis and collected in EDTA anticoagulant tubes. Red blood cell (RBC) count and red blood cell distribution width (RDW) were assessed on a Siemens Advia 2120 Hematology Analyzer. Serum iron (SI), serum iron binding capacity, serum ferritin, and HbA_2 values were determined in all children. HbA_2 was detected by high-performance liquid chromatography (Shimadzu LC-MS). SI and total iron binding capacity (TIBC) were determined calorimetrically (Siemens Advia 2400 Chemistry Analyzer), and ferritin was measured by immunoassay using a Siemens Advia XP Analyzer. Transferrin saturation was calculated as the ratio of SI to TIBC. The hematological and biochemical data of the groups are evaluated before iron replacement regimen. Those are shown in Table 1. Iron deficiency modulates HbA_2 synthesis, resulting in reduced HbA_2 levels in patients with IDA [13, 14]. The increase in HbA_2 levels (>3.5%) is the most significant parameter for identifying beta thalassemia carriers. Patients with β-TT and concomitant iron deficiency may show normal HbA_2 levels. Therefore, none of the subjects in the present study had both IDA and β-TT. All children with IDA received oral iron (3–5 mg/kg/day) for 16 weeks. HbA_2 screening was performed after completion of the 16-week iron replacement regimen.

A total of 154 children were confirmed to have β-TT. The β-TT group consisted of children with Hb levels of 9–11.46 g/dL, mean corpuscular volume (MCV) < 80 fL at age > 6 years or MCV < 70 fL at age < 6 years, serum iron level > 30 μg/dL, transferrin saturation > 16%, serum ferritin level > 12 ng/dL, and HbA_2 > 3.5%. A total of 136 children were confirmed to have IDA with serum ferritin levels ≤ 12 ng/dL. The IDA group consisted of children with Hb levels of 8.7–11.4 g/dL, mean corpuscular volume (MCV) < 80 fL at age > 6 years or MCV < 70 fL at age < 6 years, serum iron level < 30 μg/dL, transferrin saturation < 16%, and serum ferritin level ≤ 12 ng/dL. Children with Hb levels < 8.7 g/dL were excluded because these cases of severe anemia are not confused with β-TT in daily practice. None of the subjects of the present study had a combined case of β-TT and IDA. The combined cases were excluded from the early stages of the evaluation study.

The 12 discrimination indices used in the evaluation were calculated and are summarized in Table 2. Sensitivity, specificity, positive predictive value (PPV), negative predictive value (NPV), and Youden's index were calculated for each measure as follows:

$$\text{Sensitivity} = \left[\frac{\text{true positive}}{(\text{true positive} + \text{false negative})} \right] \times 100,$$

$$\text{Specificity} = \left[\frac{\text{true negative}}{(\text{true negative} + \text{false positive})} \right] \times 100,$$

$$\text{PPV} = \frac{\text{true positive}}{(\text{true positive} + \text{false positive})} \times 100,$$

$$\text{NPV} = \frac{\text{true negative}}{(\text{true negative} + \text{false negative})} \times 100,$$

$$\text{Youden's index} = (\text{sensitivity} + \text{specificity}) - 100.$$

(1)

2.1. Statistical Analysis. Data were analyzed with computerized statistical package for social sciences (SPSS) version 15.0. An independent sample t-test was performed to detect differences between the two groups of anemic children.

TABLE 2: Different RBC indices and mathematical formulas used to differentiate between β-TT and IDA.

Hematological index	Formula
Mentzer index (MI) (1973)	MCV/RBC
RDWI (1987)	MCV × RDW/RBC
Shine and Lal (S and L) (1977)	MCV × MCV × MCH/100
Srivastava (1973)	MCH/RBC
Green and King (G and K) (1989)	MCV × MCV × RDW/Hb × 100
Sirdah (2007)	MCV − RBC − (3 × Hb)
Ehsani (2005)	MCV − (10 × RBC)
England and Fraser (E and F) (1973)	MCV − (5 × Hb) − RBC − 3.4
Ricerca (1987)	RDW/RBC
MDHL (1999)	(MCH/MCV) × RBC
MCHD (1999)	MCH/MCV

MDHL index: mean density of Hb/liter of blood; MCHD index: mean cell Hb density.

P values < 0.05 were considered significant. The differential values for each discrimination index were applied as defined in the original published reports: red blood distribution width index (RDWI), Mentzer index [4], the Shine and Lal index [5], the England and Fraser index [6], the Srivastava index [7], the Green and King index [8], the Ricerca et al. index [9], and the Sirdah et al. index [10]. The Ehsani et al. index [11], mean density of hemoglobin per liter of blood (MDHL), mean cell hemoglobin density (MCHD) [12], and RBC count were evaluated and compared. The values of each index required to distinguish between β-TT and IDA and the number and proportion of correctly identified patients (true positives) calculated using these indices are shown in Table 3. Sensitivity, specificity, PPV, NPV, and Youden's index values for each index needed to distinguish between β-TT and IDA are shown in Table 4.

3. Results

Hb values in the β-TT group were 10.39 ± 0.69, and those in the IDA group were 10.23 ± 0.95 (P > 0.05). MCV was 60.11 ± 3.49 and MCHD was 18.9 ± 1.37 in the β-TT group, and these values were lower than those in the IDA group (67.49 ± 7.14 and 21.3 ± 3.09, respectively; P < 0.05). The RDWI values were increased in both groups: 17.4 ± 3.48 in the IDA group and 16.76 ± 1.83 in patients with β-TT (P > 0.05). Red cell values at various ages of study groups are shown in Table 5.

RBC count was higher in the β-TT (5.56 ± 0.4) group than that in the IDA (4.84 ± 0.59; P < 0.05) group. A high erythrocyte count (RBC > $5.0 \times 10^6/\mu$L) is a common feature of IDA and β-TT. The RBC count is one of the most accurate indices available. The RBC count provided the best sensitivity (94.8%) but had low specificity (70.5%), and Youden's index was 65.3%.

As indicated in Table 4, none of the indices studied demonstrated 100% precision in recognizing β-TT. The Ricerca

et al. and the Shine and Lal indices demonstrated the highest sensitivity (100%) but had low specificities for correctly identifying IDA (14.7%) and β-TT (10.2%). Therefore, according to our results, these indices cannot be used as screening tools for β-TT, as using them could result in a significant number of false-negative results. The England and Fraser index had the lowest sensitivity of 66.2%, and identification was wrong in about 28% of β-TT cases. The England and Fraser and the Mentzer indices demonstrated the highest specificities at 85.3% and 82.3%, respectively. Furthermore, Table 4 shows the highest and lowest PPV, which were found for the Mentzer index (86.3%) and the Shine and Lal (55%) and MCHL indices (55%), respectively. The Shine and Lal and the Ricerca et al. indices demonstrated the highest NPV at 100%, and MCHD had the lowest NPV at 52.7%. Additionally, Table 4 shows that the highest and lowest Youden's index values belonged to the Mentzer index (81%) and MCHD (5.8%). None of the indices was completely sensitive or specific in distinguishing β-TT and IDA.

The Mentzer index showed good sensitivity, specificity, and Youden's index values of 98.7%, 82.3%, and 81%, respectively. When the Mentzer index was calculated, 264 children with microcytic anemia (91%) were correctly diagnosed. Youden's index showed the following ranking with respect to the indices' ability to distinguish between β-TT and IDA: Mentzer index > Ehsani et al. index > RBC count > Sirdah et al. index > RDWI > Srivastava index > Green and King index > England and Fraser index > MDHL > Ricerca et al. index > Shine and Lal index > MCHD. The difference between the results of all of these indices and the gold standard (HbA$_2$) was significant (P < 0.001).

4. Discussion

β-TT and IDA are among the most common types of microcytic anemia encountered by pediatricians. Distinguishing β-TT from IDA has important clinical implications because each disease has an entirely different cause, prognosis, and treatment. Thalassemia is endemic in Turkey. Misdiagnosis of β-TT has consequences for potential homozygous offspring. Up to now, many investigators have used different mathematical indices to distinguish β-TT from IDA using only a complete blood count. This process helps to select appropriate individuals for a more detailed examination; however, no study has found 100% specificity or sensitivity for any of these RBC indices. Our data (Table 1) showed significant differences between the hematological and biochemical parameters of β-TT and IDA children except for Hb and RDW, but these differences were not reflected in the indices' reliability in differential diagnosis of β-TT and IDA. RBC count has been considered a valuable index [15], but we showed that RBC count had only 70.5% specificity and 65.3% Youden's index. In the 290 children with microcytic anemia, 186 children (64.1%) had a high RBC count (RBC count > $5.0 \times 10^6/\mu$L) at the time of diagnosis. However, the frequency of high RBC count was 29.4% in children with IDA. It seems that RBC alone was not a reliable tool for distinguishing β-TT from IDA. Elevated RBC count might be associated with

TABLE 3: Results obtained from each discrimination index and correctly identified number of the children.

Indices (cutoffs)	β-TT (n: 154)	IDA (n: 136)	Total number of correctly diagnosed children	Correctly diagnosed (%)
Mentzer				
β-TT < 13	152	24	264 (152 + 112)	91
IDA > 13	2	112		
RBC count ($\times 10^6$/L)				
β-TT > 5	146	40	242 (146 + 96)	83.4
IDA < 5	8	96		
RDWI				
β-TT < 220	128	32	232 (128 + 104)	80
IDA > 220	26	104		
Shine and Lal				
β-TT < 1530	154	122	168 (154 + 14)	57.9
IDA > 1530	0	14		
Srivastava				
β-TT < 3.8	132	38	230 (132 + 98)	79.3
IDA > 3.8	22	98		
Green and King				
β-TT < 65	128	36	228 (128 + 100)	78.6
IDA > 65	26	100		
Sirdah				
β-TT < 27	132	28	240 (132 + 108)	82.7
IDA > 27	22	108		
Ehsani				
β-TT < 15	146	36	246 (146 + 100)	84.8
IDA > 15	8	100		
England and Fraser				
β-TT < 0	102	20	218 (102 + 116)	75
IDA > 0	52	116		
Ricerca				
β-TT < 4.4	154	116	174 (154 + 20)	60
IDA > 4.4	0	20		
MDHL				
β-TT > 1.63	118	36	198 (118 + 80)	68.2
IDA < 1.63	36	80		
MCHD				
β-TT > 0.3045	120	98	158 (120 + 38)	54.4
IDA < 0.3045	34	38		

erythrocytosis. We observed that the RBC count increased at the initiation of iron therapy in patients with IDA and decreased by the end of therapy. A similar observation was made by Aslan and Altay, who reported an elevated RBC count in 61% of cases with mild anemia [16].

In a 2010 study, Ferrara et al. demonstrated that RDWI had the highest sensitivity (78.9%), that the England and Fraser index had the highest specificity and highest Youden's index (99.1 and 64.2%, resp.), and that the Green and King index had the highest efficiency (80.2%) in 458 children with mild microcytic anemia aged 1.8–7.5 years [17].

AlFadhli et al. compared nine discriminant functions in patients with microcytic anemia and measured validity using Youden's index. Youden's index considers both sensitivity and specificity and provides an appropriate measure of validity for

a particular question or technique. They showed that the England and Fraser index had the highest Youden's index value (98.2%) for correctly differentiating β-TT and IDA, whereas the Shine and Lal index was ineffective for differentiating microcytic anemia [18]. According to our data, the Mentzer index had the highest Youden's index for correctly distinguishing β-TT and IDA at 81%. When the Mentzer index was calculated, 91% of children with microcytic anemia were correctly diagnosed. The England and Fraser and the Shine and Lal indices had the lowest Youden's index values of 51.4% and 10.2%, respectively.

In 2009, Ehsani et al. showed that the best discrimination index according to Youden's criteria was the Mentzer index (90.1%), followed by the Ehsani et al. index (85.5%). In their study, the Mentzer and Ehsani et al. indices were able to

TABLE 4: Sensitivity, specificity, positive predictive value (PPV), negative predictive value (NPV), and Youden's index of twelve indices to discriminate between β-TT and IDA in 290 children.

Indices	Sensitivity (%)	Specificity (%)	PPV (%)	NPV (%)	Youden's index
Mentzer					
β-TT	98.7	82.3	86.3	98.2	81
IDA	82.3	98.7	98.2	86.3	
RBC count					
β-TT	94.8	70.5	78.4	92.3	65.3
IDA	70.5	94.8	92.3	78.4	
RDWI					
β-TT	83.1	76.4	80	80	59.5
IDA	76.4	83.1	80	80	
Shine and Lal					
β-TT	100	10.2	55	100	10.2
IDA	10.2	100	100	55	
Srivastava					
β-TT	85.7	72	77.6	81.6	57.7
IDA	72	85.7	81.6	77.6	
Green and King					
β-TT	83.1	73.5	77.6	79.3	56.6
IDA	73.5	83.1	79.3	77.6	
Sirdah					
β-TT	85.7	79.4	82.5	83	65
IDA	79.4	85.7	83	82.5	
Ehsani					
β-TT	94.8	73.5	80.2	92.5	68.3
IDA	73.5	94.8	92.5	80.2	
England and Fraser					
β-TT	66.2	85.3	83.6	69	51.4
IDA	85.3	66.2	69	83.6	
Ricerca					
β-TT	100	14.7	57	100	14.7
IDA	14.7	100	100	57	
MDHL					
β-TT	76	58.8	76.6	69	34.8
IDA	58.8	76	69	76.6	
MCHD					
β-TT	77.9	27.9	55	52.7	5.8
IDA	27.9	77.9	52.7	55	

correctly diagnose 94.7% and 92.9% of cases, respectively, and both are easy to calculate [11]. Similar results (Mentzer index: sensitivity, 90.9%; specificity, 80.3%) were found by Ghafouri et al. [19]. Their results overlapped those of our study.

Rahim and Keikhaei examined the diagnostic accuracy of 10 indices in 153 patients with β-TT and 170 patients with IDA. According to Youden's index, the Shine and Lal index and RBC count showed the greatest diagnostic value in patients < 10 years (89% and 82%, resp.). They found that the Mentzer index had 85% sensitivity, 93% specificity, and 79% Youden's index [20].

In 2007, Ntaios et al. reported that the Green and King index was the most reliable index, as it had the highest sensitivity (75.06%), efficiency (80.12%), and Youden's index

(70.86%) for detecting β-TT [21]. A similar result for the Green and King index (Youden's index, 80.9%) was found by Urrechaga et al. [2]. However, studies in pediatric age groups are scarce, and their results are conflicting. It may be that interpopulation differences in the effectiveness of various RBC indices for discriminating β-TT from IDA could be attributed to differences in the mutation spectrum of the thalassemia disease in different populations [22].

The diagnosis of β-TT involves measuring the HbA_2 concentration of lysed RBCs via HPLC. The HbA_2 analysis is considered the gold standard for diagnosing thalassemia. Several studies have shown that iron deficiency directly affects the rates of HbA_2 synthesis in bone marrow; therefore, 16–20 weeks of iron therapy should be instituted, after which

TABLE 5: Red cell values at various ages of study groups and mean and lower limit of normal (−2 SD).

Age	Hemoglobin (g/dL) Mean ± SD (range)	Hemoglobin (g/dL) Mean and lower limit of normal (−2 SD)	MCV (fL) Mean ± SD (range)	MCV (fL) Mean and lower limit of normal (−2 SD)
Female				
0.5–2 years	10.06 ± 0.73 (9.0–11.4)	12.0 (10.5)	63.79 ± 4.24 (56.62–69.74)	78 (70)
2–6 years	10.17 ± 0.74 (8.9–11.6)	12.5 (11.5)	62.09 ± 5.42 (49.0–69.90)	81 (75)
6–12 years	10.42 ± 0.78 (8.9–11.4)	13.5 (11.5)	62.80 ± 5.80 (53.4–77.3)	86 (77)
12–18 years	10.15 ± 0.99 (8.9–11.6)	14.0 (12.0)	65.71 ± 5.23 (56.8–71.9)	90 (78)
Male				
0.5–2 years	10.16 ± 0.74 (8.9–11.3)	12.0 (10.5)	69.90 ± 3.85 (57.0–69.4)	78 (70)
2–6 years	10.38 ± 0.75 (8.9–11.5)	12.5 (11.5)	60.92 ± 5.0 (52.0–69.7)	81 (75)
6–12 years	10.72 ± 0.71 (9.0–11.4)	13.5 (11.5)	63.25 ± 6.03 (56.7–74.3)	86 (77)
12–18 years	10.78 ± 0.78 (8.9–11.4)	14.5 (13.0)	62.46 ± 3.59 (59.6–68.7)	88 (78)

Hb: hemoglobin; MCV: mean corpuscular volume; SD: standard deviation.
From [24].

a repeat serum iron with electrophoresis is done to confirm improvement in the HbA_2 levels [23].

5. Conclusion

In conclusion, the cell-count-based indices, particularly the Mentzer index, are easily available and reliable methods for detecting β-TT. According to our results, the percentage of correctly diagnosed patients was the highest with the Mentzer index (91%) followed by the Ehsani et al. index (84.8%). The third highest one was RBC count (83.4%). Cell-count-based parameters and formulas, particularly the MCV and RBC counts and their related indices (Mentzer index and Ehsani et al. index), have good discrimination ability in diagnosing β-TT.

Conflict of Interests

The authors declare that there is no conflict of interests regarding the publication of this paper.

References

[1] D. A. Rathod, A. Kaur, V. Patel et al., "Usefulness of cell counter-based parameters and formulas in detection of β-thalassemia trait in areas of high prevalence," American Journal of Clinical Pathology, vol. 128, no. 4, pp. 585–589, 2007.

[2] E. Urrechaga, L. Borque, and J. F. Escanero, "The role of automated measurement of RBC subpopulations in differential diagnosis of microcytic anemia and β-thalassemia screening," American Journal of Clinical Pathology, vol. 135, no. 3, pp. 374–379, 2011.

[3] C. Thomas and L. Thomas, "Biochemical markers and hematologic indices in the diagnosis of functional iron deficiency," Clinical Chemistry, vol. 48, no. 7, pp. 1066–1076, 2002.

[4] W. C. Mentzer Jr., "Differentiation of iron deficiency from thalassaemia trait," The Lancet, vol. 1, no. 7808, p. 882, 1973.

[5] I. Shine and S. Lal, "A strategy to detect β thalassaemia minor," The Lancet, vol. 1, no. 8013, pp. 692–694, 1977.

[6] J. M. England and P. M. Fraser, "Differentiation of iron deficiency from thalassaemia trait by routine blood-count," The Lancet, vol. 1, no. 7801, pp. 449–452, 1973.

[7] P. C. Srivastava, "Differentiation of thalassaemia minor from iron deficiency," The Lancet, vol. 2, pp. 154–155, 1973.

[8] R. Green and R. King, "A new red cell discriminant incorporating volume dispersion for differentiating iron deficiency anemia from thalassaemia minor," Blood Cells, vol. 15, no. 3, pp. 481–495, 1989.

[9] B. M. Ricerca, S. Storti, G. d'Onofrio et al., "Differentiation of iron deficiency from thalassaemia trait: a new approach," Haematologica, vol. 72, no. 5, pp. 409–413, 1987.

[10] M. Sirdah, I. Tarazi, E. Al Najjar, and R. Al Haddad, "Evaluation of the diagnostic reliability of different RBC indices and formulas in the differentiation of the β-thalassaemia minor from iron deficiency in Palestinian population," International Journal of Laboratory Hematology, vol. 30, no. 4, pp. 324–330, 2008.

[11] M. A. Ehsani, E. Shahgholi, M. S. Rahiminejad, F. Seighali, and A. Rashidi, "A new index for discrimination between iron deficiency anemia and beta-thalassemia minor: results in 284 patients," Pakistan Journal of Biological Sciences, vol. 12, no. 5, pp. 473–475, 2009.

[12] O. A. Telmissani, S. Khalil, and T. R. George, "Mean density of hemoglobin per liter of blood: a new hematologic parameter with an inherent discriminant function," Laboratory Haematology, vol. 5, pp. 149–152, 1999.

[13] A. Mosca, R. Paleari, G. Ivaldi, R. Galanello, and P. C. Giordano, "The role of haemoglobin A(2) testing in the diagnosis of thalassaemias and related haemoglobinopathies," Journal of Clinical Pathology, vol. 62, no. 1, pp. 13–17, 2009.

[14] E. J. Harthoorn-Lasthuizen, J. Lindemans, and M. M. A. C. Langenhuijsen, "Influence of iron deficiency anaemia on

haemoglobin A(2) levels: possible consequences for β-thalassaemia screening," *Scandinavian Journal of Clinical and Laboratory Investigation*, vol. 59, no. 1, pp. 65–70, 1999.

[15] A. Demir, N. Yaralı, T. Fısgın, F. Duru, and A. Kara, "Most reliable indices in differentiation between thalassemia trait and iron deficiency anemia," *Pediatrics International*, vol. 44, no. 6, pp. 612–616, 2002.

[16] D. Aslan and Ç. Altay, "Incidence of high erythrocyte count in infants and young children with iron deficiency anemia: reevaluation of an old parameter," *Journal of Pediatric Hematology/Oncology*, vol. 25, no. 4, pp. 303–306, 2003.

[17] M. Ferrara, L. Capozzi, R. Russo, F. Bertocco, and D. Ferrara, "Reliability of red blood cell indices and formulas to discriminate between β thalassemia trait and iron deficiency in children," *Hematology*, vol. 15, no. 2, pp. 112–115, 2010.

[18] S. M. AlFadhli, A. M. Al-Awadhi, and D. AlKhaldi, "Validity assessment of nine discriminant functions used for the differentiation between Iron deficiency anemia and thalassemia minor," *Journal of Tropical Pediatrics*, vol. 53, no. 2, pp. 93–97, 2007.

[19] M. Ghafouri, L. Mostaan Sefat, and L. Sharifi, "Comparison of cell counter indices in differention of beta thalassemia trait and iron deficiency anemia," *The Scientific Journal of Iranian Blood Transfusion Organization*, vol. 2, no. 7, pp. 385–389, 2006.

[20] F. Rahim and B. Keikhaei, "Better differential diagnosis of iron deficiency anemia from beta-thalassemia trait," *Turkish Journal of Hematology*, vol. 26, no. 3, pp. 138–145, 2009.

[21] G. Ntaios, A. Chatzinikolaou, Z. Saouli et al., "Discrimination indices as screening tests for β-thalassemic trait," *Annals of Hematology*, vol. 86, no. 7, pp. 487–491, 2007.

[22] C. Rosatelli, G. B. Leoni, T. Tuveri et al., "Heterozygous β-thalassemia: relationship between the hematological phenotype and the type of β-thalassemia mutation," *American Journal of Hematology*, vol. 39, no. 1, pp. 1–4, 1992.

[23] I. El-Agouza, A. Abu Shahla, and M. Sirdah, "The effect of iron deficiency anaemia on the levels of haemoglobin subtypes: possible consequences for clinical diagnosis," *Clinical and Laboratory Haematology*, vol. 24, no. 5, pp. 285–289, 2002.

[24] P. R. Dallman, "Blood and blood-forming tissue," in *Pediatrics*, A. Rudolph, Ed., Appleton-Century-Crofts, Norwalk, Conn, USA, 16th edition, 1977.

8

The Validation of a New Visual Anaemia Evaluation Tool HemoHue HH1 in Patients with End-Stage Renal Disease

Robert M. Kalicki, Stefan Farese, and Dominik E. Uehlinger

Department of Nephrology, Hypertension and Clinical Pharmacology, Inselspital Bern, University Hospital and University of Bern, Freiburgstrasse 15, 3010 Bern, Switzerland

Correspondence should be addressed to Robert M. Kalicki; robert.kalicki@mph.unibe.ch

Academic Editor: Aurelio Maggio

In chronic haemodialysis patients, anaemia is a frequent finding associated with high therapeutic costs and further expenses resulting from serial laboratory measurements. HemoHue HH1, HemoHue Ltd, is a novel tool consisting of a visual scale for the noninvasive assessment of anaemia by matching the coloration of the conjunctiva with a calibrated hue scale. The aim of the study was to investigate the usefulness of HemoHue in estimating individual haemoglobin concentrations and binary treatment outcomes in haemodialysis patients. A prospective blinded study with 80 hemodialysis patients comparing the visual haemoglobin assessment with the standard laboratory measurement was performed. Each patient's haemoglobin concentration was estimated by seven different medical and nonmedical observers with variable degrees of clinical experience on two different occasions. The estimated population mean was close to the measured one (11.06 ± 1.67 versus 11.32 ± 1.23 g/dL, $P < 0.0005$). A learning effect could be detected. Relative errors in individual estimates reached, however, up to 50%. Insufficient performance in predicting binary outcomes (ROC AUC: 0.72 to 0.78) and poor interrater reliability (Kappa < 0.6) further characterised this method.

1. Introduction

Anaemia is a feature commonly encountered in daily medical practice especially in well-defined clinical subpopulations such as nephrologic, oncologic, or pediatric patients. Diagnosis and therapeutic monitoring of anaemia are based on blood sampling and laboratory measurements, both necessitating the presence of qualified personnel, logistic, and technical resources and generate high costs especially if repetitive measurements are required. This is particularly striking when considering end-stage renal disease patients treated with recombinant human erythropoietin (rHuEPO) [1]. The imperative to reach and stay within a narrow haemoglobin concentration target range [2, 3], the peculiar pharmacokinetic and pharmacodynamic properties of rHuEPO [4–8], making its use difficult even in hands of experienced nephrologists, has led to the general acceptance of systematic and frequent monitoring of the haemoglobin concentration levels during therapy with rHuEPO.

Although in developed countries laboratory facilities are easily accessible, the availability of a simple, cheap, noninvasive, and reproducible bedside method to assess the degree of anaemia in patients necessitating serial measurements would be very suitable [9, 10].

Severe anaemia may be detected by the naked-eye in the presence of significant skin pallor, pale nail beds and palms, whereas the examination of the conjunctiva provides in general a more sensitive and accurate estimation independent of the skin pigmentation [9–13]. However, this method remains crude and largely observer-dependent since the intensity of the conjunctiva colour is not matched with a reference hue [10].

The HemoHue HH1 device (HemoHue Ltd) consists of a credit card-like small tool with an imprinted red hue consisting in seven red spots with increasing colour intensity matched with increasing haemoglobin concentrations (Figure 1).

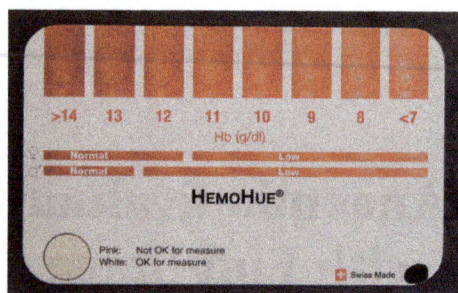

FIGURE 1: HemoHue HH1, HemoHue Ltd. Credit card sized device with an imprinted red hue, corresponding Hb levels, and a white luminescent control spot.

The aim of the present prospective, comparative, and blinded study was to assess the validity of the HemoHue HH1 device in detecting and scaling the degree of anaemia in chronic haemodialysis patients. Eventual effects of an increased observer practice, formation, and general characteristics such as age and gender, on estimation of the haemoglobin concentration were evaluated. The ability of this new method in correctly detecting patients' haemoglobin concentrations inside and outside the therapeutic range was also assessed.

2. Subjects and Methods

2.1. Patients. Eighty chronic haemodialysis patients from our dialysis ward were enrolled in the study. Inclusion criteria were age over eighteen and capacity to understand the aim of the study and to give verbal consent. Any of the following excluded the patient from participating in study: acute or chronic affection of the anterior segment of the eye and the unavailability of a laboratory measurement of haemoglobin within two weeks of the visual assessment or the presence of a clinically relevant bleeding and/or transfusion requirements. The study was approved by the local ethics committee board, Kantonale Ethikkommission Bern, Universität Bern, Switzerland.

2.2. Study Design and Methods. Patients were assessed in decubitus or semidecubitus position on the dialysis chair within the first two hours of their usual treatment session. Localization of the patient in the dialysis room in relation to the natural light intensity (next to the window, intermediary, next to the door), the day time, and the ultrafiltration performed at the time of measurement was recorded. Two commercially available polychromatic neon tubes providing natural light, fixed perpendicularly on a rolling tripod, were used to ensure optimal lighting conditions as indicated by the whitening of the control luminescent spot on the HemoHue HH1 card.

The visual estimation of the haemoglobin concentration was performed as follows: the inferior lid was retracted, and the most intensely colored spot of the conjunctival sack was compared with the colored spots on the HemoHue HH1 card and matched. This procedure was repeated independently

by all seven observers: one medical student (*med stud*), one dialysis nurse (*nurse*), three physicians with increasing age and degree of clinical experience (*phys A, phys B, and phys C*), and two administrative employees (*desk A and desk B*). The sequence in which the estimations were performed was randomized each time. Every observer was blinded for the estimates of all coobservers and the measured haemoglobin values during the whole study.

The procedure mentioned above was repeated on two nonconsecutive haemodialysis sessions at a two-week interval (*1st and 2nd session*). In the meantime, the laboratory measurement of haemoglobin was performed in all subjects at the beginning of a haemodialysis session, hence providing one individual reference value. Some observers participated to both sessions and were, therefore, considered to be *skilled* as opposed to those who assisted only punctually to the first or the second session (*novice*).

2.3. Statistics. The software package Systat 12 (SPSS Inc., Chicago, IL) and R.2.8.1 (R Development Core Team) were used for statistical analyses and graphical presentation. Values are given as mean ± standard deviation (SD) if not indicated otherwise. Intergroup analysis was performed by one-way ANOVA with Bonferroni post-hoc analysis. The package "irr" v. 0.7 (R Development Core Team) was used to compute the Cohen's and Fleiss' Kappa test [14] for the interobserver reliability. The overall agreement between the visual and the standard method was assessed with the Bland-Altman plot [15].

According to our preliminary statistical analysis, 68 patients were necessary to reject the null hypothesis in discriminating between both methods (measured haemoglobin-estimated haemoglobin concentration $= \pm 5$ g/L) to reach a power of 90% at a significance level of 5%.

3. Results

From the initially evaluated 80 patients during the first session, 75 were still available for visual estimations during the second session. Five dropouts were recorded (3 absences and 2 missing laboratory data). Patient characteristics are summarized in Table 1.

3.1. Pooled Data Analysis. The estimated population mean was close to the measured one (11.06 ± 1.67 versus 11.32 ± 1.23 g/dL, $P < 0.0005$), and the slight underestimation could be improved during the second session as indicated by the reduced absolute residuals (estimated and measured Hb concentration, *1st session* versus *2nd session*: -0.47 ± 0.07 versus -0.06 ± 0.07 g/dL, $P < 0.0005$).

The analysis of the Bland-Altman plots (mean of estimated and measured haemoglobin values versus absolute residuals consisting of estimated and measured values) provided further information concerning the performance of this method (Figure 2). As may be easily seen from these plots, a poor agreement between the estimated and the measured values was found, highlighting a clear systematic error (misspecification) with underestimation in the low concentration range and overestimation in the higher range. In

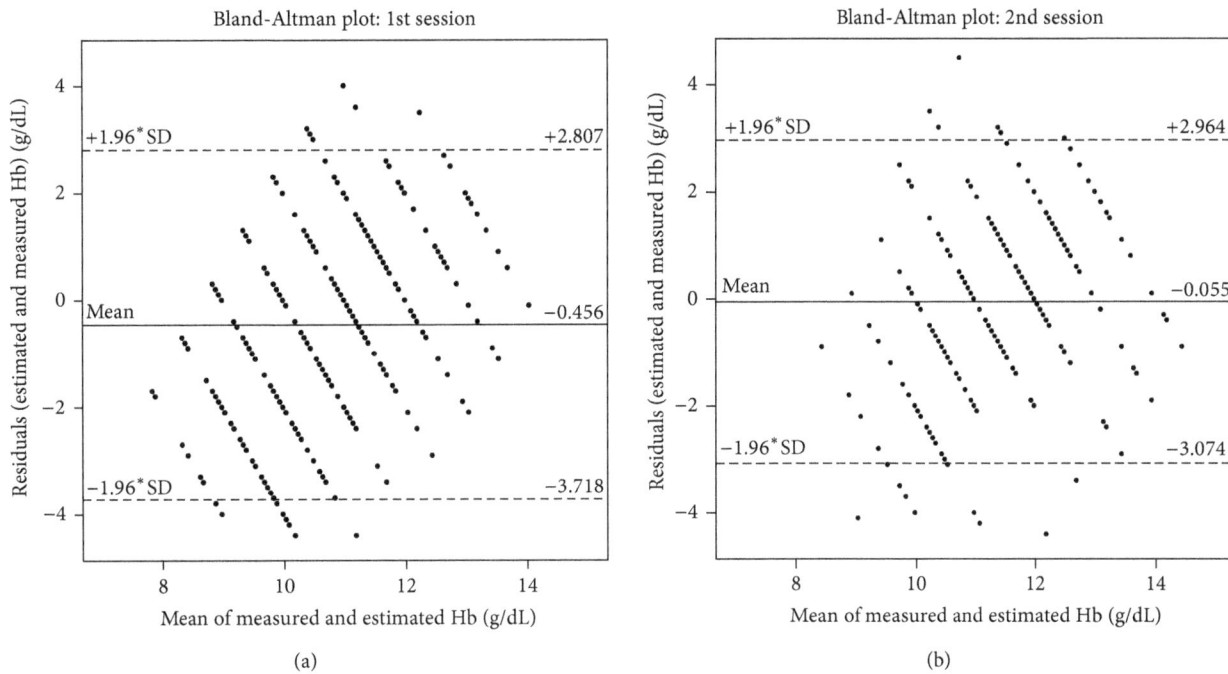

FIGURE 2: Bland-Altman plot highlighting the results of the first (a) and second (b) session. On the X-axis, is plotted the mean of the measured and estimated Hb values. The absolute residuals (estimated and measured) are plotted on the Y-axis. The plain line represents the mean residual, the mean $\pm 1.96 * SD$ is represented by the dotted lines, respectively.

TABLE 1: Patients characteristics (pooled sessions) ($N = 80$ on 1st session and $N = 75$ on 2nd session).

Age, years	66.0 ± 14.4	(70^*)		
Race, white versus black	$76:4$			
Gender, male versus female	$47:33$			
Measured hemoglobin level, g/dL	11.32 ± 1.23	(11.3^*)	$Q_{25-75} = [10.6; 12.1]$	
Estimated haemoglobin level, g/dL (pooled)	11.06 ± 1.67	(11.0^*)	$Q_{25-75} = [10.0; 12.0]$	$Q_{25-75} = [10.21; 12.00]^\dagger$

Values are mean $\pm$ SD.
* Indicates the median.
† Quartiles based on the mean of all observers per patient.

accordance with the previous statement, the linear regression performed on pooled values yielded a rather flat line with a high intercept: $[Hb]_{Measured} = 0.302 \cdot [Hb]_{Estimated} + 7.984$ in [g/dL]; $R = 0.1692$, $P < 0.001$. Further, for the same measured value, very high dispersion of the estimates could be noticed with relative error reaching nearly 50%.

3.2. Interobserver Differences and Multivariate Analysis. Dichotomizing the observers into two groups: medical student and physicians (*physicians*) versus nurse and administrative employees (*nonphysicians*) permitted to show an improved accuracy of the estimate in the *physicians* versus the *nonphysicians* group (ΔResidual = 0.626 g/dL, $P < 0.0005$). *Skilled* observers gave a more accurate estimation of Hb concentrations as compared with *novices* (ΔResidual = 0.341 g/dL, $P < 0.001$). Crossing both categories provided further significant results for all subcategories with the exception of the "*physicians $\times$ skilled*" versus "*physicians $\times$ novice*" pair.

Cofactors interfering with the lighting conditions such as the position of the patient in the dialysis room in relation to

the windows or the day time did not influence significantly the accuracy of the estimates. The same was observed if the estimates were corrected by the actual amount of ultrafiltration at the time of measurement. A trend towards better estimates in younger patients with presumed less degenerative conjunctival affections (*<40 years*) compared to older ones (*>80 years*) (+0.032 versus −0.544 g/dL, $P = 0.064$) as well as the providing of higher estimates by the two last observers due to the hyperthermic effect of the manipulation on the conjunctiva (*observers [1–5] versus observers [6, 7]*) (−0.327 versus −0.127 g/dL, $P = 0.066$) were noted. The correction with the confounding factor (*observer*) failed, however, in achieving the significance level. The gender of the patients and the observers was not associated with any difference in the accuracy of the estimates.

3.3. Test Specificities and Interrater Agreement in Binary Outcomes. Besides the aptitude of the HemoHue HH1 tool to improve visual estimation of individual haemoglobin values, we, furthermore, tested its performance in providing

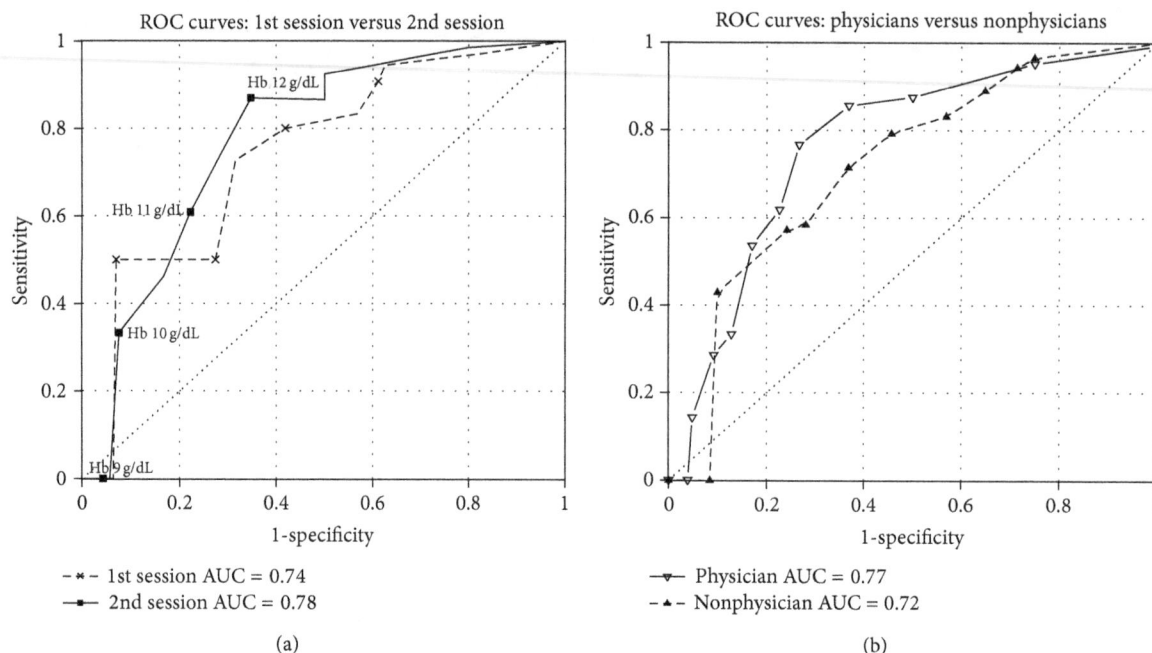

FIGURE 3: Receiver operating characteristic (ROC) curves for detecting anaemia at different cutoff values. First versus second session with corresponding haemoglobin concentration cutoff values and ROC AUC (a). Physicians versus nonphysicians and corresponding ROC AUC (b).

TABLE 2: Test specificities in detecting binary outcomes.

Outcome	Sens.	Spec.	PPV	NPV	Kappa	Sens.	Spec.	PPV	NPV	Kappa
	1st session					2nd session				
Hb < 10 g/dL	50	73	29	89	0.34	33	92	38	91	0.29
10 g/dl ≤ Hb ≤ 12 g/dL	53	48	60	42	0.22	74	56	70	62	0.31
Hb > 12 g/dL	39	91	58	82	0.45	65	87	71	83	0.46
	Physicians					Non-physicians				
Hb < 10 g/dL	32	87	29	88	0.44	55	76	29	90	0.39
10 g/dL ≤ Hb ≤ 12 g/dL	64	51	64	51	−0.01	59	46	60	45	−0.04
Hb > 12 g/dL	63	86	63	86	0.58	35	89	54	79	0.41

Sensitivity, specificity, and positive and negative predictive values are given in percents.

estimation of binary treatment outcomes. According to KDOQI guidelines, the therapeutic haemoglobin target for rHuEPO treated patients should be in the range of 11.0 to 12.0 g/dL [2, 16]. Since the proposed range is very narrow and reaches the discrimination limit of the HemoHue HH1 device of ±1 g/dL, we arbitrarily defined the outcomes (*undertreatment*) as a haemoglobin concentration below 10 g/dL, (*within therapeutic range*) as a haemoglobin concentration between 10 and 12 g/dL, respectively, whereas (*overtreatment*) was set above 12 g/dL. In Table 2, the test specificities (sensitivity, specificity, positive and negative predictive values) and the interobserver agreement (reliability) in detecting the three scenarios described above are shown. As may be easily seen, the predictive performance of the method was slightly better at extreme haemoglobin values, especially in correctly rejecting *undertreatment*, without reaching, however, the standards

to qualify as a good screening test. These findings are visually summarized with the receiver operating characteristic (ROC) curves in Figure 3. Furthermore, the reported values across subgroups (1st versus 2nd session, physician versus nonphysician) were not substantially different. A slight to moderate interobserver agreement (reliability) for the outcome *undertreatment* and *overtreatment* could be noted (Kappa's ranging from 0.29 to 0.58), whereas a striking poor reliability could be observed for the *within therapeutic range* outcome.

4. Discussion

To our knowledge, this is the first clinical trial which systematically assesses the validity of the novel visual bedside tool HemoHue HH1 for the estimation of haemoglobin concentration in chronic haemodialysis patients.

Despite its simple use as a noninvasive and inexpensive test, convincing theoretical aspects and practical experience from previous clinical trials, this study clearly demonstrated the poor performance of the HemoHue HH1 tool in predicting visually the actual haemoglobin concentration in dialysis patients. This failure is evidenced by (1) the inability to estimate the actual haemoglobin level accurately based on one-observer guess, (2) no further consistent improvement of the accuracy when averaging the estimates of different observers, and finally (3) poor performance in estimating the binary treatment outcomes.

Although the estimated population mean was rather close to the measured population mean, individual estimates (one-observer estimation of one patient value) were crude with relative error ranging up to 50%. Further, as pointed out by the Bland-Altman plot, the presence of a systematic error with underestimation in lower Hb range and overestimation in the higher range was found.

In the analysis of variance, a leaning effect with decreased residuals during the second session could be detected. The same feature was seen when comparing skilled with novice observers. It appears, however, improbable that this effect could be further substantially extended with practice. Assuming that the provided estimation is a sum of the true estimated value and an error which is largely due to interobserver discrimination aptitude, increasing the number of raters per item, should theoretically improve the precision of the estimates by lowering the noise component due to the error. However, this approach is hampered by the relative poor gain in accuracy over the individual approach and the difficulties in clinical implementation.

The estimation of the binary treatment outcomes was also characterized by an overall poor performance, especially by a very poor interobserver agreement in the therapeutic range. The test specificities for binary outcomes at the haemoglobin level of 11 g/dL were comparable with those described in previous works in nonnephrologic patients [10, 11].

There are different possible explanations of this failure. First, the achieved haemoglobin values in this particular population are within a narrow therapeutic range of 1 to 2 g/dL. When considering the density plot of the measured haemoglobin values, most of the patients were within the therapeutic range of 11 to 12 g/dL. The HemoHue HH1 device based on a visual estimation with a discrimination power of 1 g/dL could be not precise enough in this setting.

Further, the inclusion of nephrologists aware of treatment goals and outcomes provides certainly a bias. The analysis of the density plots of the estimated values shows a narrow curve centred at known treatment targets in nephrologists. The curves in nonmedical staff were more dispersed about the theoretical mean and left skewed (tendency to provide low values). This may be underlined by the fact that there was no statistically significant difference in estimates between skilled and novice medical observers.

On the other side, our study population consisting principally of aged, chronic haemodialysis patients with some degree of degenerative ocular affection and vascular dysfunction could account in part for the discrepancy between the estimated and the measured haemoglobin level. So far,

the visual anaemia evaluation was principally assessed and validated in paediatric and gynaecologic patients as a raw screening test. Although not significant, a trend toward decreased accuracy of the estimates in older patients was noted.

There are several limitations to this study including among others the lack of a real training component. Indeed, the observers in our study were neither aware of real results nor could they train themselves against reference values. However, the effect of training on the use of the HemoHue HH1 reference card for the visual estimation of hemoglobin values was not the aim of this study. As a matter of fact, the study was designed to prevent a carryover effect of education on the outcome by not providing the testers with a feedback on their performance. According to the manufacturer, the device can be used even by untrained people and still produce good results provided that adequate lighting conditions are fulfilled as indicated by the whitening of the control spot. In other words, appropriate estimation would have been ensured by the correct matching of the hue between the card and the conjunctiva, primary implicating skills in discriminating colors, rather than by conditioning the response of the observer with a reference value.

Finally, training observers against reference values in the dialysis setting would have been impracticable. The time required to obtain laboratory results is much too long to permit the required simultaneous comparison since time delay may preclude correct estimation due to hemoconcentration induced by ultrafiltration during the dialysis procedure.

When we designed the study, available preliminary data clearly confirmed the superiority of the HemoHue HH1 reference card over the naked-eye estimation, and we assumed to achieve a comparable increase in accuracy in hemodialysis patients.

Despite undeniable further improvement in estimating visually the haemoglobin level as compared with the crude, naked-eye assessment, this method failed in estimating with acceptable accuracy the individual haemoglobin level as well as the individual binary treatment outcomes. The validity of these findings should be, however, limited to the studied particular haemodialysis population and not preclude the further deployment and validation of this method in other clinical groups.

5. Conclusions

Despite undeniable additional improvement in estimating visually the haemoglobin levels as compared with the crude, naked-eye assessment, this method failed in predicting with acceptable accuracy the individual haemoglobin level as well as the individual binary treatment outcomes.

Acknowledgments

The authors of the present study would like to thank Hemo-Hue Ltd., for having provided the HemoHue HH1 cards free from charge. The first author was supported by a grant from the Swiss National Science Foundation (PBBEB-121518).

References

[1] D. N. Churchill, D. Macarios, C. Attard, J. Kallich, and R. Goeree, "Costs associated with erythropoiesis-stimulating agent administration to hemodialysis patients," *Nephron - Clinical Practice*, vol. 106, no. 4, pp. c193–c198, 2007.

[2] KDOQI, "KDOQI Clinical Practice Guideline and Clinical Practice Recommendations for anemia in chronic kidney disease: 2007 update of hemoglobin target," *American Journal of Kidney Diseases*, vol. 50, pp. 471–530, 2007.

[3] I. C. Macdougall, K. U. Eckardt, and F. Locatelli, "Latest US KDOQI Anaemia Guidelines update—what are the implications for Europe?" *Nephrology Dialysis Transplantation*, vol. 22, no. 10, pp. 2738–2742, 2007.

[4] R. M. Kalicki and D. E. Uehlinger, "Red cell survival in relation to changes in the hematocrit: more important than you think," *Blood Purification*, vol. 26, no. 4, pp. 355–360, 2008.

[5] J. J. Perez-Ruixo, H. C. Kimko, A. T. Chow, V. Piotrovsky, W. Krzyzanski, and W. J. Jusko, "Population cell life span models for effects of drugs following indirect mechanisms of action," *Journal of Pharmacokinetics and Pharmacodynamics*, vol. 32, no. 5-6, pp. 767–793, 2005.

[6] R. Ramakrishnan, W. K. Cheung, M. C. Wacholtz, N. Minton, and W. J. Jusko, "Pharmacokinetic and pharmacodynamic modeling of recombinant human erythropoietin after single and multiple doses in healthy volunteers," *Journal of Clinical Pharmacology*, vol. 44, no. 9, pp. 991–1002, 2004.

[7] D. Richardson, "Clinical factors influencing sensitivity and response to epoetin," *Nephrology Dialysis Transplantation*, vol. 17, supplement 1, pp. 53–59, 2002.

[8] D. E. Uehlinger, F. A. Gotch, and L. B. Sheiner, "A pharmacodynamic model of erythropoietin therapy for uremic anemia," *Clinical Pharmacology and Therapeutics*, vol. 51, no. 1, pp. 76–89, 1992.

[9] M. G. N. Spinelli, J. M. P. Souza, S. B. de Souza, and E. H. Sesoko, "Reliability and validity of palmar and conjunctival pallor for anemia detection purposes," *Revista de Saude Publica*, vol. 37, no. 4, pp. 404–408, 2003.

[10] M. E. E. K. Chowdhury, V. Chongsuvivatwong, A. F. Geater, H. H. Akhter, and T. Winn, "Taking a medical history and using a colour scale during clinical examination of pallor improves detection of anaemia," *Tropical Medicine and International Health*, vol. 7, no. 2, pp. 133–139, 2002.

[11] J. P. Chalco, L. Huicho, C. Alamo, N. Y. Carreazo, and C. A. Bada, "Accuracy of clinical pallor in the diagnosis of anemia in children: a meta-analysis," *BMC Pediatrics*, vol. 5, article 46, 2005.

[12] S. S. Yalçin, S. Ünal, F. Gümrük, and K. Yurdakök, "The validity of pallor as a clinical sign of anemia in cases with beta-thalassemia," *Turkish Journal of Pediatrics*, vol. 49, no. 4, pp. 408–412, 2007.

[13] R. S. Strobach, S. K. Anderson, D. C. Doll, and Q. S. Ringenberg, "The value of the physical examination in the diagnosis of anemia. Correlation of the physical findings and the hemoglobin concentration," *Archives of Internal Medicine*, vol. 148, no. 4, pp. 831–832, 1988.

[14] A. J. Viera and J. M. Garrett, "Understanding interobserver agreement: the kappa statistic," *Family Medicine*, vol. 37, no. 5, pp. 360–363, 2005.

[15] J. M. Bland and D. G. Altman, "Agreement between methods of measurement with multiple observations per individual," *Journal of Biopharmaceutical Statistics*, vol. 17, no. 4, pp. 571–582, 2007.

[16] I. C. Macdougall, K. U. Eckardt, and F. Locatelli, "Latest US KDOQI Anaemia Guidelines update—what are the implications for Europe?" *Nephrology Dialysis Transplantation*, vol. 22, no. 10, pp. 2738–2742, 2007.

9

Diagnosis of Fanconi Anemia: Mutation Analysis by Multiplex Ligation-Dependent Probe Amplification and PCR-Based Sanger Sequencing

Johan J. P. Gille, Karijn Floor, Lianne Kerkhoven, Najim Ameziane, Hans Joenje, and Johan P. de Winter

Department of Clinical Genetics, VU University Medical Center, Van der Boechorststraat 7, 1081 BT Amsterdam, The Netherlands

Correspondence should be addressed to Johan J. P. Gille, jjp.gille@vumc.nl

Academic Editor: Stefan Meyer

Fanconi anemia (FA) is a rare inherited disease characterized by developmental defects, short stature, bone marrow failure, and a high risk of malignancies. FA is heterogeneous: 15 genetic subtypes have been distinguished so far. A clinical diagnosis of FA needs to be confirmed by testing cells for sensitivity to cross-linking agents in a chromosomal breakage test. As a second step, DNA testing can be employed to elucidate the genetic subtype of the patient and to identify the familial mutations. This knowledge allows preimplantation genetic diagnosis (PGD) and enables prenatal DNA testing in future pregnancies. Although simultaneous testing of all FA genes by next generation sequencing will be possible in the near future, this technique will not be available immediately for all laboratories. In addition, in populations with strong founder mutations, a limited test using Sanger sequencing and MLPA will be a cost-effective alternative. We describe a strategy and optimized conditions for the screening of *FANCA, FANCB, FANCC, FANCE, FANCF,* and *FANCG* and present the results obtained in a cohort of 54 patients referred to our diagnostic service since 2008. In addition, the follow up with respect to genetic counseling and carrier screening in the families is discussed.

1. Introduction

Fanconi anemia (FA) is a rare inherited syndrome with diverse clinical symptoms including developmental defects, short stature, bone marrow failure, and a high risk of malignancies. Fifteen genetic subtypes have been distinguished: FA-A, -B, -C, -D1, -D2, -E, -F, -G, -I, -J, -L, -M, -N, -O, and -P. [1–4]. The majority of patients (~85%) belong to the subtypes A (~60%), C (~10–15%), or G (~10%), while a minority (~15%) is distributed over the remaining 12 subtypes, with relative prevalences between <1 and 5%. These percentages may differ considerably within certain ethnic groups, due to founder effects. All subtypes seem to fit within a "classical" FA phenotype, except for D1 and N (mutated in *BRCA2/FANCD1* and *PALB2/FANCN*), which are associated with a distinct, more severe, syndromic association. The mode of inheritance for all subtypes is autosomal recessive, except for FA-B, which is X-linked. These two different modes of inheritance have important consequences for the counseling of FA families. The relative prevalence of FA-B amongst unselected FA patients is estimated at 1.6% [5]. For all genetic subtypes disease genes have been identified (Table 1). Many mutations found in the various subtypes are private, but recurrent mutations are known, particularly in specific ethnic backgrounds (Table 2).

Most FA genes encode orphan proteins with no known molecular function. At least eight FA proteins (FANCA, -B, -C, -E, -F, -G, -L, and -M) assemble into a nuclear multiprotein core complex, which is required to activate FANCD2 and FANCI by monoubiquitination [6]. FANCL, which carries a RING finger domain, is supposed to represent the ubiquitin E3 ligase in this activation [7]. FANCM probably acts as a sensor of DNA damage and recruits the FA core complex to the site of damage, but FANCM also interacts with other proteins including Blm [6]. Monoubiquitination of FANCD2 and FANCI directs these proteins to areas of damaged chromatin where they interact with other proteins, resulting in repair of the damage [6]. The remaining FA

TABLE 1: Fanconi anemia complementation groups, genes, and proteins.

Group	Gene symbol(s)[a]	Cytogenetic location	Protein (amino acids)	Domain structure (references)
A	FANCA	16q24.3	1455	HEAT repeats [8]
B	FANCB	Xp22.31	859	—
C	FANCC	9q22.3	558	HEAT repeats [8]
D1[b]	BRCA2	13q12.3	3418	RAD51- and DNA-binding motifs [9]
D2	FANCD2	3p25.3	1451	—
E	FANCE	6p21.3	536	—
F	FANCF	11p15	374	—
G	FANCG	9p13	622	Tetratricopeptide repeats (TPR) [10]
I	FANCI	15q26.1	1328	—
J[b]	BRIP1	17q22	1249	DNA helicase [11, 12]
L	FANCL	2p16.1	375	RING finger motif (E3 ligase) [7, 8]
M	FANCM	14q21.3	2014	DNA helicase, nuclease [13]
N[b]	PALB2	16p12.1	1186	—
O[b]	RAD51C	17q25.1	376	—
P[b]	SLX4	16p13.3	1834	Endonuclease scaffold [3, 4]

[a] For gene nomenclature see http://www.genenames.org/.
[b] The proteins defective in groups D1, J, N, O, and P (boldface) act downstream or independent of the monoubiquitination of FANCD2; all other FA proteins act upstream of this process.

TABLE 2: Major recurrent mutations in FA.

Gene	Mutation*	Geographic/ethnic background	Comment	References
FANCA	c.3788_3790del (p.Phe1263del)	European, Brazilian	Relatively mild	[14, 15]
	c.1115_1118delTTGG (p.Val372fs)	European	Relatively mild	[16]
	Exon 12–17del Exon 12–31del	South-African	Relatively common in Afrikaners	[17]
	c.295C>T (p.Gln99X)	Spanish Gypsy population	Worldwide highest prevalence of mutant FANCA allele	[18]
FANCC	c.711+4A>T (originally reported as IVS4+4A>T)	Homozygous in 80% of Ashkenazi Jewish FA; relatively common in Japan.	Severe phenotype in Jews, milder in Japanese.	[19–22]
	c.67delG (originally reported as 322delG)	Homozygous in approx. 50% of Dutch FA patients	Like other exon 1 mutations, relatively mild phenotype.	[19, 23–25]
FANCD2	c.1948-16T>G	Turkish	Founder mutation	[26]
FANCG	c.313G>T (p.Glu105X)	European	44% of mutated FANCG alleles in Germany.	[27]
	c.1077-2A>G	Portuguese/Brazilian	Founder mutation	[27, 28]
	c.1480+1G>C	French-Canadian	Founder mutation	[28]
	c.307+1G>C	Japanese	Founder mutation	[28, 29]
	c.1794_1803del (p.Trp599fs)	European		[28]
	c.637_643del (p.Tyr213fs)	Sub-Saharan Africa	82% of all black FA patients	[30]
FANCJ	c.2392C>T (p.Arg798X)		Found in ca. 50% of FA-J patients of diverse ancestry; ancient mutation or hot spot.	[11, 12]

Nucleotide numbering based on <u>A</u>TG = +1.
Published sequence variations in FA genes, with their descriptions conforming to the current nomenclature rules, are listed at http://www.rocke-feller.edu/fanconi/.

proteins function downstream of or parallel to the FANCD2 activation step [6]. The exact nature of the DNA damage response, which when defective causes FA, remains to be defined. FANCJ/BRIP1 and FANCM possess DNA helicase motifs, which strongly suggests that the FA pathway acts through a direct interaction with DNA, presumably to resolve or remodel blocked DNA replication forks resulting from DNA interstrand cross-link damage [6]. This idea is strengthened by the recent extension of the FA pathway with SLX4, a scaffold protein for structure-specific endonucleases involved in unhooking the DNA cross-link [3, 4].

2. Laboratory Diagnostics in FA

Cells derived from FA patients are—by definition—hypersensitive to chromosomal breakage induced by DNA cross-linking agents such as mitomycin C (MMC) or diepoxybutane (DEB) [31]. This cellular phenotype is ascertained using stimulated blood T lymphocytes. The indications for FA laboratory testing are rather broad [32]. As a consequence, in only a small proportion of patients (about 10%) the chromosomal breakage test is positive, and an FA diagnosis is established. Since mutation testing by Sanger sequencing and MLPA is rather laborious, time consuming and therefore expensive, a positive chromosomal breakage test is a prerequisite for starting mutation screening. Confirmation of the FA diagnosis at the DNA level is important in patients in whom the chromosomal breakage test was inconclusive. Furthermore, knowledge about the FA subtype is relevant for the treatment and prognosis of the patients. In addition, identification of mutations allows carrier testing in the family and will enable prenatal DNA testing and preimplantation genetic diagnosis (PGD) in future pregnancies. Finally, this information can be used to rule out FA in potential donors for bone marrow transplantation.

Although simultaneous testing of all FA genes by next generation sequencing will be possible in the near future, this technique will not be available immediately for all laboratories worldwide. In addition, in populations with strong founder mutations, a limited test using Sanger sequencing and MLPA will be a cost-effective alternative [33]. The strategy outlined below has been developed at our DNA diagnostics laboratory to provide a molecular diagnosis of FA. It is recognized that mutations in *FANCA* account for 60–70% of all FA cases and that about 15–20% of the mutations in this gene are large deletions [33, 34]. Therefore, DNA testing usually starts with a screen for deletions in *FANCA*. However, depending on the circumstances strategies may differ from case to case.

2.1. Materials. Genomic DNA (from e.g., leukocytes or fibroblasts derived from the proband or the parents) is adequate for most mutation screening assays. Screening on cDNA is more efficient but has several drawbacks: for high-quality cDNA, growing cells (stimulated leukocytes, lymphoblastoid cell lines, or fibroblasts) are necessary. In addition, common alternative splice variants will hamper

the evaluation of DNA sequences. Therefore, screening on gDNA is the preferred method for mutation screening. However, during the diagnostic process, growing cells from the proband will be helpful in a couple of situations. Growing cells are indispensable for studying the effect of unclassified variants on splicing or to verify the disease gene by functional complementation of the cellular phenotype with a construct expressing a wild type copy of the suspected gene [35–37]. Finally, if no mutations can be de detected, growing cells can be used to reconfirm the diagnosis FA by checking MMC sensitivity in cell growth or G2-arrest assays [38, 39].

2.2. Mutation Screening Strategy

2.2.1. Hints from Ethnic Background or Phenotype. Information on the ethnic background of the proband may provide a clue for a specific pathogenic mutation that most likely causes the disease, such as c.711 + 4A>T (IVS4 + 4A>T) in *FANCC*, a mutation present in homozygous state in 80% of all FA cases of Ashkenazi Jewish ancestry, and c.295C >T in *FANCA*, which was present homozygously in all 40 FA cases of Spanish Gypsy ancestry so far investigated. More examples of recurrent mutations are shown in Table 3. The distinct clinical phenotype of D1 and N patients (severely affected, often combined with leukemia or solid tumors below the age of 5 years) may provide a clue to favor *BRCA2/FANCD1* and *PALB2/FANCN* as the first gene to be screened [40–44]. This is especially worthwhile if confirmed by the cellular phenotype: in contrast to cells from all other known FA subtypes, cells from D1, N and O patients are unable to form RAD51 foci upon exposure to X rays or MMC [43–45].

2.2.2. No Clues Available

(1) In the absence of any clue to the disease gene, mutation screening starts with a search for deletions in *FANCA*, as this type of mutation accounts for 40% of all mutant *FANCA* alleles. The quantitative multiplex ligation-dependent probe amplification (MLPA) method [46] is used for this initial screen, which identifies *FANCA* as the most likely disease gene in 1 out of 4 patients by the detection of a—usually hemizygous-deletion. In parallel, the *FANCA* gene is completely sequenced. The combination of these two approaches identifies 60–70% of all FA patients as FA-A.

(2) Next, *FANCC, -E, -F*, and *-G* are screened by DNA sequencing.

(3) Only if the proband is a male, *FANCB* is screened by MLPA and DNA sequencing,

In Table 4, optimized conditions are provided for the PCR amplification of *FANCA, -C, -E, -F, -G, and -B*. Most PCRs can be performed under standard conditions. The PCR primers have M13 extensions which allow sequencing of all fragments with universal sequencing primers. MLPA was performed according to the instructions of the supplier. Detailed information about the sequences of the MLPA probes is available from the website of the

TABLE 3: Mutations detected in a cohort of 54 patients by screening *FANCA*, *FANCC*, *FANCE*, *FANCF* and *FANCG*.

	Country of origin[1]	Gene	Allele 1			Allele 2		
			DNA change	Effect	Number of database entries	DNA change	Effect	Number of database entries
1	ES	FANCA	ex16_17del	del	12x	c.1115_1118del	p.Val372fs	62x
2	PT	FANCA	c.718C>T	p.Gln240X	2x	c.2870G>A	W957X	1x
3	NL	FANCA	ex15del	del	3x	ex15del	del	3x
4	NL	FANCA	c.3788_3790del	p.Phe1263del	215x	c.3788_3790del	p.Phe1263del	215x
5	CA	FANCA	c.718C>T	pGlnx240X	2x	c.1085T>C	p.Leu362Pro	novel
6	PT	FANCA	c.3788_3790del	p.Phe1263del	215x	c.4130C>G	p.Ser1377X	1x
7	IE	FANCA	c.2812_2830dup	p.Asp944fs	3x	c.2812_2830dup	p.Asp944fs	3x
8	AU	FANCA	c.2303T>C	p.Leu768Pro	5x	c.2303T>C	p.Leu768Pro	5x
9	NL	FANCA	c.862G>T	p.Glu288X	1x	c.862G>T	p.Glu288X	1x
10	NL	FANCA	ex11_33del	del	1x	c.2121delC	p.Asn707fs	novel
11	DK	FANCA	ex1_8del	del	1x	c.3788_3790del	p.Phe1263del	215x
12	UK	FANCA	c.337_338del	p.Ala114fs	1x	c.3349A>G	p.Arg1117Gly	2x
13	UK	FANCA	c.3568C>T	p.Gln1190X	novel	c.3568C>T	p.Gln1190X	novel
14	NL	FANCA	c.487delC	p.Arg163fs	1x	c.2851C>T	p.Arg951Trp	11x
15	SE	FANCA	c.88delG	p.Val30fs	novel	c.100A>T	p.Lys34X	2x
16	NL	FANCA	c.862G>T	p.Glu288X	9x	c.1771C>T	p.Arg591X	9x
17	PT	FANCA	c.1709_1715+4del	p.Glu570fs	novel	c.3430C>T	p.Arg1144Trp	novel
18	NO	FANCA	c.100A>T	p.Lys34X	2x	c.1378C>T	p.Arg460X	novel
19	PT	FANCA	ex15_17del	del	2x	ex15_17del	del	2x
20	NL	FANCA	c.2982-192A>G	splice[2]	novel	ex7_31del	del	
21	AU	FANCA	c.427-8_427-5del	splice	novel	c.1771C>T	p.Arg591X	9x
22	AU	FANCA	c.3491C>T	p.Pro1164Leu	novel	c.3491C>T	p.Pro1164Leu	novel
23	CA	FANCA	ex4_29del	del	novel	ex31del	del	6x
24	NL	FANCA	c.3391A>G	p.Thr1131Ala	15x	c.3391A>G	p.Thr1131Ala	15x
25	GR	FANCA	c.2T>C	p.Met1?	1x	c.3788_3790del	p.Phe1263del	215x
26	IE	FANCA	c.851dup	p.Val285fs	novel	c.2534T>C	p.Leu845Pro	4x
27	NL	FANCA	c.2852G>A	p.Arg951Gln	6x	c.3624C>T	p.= (splice)	2x
28	AU	FANCA	c.331_334dup	p.Leu112fs	novel	ex22_29del	del	novel
29	NL	FANCA	c.862G>T	p.Glu288X	9x	c.3920delA	p.Gln1307fs	2x
30	IR	FANCA	ex21del	del	novel	ex21del	del	novel
31	SE	FANCA	ex1_12del	del	novel	ex22_29del	del	novel
32	NL	FANCB	c.755_767del	p.Leu252fs	novel	—	—	—
33	NL	FANCC	c.67delG	p.Asp23fs	50x	c.553C>T	p.Arg185X	14x
34	NL	FANCC	c.67delG	p.Asp23fs	50x	c.67delG	p.Asp23fs	50x
35	CA	FANCC	c.67delG	p.Asp23fs	50x	c.553C>T	p.Arg185X	14x
36	NL	FANCC	c.67delG	p.Asp23fs	50x	c.1155-1G>C	splice	novel
37	NL	FANCC	c.67delG	p.Asp23fs	50x	c.67delG	p.Asp23fs	50x
38	NL	FANCC	c.67delG	p.Asp23fs	50x	c.467delC	p.Ser156fs	novel
39	PT	FANCE	c.1111C>T	p.Arg371Trp	6x	c.1111C>T	p.Arg371Trp	6x
40	UK	FANCF	c.496C>T	p.Gln166X	4x	c.496C>T	p.Gln166X	4x
41	UK	FANCG	c.307+2delT	splice	novel	c.307+2delT	splice	novel
42	UK	FANCG	c.1471_1473delinsG	p.Lys491fs	novel	c.1471_1473delinsG	p.Lys491fs	novel
43	NL	FANCG	c.65G>C	p.Arg22Pro	6x	c.65G>C;	p.Arg22Pro	6x
44	IR	FANCG	c.307+1G>C	splice	21x	c.307+1G>C	splice	21x
45	NL	FANCG	c.85-1G>A	splice	novel	c.85-1G>A	splice	novel

[1] Country of origins: AU: Australia; CA: Canada; DK: Denmark; ES: Spain; GR: Greece; IE: Ireland; IR: Iran; NL: Netherlands; PT: Portugal; SE: Sweden; UK: United Kingdom

Number of database entries refers to the FA database at: http://www.rockefeller.edu/fanconi/.

The pathogenic state of novel missense mutations is based upon *in silico* prediction algorithms (SIFT, POLYPHEN2, Align GVGD), the presence of a second clearly pathogenic mutation in the same gene and segregation in the family.

[2] Effect c.2982-192A>G: by studying cDNA it was shown that the mutation created a new splice donor site resulting in an aberrant mRNA.

TABLE 4: Primers and conditions for PCR on genomic DNA of the coding sequence plus intron/exon boundaries of *FANCA, FANCC, FANCE, FANCF, FANCG,* and *FANCB*.

(a)

FANCA		
Primer name	Sequence (5′ > 3′)	Product length (bp)
FANCA_ex1F	gtaaaacgacggccag GCGCCTCCCCCAGGACCAACA	362
FANCA_ex1R	caggaaacagctatga AGGCTCTGGCGGGAAGGGATCGG	
FANCA_ex2F	gtaaaacgacggccag CTCTTCGGGAGGGTGTCGCTGGT	328
FANCA_ex2R	caggaaacagctatga CTCTTCGGGAGGGTGTCGCTGGT	
FANCA_ex3F	gtaaaacgacggccag GCCTGGCCTGGAGCTTGAAT	392
FANCA_ex3R	caggaaacagctatga CGCAGGTTGAATCAGACGCTGTT	
FANCA_ex4F	gtaaaacgacggccag TAAGGCATTTTAAACAGCAAGTC	430
FANCA_ex4R	caggaaacagctatga TGCCAATAAATACTGAGCAAACT	
FANCA_ex5F	gtaaaacgacggccag AGTATTGTTTCAGGTAATTTGTT	356
FANCA_ex5R	caggaaacagctatga TGAAGGTACTTCTTTCCAATCCA	
FANCA_ex6F	gtaaaacgacggccag AGATGTGTTTCAGGCTCTAAGTT	402
FANCA_ex6R	caggaaacagctatga GCAATGCAATCTAGTCTAGTACA	
FANCA_ex7F	gtaaaacgacggccag TGGGATTTAGTTGAGCCTTACGTCTGC	421
FANCA_ex7R	caggaaacagctatgaAAGGTGAATGGAAACACTTAAACTCATGTCA	
FANCA_ex8F	gtaaaacgacggccag GTGGTCAGGTGAGCAGTAACTTC	401
FANCA_ex8R	caggaaacagctatga TAAATAGGTACAAACAGCACGTT	
FANCA_ex9F	gtaaaacgacggccag TTCTCTTGTGTGATGCAGGTATC	332
FANCA_ex9R	caggaaacagctatga TGACCCACAGATTCATGAGGTAT	
FANCA_ex10F	gtaaaacgacggccag TTTTGATTAAGGCCTACAGATTG	406
FANCA_ex10R	caggaaacagctatga CCTCCTCCTCACGCACGTTATCG	
FANCA_ex11F	gtaaaacgacggccag TTTCAAGTCTGTGGTTATAGTGG	410
FANCA_ex11R	caggaaacagctatga AGACGTAAAAGAGGTCCTAGAAT	
FANCA_ex12F	gtaaaacgacggccag CTGTGGGGCTGGTCCTTAACAAA	236
FANCA_ex12R	caggaaacagctatga AGGCAGCATGACAAGTACTAGGC	
FANCA_ex13F	gtaaaacgacggccag ACATTGGTTTGCTTGGATATTGA	377
FANCA_ex13R	caggaaacagctatga CTGACAAAGAATGTTCCATCGAC	
FANCA_ex14F	gtaaaacgacggccag TGCTGTAATTGCTGTGTAGTCTT	411
FANCA_ex14R	caggaaacagctatga ACTCACATGACAGAGAATCAGGT	
FANCA_ex15F	gtaaaacgacggccag ACTACAGCAGCCGCCCGGACACT	430
FANCA_ex15R	caggaaacagctatga GCAGATCTGCAGGAGGCTCTTGG	
FANCA_ex16F	gtaaaacgacggccag TCCCAGGCAGTTCCCAGACTAAC	312
FANCA_ex16R	caggaaacagctatga AGCTGATGACAAATCCTCGTAGA	
FANCA_ex17F	gtaaaacgacggccag ACCGCTCCCTCCTCACAGACTAC	334
FANCA_ex17R	caggaaacagctatga AAGGCTGAAAAACTCAACTCAAG	
FANCA_ex18F	gtaaaacgacggccag GCGCACAGCATGTGGGCCTTTAC	397
FANCA_ex18R	caggaaacagctatga GCAGCTGCTAGAGGCCTTTTCGG	
FANCA_ex19F	gtaaaacgacggccag GTGCACAAGAAGACTTCATAATG	284
FANCA_ex19R	caggaaacagctatga AGTCCTTGCTTTCTACACAACTG	
FANCA_ex20F	gtaaaacgacggccag CTTCTCTGTGTTGCAGCATATTC	298
FANCA_ex20R	caggaaacagctatga AGAAGAAACCTGGAAGTAGTCAT	
FANCA_ex21F	gtaaaacgacggccag ATAATAGATTTGGGGATTGTAAT	255
FANCA_ex21R	caggaaacagctatga CAACAGACACTCAAGGTTAGGAA	
FANCA_ex22F	gtaaaacgacggccag TGCAGTGAAGAGTCCTGTTGAGT	305
FANCA_ex22R	caggaaacagctatga ACACACCAGCCTGATGTCACTAT	
FANCA_ex23F	gtaaaacgacggccag CAGTCAGCAGGATCCGTGGAATC	416

(a) Continued.

FANCA

Primer name	Sequence (5′ > 3′)	Product length (bp)
FANCA_ex23R	caggaaacagctatga GGCCCTGGAACATCTGATACGAC	
FANCA_ex24F	gtaaaacgacggccag CCTTCCTGCTGCTCCCGTCC	229
FANCA_ex24R	caggaaacagctatga CAGACTTGGCCCAGCAAGAG	
FANCA_ex25F	gtaaaacgacggccag CCGCTGGTGGTTGGATTAGCTGT	296
FANCA_ex25R	caggaaacagctatga TTTCCAGGGCACTGAAGACGAAT	
FANCA_ex26F	gtaaaacgacggccag AGCTTGGAAGAGGGCAGTCTGCT	347
FANCA_ex26R	caggaaacagctatga CTCTTCTAATTTTATCAAACGAG	
FANCA_ex27F	gtaaaacgacggccag AGACTGTCTCACAACAAACGAAC	356
FANCA_ex27R	caggaaacagctatga CGGTCCGAAAGCTGCGTAAAC	
FANCA_ex28F	gtaaaacgacggccag GTTGATGGTCTGTTTCCACCTGA	401
FANCA_ex28R	caggaaacagctatga GAAGGAACGGTCACCTACGTGCT	
FANCA_ex29F	gtaaaacgacggccag GACATGGAGGACTGCGTATGAGA	411
FANCA_ex29R	caggaaacagctatga GTGGCTGTGATGACTGGAACGTG	
FANCA_ex30F	gtaaaacgacggccag CCCGAGCCGCCAGTCTCAACCCA	411
FANCA_ex30R	caggaaacagctatga AAAGGCAGACCCACCCTAAGCTA	
FANCA_ex31F	gtaaaacgacggccag GATAAGCCTCCTTGGTCATGGTA	406
FANCA_ex31R	caggaaacagctatga TGGCAATAAATATCTTAATAGCA	
FANCA_ex32F	gtaaaacgacggccag TTCCTGTGCCAGCATACTGCTCT	359
FANCA_ex32R	caggaaacagctatga GGGTGGGGACACACAGACAAGTA	
FANCA_ex33F	gtaaaacgacggccag TGGGTTTCAGGGTGGTGGTTGCT	356
FANCA_ex33R	caggaaacagctatga GAACCCTTTCCTCAGTAATTCAC	
FANCA_ex34F	gtaaaacgacggccag CGCCCAGGGAAGCCGTTAAGTTT	333
FANCA_ex34R	caggaaacagctatga GCGTTCTGAGAAGGCCACGAGAG	
FANCA_ex35F	gtaaaacgacggccag TTCCTTCACTCTACTAGTTGTGG	311
FANCA_ex35R	caggaaacagctatga TGAGATGGTAACACCCGTGATGG	
FANCA_ex36F	gtaaaacgacggccag CCATCTCAGCCACCCTCATCTGT	350
FANCA_ex36R	caggaaacagctatga AGGCGCCCACCACCACGAGAACT	
FANCA_ex37F	gtaaaacgacggccag GACTTGGTTTCTATGGCGTGGTT	310
FANCA_ex37R	caggaaacagctatga CCCAGAGAAATAGCACTGATTGA	
FANCA_ex38F	gtaaaacgacggccag GTTTTCTAAGATCCACTTAAAGG	362
FANCA_ex38R	caggaaacagctatga CTCACTCACACTTCCGCAAACAC	
FANCA_ex39F	gtaaaacgacggccag CTGTCCAGAGGCCCAGTATTACC	387
FANCA_ex39R	caggaaacagctatga AGGAGGGCTCGTTCTTAACCATT	
FANCA_ex40F	gtaaaacgacggccag GGTGTCCCCAGCACTGATAATAG	353
FANCA_ex40R	caggaaacagctatga AGACATAGTGACAAATGGCTACA	
FANCA_ex41F	gtaaaacgacggccag CCCTTGGCATCACCTGCTACCTT	403
FANCA_ex41R	caggaaacagctatga AACAGGCAAACTCACAGGTTAGA	
FANCA_ex42F	gtaaaacgacggccag ACCAGCCCTGTTTCTGTATGTCT	248
FANCA_ex42R	caggaaacagctatga ACATGGCCCAGGCAGCTGTCAAT	
FANCA_ex43F	gtaaaacgacggccag TGTGGGGGACATGAGAATTGACA	378
FANCA_ex43R	caggaaacagctatga GTAATCCACTTTTTAGTGCAACA	
FANCAIVS10F	gtaaaacgacggccag TTTACATGTGCATCAGTTAGCTT	184
FANCAIVS10R	caggaaacagctatga CATGAAGACACAGAAAAAGTAGGT	

(b)

FANCC

Primer name	Sequence (5′ > 3′)	Product length (bp)
FANCC_ex1F	gtaaaacgacggccag ACCATTCCTTCAGTGCTGGACA	378
FANCC_ex1R	caggaaacagctatga CCATCGGCACTTCAGTCAATACC	

(b) Continued.

FANCC

Primer name	Sequence (5′ > 3′)	Product length (bp)
FANCC_ex2F	gtaaaacgacggccag CTAAACAAGAAGCATTCACGTTC	303
FANCC_ex2R	caggaaacagctatga GGAGAAAGGTTCATAATGTAAGC	
FANCC_ex3F	gtaaaacgacggccag TCAGCAGAAAGAGAATGTGCAAA	405
FANCC_ex3R	caggaaacagctatga AACATCATAGAACTGGATTCCAC	
FANCC_ex4F	gtaaaacgacggccag TGTACATAAAAGGCACTTGCATT	380
FANCC_ex4R	caggaaacagctatga TCCCATCTCACATTTCTTCCGTA	
FANCC_ex5F	gtaaaacgacggccag AGAACTGATGTAATCCTGTTTGC	367
FANCC_ex5R	caggaaacagctatga TTACTGCTCTGTGAGAGTTGAGA	
FANCC_ex6F	gtaaaacgacggccag GTCTTTGACCTTTTTAGCATGAA	387
FANCC_ex6R	caggaaacagctatga AACGTTTGGACACTGCTGTCGTA	
FANCC_ex7F	gtaaaacgacggccag ATTAGTGATTGCATTTTGAACTT	422
FANCC_ex7R	caggaaacagctatga CAAAAATAAAATGTAAATACACG	
FANCC_ex8F	gtaaaacgacggccag CTCCTTTGGCTGATAATAGCAAG	336
FANCC_ex8R	caggaaacagctatga CTGATTTTTGAGTTTTTACCTCT	
FANCC_ex9F	gtaaaacgacggccag ATACTGCTGAAGCTTATGGCACA	400
FANCC_ex9R	caggaaacagctatga TAACCTTTGTTGGGGCACTCATT	
FANCC_ex10F	gtaaaacgacggccag TATGAGGTTATTGGGAGCTTATT	382
FANCC_ex10R	caggaaacagctatga CTGTCTCCCTCATGCTGTAGATA	
FANCC_ex11F	gtaaaacgacggccag GAACCAGAAGTAAAGGGCGTCTC	416
FANCC_ex11R	caggaaacagctatga CTGACCTGCTCCAAGCCATCCGT	
FANCC_ex12F	gtaaaacgacggccag AAGTACAATTTAAGCCAACCGTT	451
FANCC_ex12R	caggaaacagctatga AGGTTGCCATGACATATGCCATC	
FANCC_ex13F	gtaaaacgacggccag CCTCTCTCAGGGGCCAGTGCTTA	435
FANCC_ex13R	caggaaacagctatga AGACCCTCGGACAGGTAACCCAC	
FANCC_ex14F	gtaaaacgacggccag ACTTGCTATGCTAATCACCTTGC	437
FANCC_ex14R	caggaaacagctatga AATGCGTGGCCACAGGTCATCAC	

(c)

FANCE

Primer name	Sequence (5′ > 3′)	Product length (bp)
FANCE_ex1F	gtaaaacgacggccag CGCCTCCCTCCTTCCCTTTC	540
FANCE_ex1R	caggaaacagctatga CCCGCCTCCCATACCTGCTAA	
FANCE_ex2aF	gtaaaacgacggccag GCTCTGCCCAGTCTGCCTTGTGC	469
FANCE_ex2aR	caggaaacagctatga CTCTGAGTCCTTTCTGCGTTTCC	
FANCE_ex2bF	gtaaaacgacggccag GCCAGAGACAGCTCCAAAGTCTA	479
FANCE_ex2bR	caggaaacagctatga CAGCCTTCCCCATGGATAAAGCC	
FANCE_ex3F	gtaaaacgacggccag GCCTCTTGACTTTCTTGAATCAT	352
FANCE_ex3R	caggaaacagctatga ACTGTCCTCAGACCTTTACTCCA	
FANCE_ex4F	gtaaaacgacggccag TTGAACCAAGTGTAGACTTACCA	436
FANCE_ex4R	caggaaacagctatga GGGAAGGAACCAAGGGCTAAAAG	
FANCE_ex5F	gtaaaacgacggccag GTATCTTTTAGCCCTTGGTTCCT	431
FANCE_ex5R	caggaaacagctatga GAATCCCCTCTCTCAAGTACCAC	
FANCE_ex6F	gtaaaacgacggccag TTTCCTTTGTAACATGTATCATC	433
FANCE_ex6R	caggaaacagctatga AGCAGAAAGCAGGGAGGCGGTAA	
FANCE_ex7F	gtaaaacgacggccag ACAGGCTGGGCATTCTGTTACCG	425
FANCE_ex7R	caggaaacagctatga AGTGAGACACAAGGATCCCCTAA	
FANCE_ex8F	gtaaaacgacggccag TTGGAGCAGCAGATAGATACTCA	380
FANCE_ex8R	caggaaacagctatga AGAGGTGGAGCTGAAGTGACCAT	
FANCE_ex9F	gtaaaacgacggccag GTTACCTGCCCAGGGTCACCTAG	388
FANCE_ex9R	caggaaacagctatga CTGGCCAGCACTCAGGGTTTTAT	

(c) Continued.

FANCE

Primer name	Sequence (5′ > 3′)	Product length (bp)
FANCE_ex10F	gtaaaacgacggccag TGGCCTCCTCTCTCCTCAATAGA	369
FANCE_ex10R	caggaaacagctatga AACAGGGAGGCAGTTGCAATCTG	

(d)

FANCF

Primer name	Sequence (5′ > 3′)	Product length (bp)
FANCF_ex1aF	gtaaaacgacggccag TTTCGCGGATGTTCCAATCAGTA	449
FANCF_ex1aR	caggaaacagctatga CTGCACCAGGTGGTAACGAGCTG	
FANCF_ex1bF	gtaaaacgacggccag AGTGGAGGCAAGAGGGCGGCTTT	456
FANCF_ex1bR	caggaaacagctatga GCTATCACCTTCAGGAAGTTGTT	
FANCF_ex1cF	gtaaaacgacggccag CCCAAATCTCCAGGAGGACTCTC	444
FANCF_ex1cR	caggaaacagctatga TTTCTGAAGGTCATAGTGCAAAC	
FANCF_ex1dF	gtaaaacgacggccag GCTTTTGACTTTAGTGACTAGCC	456
FANCF_ex1dR	caggaaacagctatga ATTTGGTGAGAACATTGTAATTT	

(e)

FANCG

Primer name	Sequence (5′ > 3′)	Product length (bp)
FANCG_ex1F	gtaaaacgacggccag AGCCTGGGCGGGTGGATTGGGAC	389
FANCG_ex1R	caggaaacagctatga TCATTTCTGGCTCTTTGGTCAAG	
FANCG_ex2F	gtaaaacgacggccag CAGGCCAAGGTAACACGGTTGCT	460
FANCG_ex2R	caggaaacagctatga CCAGTCTCCTCTGTGCCTTAAAC	
FANCG_ex3F	gtaaaacgacggccag TATTGTAGCTGTTTTGGTTGGAG	362
FANCG_ex3R	caggaaacagctatga GGTGACAGATGTTGTTTATCCTC	
FANCG_ex4F	gtaaaacgacggccag GGAGATGGAGGATGAGGTGCTAC	411
FANCG_ex4R	caggaaacagctatga CGACCACCAACCCAGCCGCCTGT	
FANCG_ex5F	gtaaaacgacggccag AGATGGAGATAGGAGAAGACGAG	454
FANCG_ex5R	caggaaacagctatga GCTTCATGAAGGCTGCTTAGTGC	
FANCG_ex6F	gtaaaacgacggccag CAGTTCCATGGGCTTCTTAGACC	393
FANCG_ex6R	caggaaacagctatga TCAGGGCTGCAACCAAGTACAAC	
FANCG_ex7F	gtaaaacgacggccag GCACTGGGGTCCTGTCACCGTAA	418
FANCG_ex7R	caggaaacagctatga ATAATCTTTGGGAGCCATACTTC	
FANCG_ex8F	gtaaaacgacggccag GCTTGTGATGGGGTGACTTGACT	438
FANCG_ex8R	caggaaacagctatga AGTTCAGGTCTAGAAGCAAGGTA	
FANCG_ex9F	gtaaaacgacggccag CCTCCTCAGGGCCCATGAACATC	400
FANCG_ex9R	caggaaacagctatga GCAGTGTCTTGAAAGGCATGAGC	
FANCG_ex10F	gtaaaacgacggccag CAGGACTCTGCATGGTACCAG	460
FANCG_ex10R	caggaaacagctatga CCAATCAGAAAATCATCCCTC	
FANCG_ex11F	gtaaaacgacggccag AGCTCCATGTTCACCTACTTACC	397
FANCG_ex11R	caggaaacagctatga CAGTGCCGCATCTGACTTACATC	
FANCG_ex12F	gtaaaacgacggccag AGGATTTGGGGTTTTGGTGACTG	445
FANCG_ex12R	caggaaacagctatga AACTCTTGGGAGCCCTGCATACA	
FANCG_ex13F	gtaaaacgacggccag CCGCTTCCATATGTGAGTGTAGG	340
FANCG_ex13R	caggaaacagctatgaC CACAATAGGTCCAAGGACTCTA	
FANCG_ex14F	gtaaaacgacggccag CCAAACTAAGGGGTCACATGAAG	405
FANCG_ex14R	caggaaacagctatga GATGGTGAAGCAGAAAGCCCTCC	

(f)

FANCB

Primer name	Sequence (5′ > 3′)	Product length (bp)
FANCB_ex3AF	gtaaaacgacggccag	721
FANCB_ex3AR	GATATGGTTATTTGAATTCTTAGCAcaggaaacagctatga	
	GCCATCCTTCATCTCATAGCCTAGT	

(f) Continued.

FANCB

Primer name	Sequence (5′ > 3′)	Product length (bp)
FANCB_ex3BF FANCB_ex3BR	gtaaaacgacggccag ATTAACCTCCCTTACATTGTGATAGcaggaaacagctatga CAATAAGACTCCAGAATGAACTCTA	811
FANCB_ex4F FANCB_ex4R	gtaaaacgacggccag TTTACAAATGACAACTACATGAcaggaaacagctatga TTAAGTATAAAACCACCAATAT	391
FANCB_ex5F FANCB_ex5R	gtaaaacgacggccag ACTGCATCTGGCCTATAGTTcaggaaacagctatga AATACCATTTTTACCCAAGC	411
FANCB_ex6F FANCB_ex6R	gtaaaacgacggccag GTATTTCCTGAATTATTGGTATGTC caggaaacagctatga CATAAAAGTCCACCATTATAACCTC	395
FANCB_ex7F FANCB_ex7R	gtaaaacgacggccag TGTTTGGGCCATAAGCCCTA caggaaacagctatga TTCTGGAGCATCAAGACAGT	355
FANCB_ex8F FANCB_ex8R	gtaaaacgacggccag GTTGTTTGTATGACATTTAATCATC caggaaacagctatga ATCATTAAACTCTGCCCATTATCAG	636
FANCB_ex9F FANCB_ex9R	gtaaaacgacggccag AGGTAATTTTGTTGGCACTT caggaaacagctatga ATGCGTTCATTCATGCTAGG	531
FANCB_ex10F FANCB_ex10R	gtaaaacgacggccag AATTGGTTCTGTTTATCATTATGGT caggaaacagctatga CTACTACAGTAAGCCTCGGTGTTTA	686

PCR conditions:

PCR was performed in Applied Biosystems PE9700 system using 96-well plates. PCR reactions (final volume 25 μl) contained 0.5 units Platinum Taq polymerase (Invitrogen), 1,5 mM MgCl$_2$, 0.2 mM NTPs (Invitrogen), and 10 pmol primer.

For the large majority of amplicons, standard PCR conditions were used: preheat 95°C, 5 min, denaturation 95°C, 30 sec, annealing 60°C, 30 sec., elongation 72°C, 1 min, number of cycles: 33.

Fragments with a different annealing temperature were *FANCA* exons 5, 7, 13, 21, 26, 31, and 38, *FANCC* exon 7, *FANCF* fragment 1d and *FANCE* exon 1 : 55°C; *FANCA* exon 1 : 64°C. For *FANCE* exon 1 the PCR mix was supplemented with 10% DMSO.

For *FANCB* different PCR conditions were used: preheat 95°C, 5 min, denaturation 95°C, 1 min, annealing 50°C, 1 min., elongation 72°C, 1 min., number of cycles 30. For *FANCB* exon 7 and 9 the annealing temperature was 55°C. For sequencing of exon 7 forward, a special sequencing primer was used: 5′-TTTTTAGAAGGAATGTCTTG-3′.

FA gene specific part of the primer is indicated in capitals. Primers are extended with M13 sequence (indicated in normal letter type), which is used for the sequencing reaction.

supplier (www.mlpa.com). In a well-equipped laboratory with sufficient dedicated personal, testing of *FANCA, -C, -E, -F, -G and -B* can be completed within 1-2 weeks.

After screening *FANCA, -C, -E, -F, -G, and –B*, a molecular diagnosis is obtained for ~85% of the patients [34]. In our cohort of 54 patients, referred to our diagnostic service since 2008, mutations were detected in 45 patients (83%). *FANCA* mutations were found in 31 of the patients (57%), *FANCC* mutations in 6 patients (11%), and *FANCG* mutations in 5 patients (9%). *FANCB, FANCE,* and *FANCF* mutations were found in single families (Table 3). In the small group of patients without mutations no complementation analysis or FANCD2 western blotting was performed. Therefore, we do not know if we missed *FANCA, -C, -E, -F, -G, and -B* mutations in these patients or that these patients have mutations in other FA genes. Table 3 does not include prenatal cases, because prenatal testing is only offered in couples in which the FA-causing mutations are already established. Testing was offered as a diagnostic service for which a fee was charged.

For the patients negative for *FANCA, -C, -E, -F, -G, and -B* mutations, next generation sequencing can be used to analyze all other FA genes. If this technique is not available, further analysis will depend on the availability of growing cells from the proband. In that case a western blot should

reveal whether both FANCD2 isoforms are present at normal levels.

(1) If both FANCD2 bands are absent or very weak, *FANCD2* is sequenced. Because of the presence of *FANCD2* pseudogene sequences in the genome, this testing must be performed on cDNA or gDNA using specially designed primers [26].

(2) If only the short isoform of FANCD2 is present, *FANCL* and *FANCM* are sequenced. If no mutations are found, the patient may be mutated in *FANCI* or in another unidentified FA gene acting upstream of FANCD2.

(3) If both isoforms are present, and if the clinical phenotype is compatible with FA-D1 or FA-N, *BRCA2/FANCD1* and *PALB2/FANCN* are screened by MLPA and DNA sequencing.

(4) If negative, *BRIP1/FANCJ, PALB2/FANCN, RAD51C/FANCO,* and *SLX4/FANCP* are sequenced.

(5) If negative again, the patient should be screened for mutations in *NBS1, ESCO2* and *DDX11* to test for Nijmegen breakage syndrome, Roberts syndrome and Warsaw Breakage syndrome, respectively [47, 48]. The latter two syndromes can also be

excluded by analyzing metaphase spreads for sister chromatid cohesion defects. If again negative, the patient is likely to be mutated in a novel FA gene acting downstream of FANCD2 ubiquitination.

3. Notes

3.1. Mutation Screening in Mosaic Patients. If an available lymphoblastoid cell line from an FA patient is phenotypically normal due to genetic reversion at the disease locus, mutation screening is still possible in the reverted cell line, since at least one mutation will be present [49–51]. The second mutation may be identified through investigating the parents.

3.2. Unclassified Variants. Missense mutations or *in-frame* deletions or insertions should be judged using *in silico* prediction algorithms (SIFT, POLYPHEN2, Align GVGD). Alternatively, they can be tested for pathogenicity in a cellular transfection assay to check the ability of the variant gene product to complement the cellular FA defect in a deficient cell line (see e.g., [10, 35, 52]). Generally, these tests are only feasible in a setting where a diagnostic laboratory is equipped with a research laboratory with all necessary technology.

3.3. Functional Assignment to Genetic Subtypes. Retroviral constructs have been used to identify the FA subtype by functional complementation, as an intermediate step before a mutation screen is undertaken [36]. Although knowing the disease gene facilitates mutation screening, retroviral transduction has some drawbacks in comparison to direct mutation screening: (i) growing, MMC-sensitive cells either from a cell line or fresh blood sample are required, which are not always easy to obtain; (ii) overexpression of some FA proteins (e.g., FANCM and FANCP) may be toxic for cells; (iii) novel genetic subtypes that emerge after all known groups have been excluded and cannot be readily distinguished from false negatives, that is, transductions that for some unknown reason have failed to cause complementation; (iv) the method requires relatively advanced laboratory facilities and technology. However, functional assignment of complementation group can rapidly be provided by laboratories with capability for this type of analysis [37], which has greatly facilitated reliable genotyping for over 95% of FA patients for which viral constructs are available.

3.4. Genetic Counseling. All patients with a diagnosis of FA confirmed by mutation analysis should be referred for genetic counselling, together with their parents and siblings. Mutation testing should be performed in all sibs regardless of any clinical symptoms. A complete pedigree, including a cancer history anamnesis, should be prepared. Mutation carriers might be at increased cancer risk (see Section 3.7) whose aspect should be included in the counseling (see Section 3.7).

FA patients themselves usually have decreased fertility. Women usually have late menarche, irregular menses, and early menopause. However, pregnancies in women with FA have been described, and therefore women should be adequately informed about the risks for their offspring, which is mainly related to an increase in pregnancy-related complications [53].

Sibs of the parents of an FA patient often request carrier screening to assess their risk of getting a child with FA. If a sib appears to be carrier, this risk is still minimal because of the very low carrier frequency in the population. In the US the carrier frequency has been estimated to be about 1 in 181 [54]. The risk of a proven carrier to get a child with FA is therefore about 1 in 724. However, in small communities or in consanguineous couples this risk is much higher, and mutation screening in spouses of proven carriers may be indicated.

3.5. Prenatal Diagnosis. Prenatal diagnosis of FA is relatively straightforward after the pathogenic mutations in a given family have been identified. Fetal cells can be obtained by chorionic villus sampling (CVS) during weeks 10–12 of the pregnancy or by amniocentesis, which is performed between weeks 14 and 16. However, CVS may be preferred as the diagnosis will be known at an earlier stage. If the mutation is not known, a chromosomal breakage test on fetal material may be performed [55], but this test may be considered less reliable than screening for mutations in the fetal material. Alternatively, flow cytometric testing of MMC sensitivity in amniotic cell cultures might be an option; however this technique is only available in a limited number of specialized laboratories [56]. Occasionally, FA may be suspected by fetal ultrasound imaging and confirmed by parental carrier testing when the family is not yet known to carry a risk for FA [57].

3.6. Genotype-Phenotype Correlation. FA is considered as one disease, and the question may be raised whether all fifteen genetic subtypes equally conform to the clinical FA phenotype. Genotype-phenotype correlation studies comparing the 3 most common groups A, C, and G indicated modest phenotypic differences, which were rather correlated with the relative severity of the mutations [23]. However, bias due to the ethnic distribution of the studied population is very well possible. Other studies reported significant differences between FA-A/G versus FA-C [58]. Cases in group FA-D1 (mutated in BRCA2) and FA-N (mutated in *PALB2*) present with a distinct, relatively severe, phenotype that is characterized by the development of leukemia at very young age (median 2.2 years) and by pediatric cancers such as nephroblastoma (Wilms tumor) or medulloblastoma [40–44]. The observations that one of the pathogenic mutations in *BRCA2* in FA-D1 patients is hypomorphic and that mice with biallelic null alleles in *Brca2* are embryonic lethals suggest that the BRCA2 protein serves a function that is essential for survival.

Different mutations in the same gene may be associated with divergent phenotypes, as illustrated by the two *FANCC* mutations, c.711+4A>T and c.67delG. The former (splice-site) mutation is associated with a relatively severe phenotype in Ashkenazi Jewish people [19] although the associated phenotype was reportedly less severe in patients of Japanese ancestry [20]. The carrier frequency for this mutation in the Ashkenazi population is relatively high (1 in 87), which has led to the recommendation of carrier detection to prevent disease [59]. In the Netherlands more than 50% of FA cases are homozygous for the *FANCC* frameshift mutation c.67delG. The phenotype associated with this mutation, like other exon 1 mutations, seems relatively mild, as these patients rarely have skeletal abnormalities and show a relatively late age of onset of their marrow failure [24]. Awareness of such genetically determined phenotypic differences may help in clinical decision making, including the counselling of patients and families.

3.7. Cancer Risk in Heterozygous Mutation Carriers. An important issue is whether FA mutation carriers are at increased risk to develop cancer or other types of disease. Overall, there is no increased risk for cancer among FA heterozygotes [60, 61]. However, the situation is different in some of the less prevalent FA subtypes. The FA-D1 subtype is caused by mutations in *BRCA2* [62] which is a well-known breast and ovarian cancer predisposition gene [63]. In FA-D1 one of the mutations will be hypomorphic because biallelic "severe" mutations are supposed to be lethal [26]. Therefore, one of the parents of a FA-D1 patient will be a heterozygous carrier of a "severe" inactivating *BRCA2* mutation and may thus have an increased risk for breast cancer and other BRCA2-associated cancers. Whether the parent with the hypomorphic mutation is also at increased risk is unknown: in breast cancer families these hypomorphic mutations are considered as variants with unknown clinical significance. Two other genes involved in FA and related to breast or ovarian cancer predisposition are *PALB2/FANCN* [64, 65] and *RAD51C/FANCO* [66]. Although cancer patients have been identified with germ-line mutations in these genes, an accurate estimate of the relative cancer risk for mutation carriers is still lacking.

Another special case is represented by female *FANCB* mutation carriers, who are supposed to consist of 50% FA-like cells due to silenced expression of the wild type *FANCB* allele by the random process of X inactivation that occurs during early embryonic development. Nevertheless, in the few female *FANCB* mutation carriers studied so far, inactivation appeared strongly skewed towards the mutated allele [67]. This suggests that FA cells have a poor chance to survive next to unaffected cells in the same tissue, and these FA cells may therefore not give an increased cancer risk. However, the data are scarce at present so that no firm conclusions can be drawn regarding the cancer risk of female *FANCB* mutation carriers [60].

Conflict of Interests

The authors do not declare any conflict of interests related to this study.

Acknowledgments

The authors thank the Fanconi Anemia Research Fund, Inc., Eugene, OR, the Netherlands Organization for Health and Development, and the Dutch Cancer Society, for financial support.

References

[1] J. P. de Winter and H. Joenje, "The genetic and molecular basis of Fanconi anemia," *Mutation Research*, vol. 668, no. 1-2, pp. 11–19, 2009.

[2] F. Vaz, H. Hanenberg, B. Schuster et al., "Mutation of the RAD51C gene in a Fanconi anemia-like disorder," *Nature Genetics*, vol. 42, no. 5, pp. 406–409, 2010.

[3] C. Stoepker, K. Hain, B. Schuster et al., "SLX4, a coordinator of structure-specific endonucleases, is mutated in a new Fanconi anemia subtype," *Nature Genetics*, vol. 43, no. 2, pp. 138–141, 2011.

[4] Y. Kim, F. P. Lach, R. Desetty, H. Hanenberg, A. D. Auerbach, and A. Smogorzewska, "Mutations of the SLX4 gene in Fanconi anemia," *Nature Genetics*, vol. 43, no. 2, pp. 142–146, 2011.

[5] M. Levitus, H. Joenje, and J. P. de Winter, "The Fanconi anemia pathway of genomic maintenance," *Cellular Oncology*, vol. 28, no. 1-2, pp. 3–29, 2006.

[6] A. J. Deans and S. C. West, "DNA interstrand crosslink repair and cancer," *Nature Reviews Cancer*, vol. 11, no. 7, pp. 467–480, 2011.

[7] A. R. Meetei, J. P. de Winter, A. L. Medhurst et al., "A novel ubiquitin ligase is deficient in Fanconi anemia," *Nature Genetics*, vol. 35, no. 2, pp. 165–170, 2003.

[8] E. Blom, "Evolutionary clues to the molecular function of Fanconi anemia genes," in *Thesis*, VU University Medical Center, Amsterdam, The Netherlands, 2006.

[9] S. C. West, "Molecular views of recombination proteins and their control," *Nature Reviews Molecular Cell Biology*, vol. 4, no. 6, pp. 435–445, 2003.

[10] E. Blom, H. J. van de Vrugt, Y. de Vries, J. P. de Winter, F. Arwert, and H. Joenje, "Multiple TPR motifs characterize the Fanconi anemia FANCG protein," *DNA Repair*, vol. 3, no. 1, pp. 77–84, 2004.

[11] M. Levitus, Q. Waisfisz, B. C. Godthelp et al., "The DNA helicase BRIP1 is defective in Fanconi anemia complementation group J," *Nature Genetics*, vol. 37, no. 9, pp. 934–935, 2005.

[12] O. Levran, C. Attwooll, R. T. Henry et al., "The BRCA1-interacting helicase BRIP1 is deficient in Fanconi anemia," *Nature Genetics*, vol. 37, no. 9, pp. 931–933, 2005.

[13] A. R. Meetei, A. L. Medhurst, C. Ling et al., "A human ortholog of archaeal DNA repair protein Hef is defective in Fanconi anemia complementation group M," *Nature Genetics*, vol. 37, no. 9, pp. 958–963, 2005.

[14] O. Levran, T. Erlich, N. Magdalena et al., "Sequence variation in the Fanconi anemia gene FAA," *Proceedings of the National Academy of Sciences of the United States of America*, vol. 94, no. 24, pp. 13051–13056, 1997.

[15] N. Magdalena, D. V. Pilonetto, M. A. Bitencourt et al., "Frequency of Fanconi anemia in Brazil and efficacy of screening for the FANCA 3788-3790del mutation," *Brazilian Journal of Medical and Biological Research*, vol. 38, no. 5, pp. 669–673, 2005.

[16] O. Levran, R. Diotti, K. Pujara, S. D. Batish, H. Hanenberg, and A. D. Auerbach, "Spectrum of sequence variations in the FANCA gene: an International Fanconi Anemia Registry (IFAR) study," *Human Mutation*, vol. 25, no. 2, pp. 142–149, 2005.

[17] A. J. Tipping, T. Pearson, N. V. Morgan et al., "Molecular and genealogical evidence for a founder effect in Fanconi

anemia families of the Afrikaner population of South Africa," *Proceedings of the National Academy of Sciences of the United States of America*, vol. 98, no. 10, pp. 5734–5739, 2001.

[18] E. Callen, J. A. Casado, M. D. Tischkowitz et al., "A common founder mutation in FANCA underlies the world's highest prevalence of Fanconi anemia in Gypsy families from Spain," *Blood*, vol. 105, no. 5, pp. 1946–1949, 2005.

[19] A. P. Gillio, P. C. Verlander, S. D. Batish, P. F. Giampietro, and A. D. Auerbach, "Phenotypic consequences of mutations in the Fanconi anemia FAC gene: an international Fanconi anemia registry study," *Blood*, vol. 90, no. 1, pp. 105–110, 1997.

[20] M. Futaki, T. Yamashita, H. Yagasaki et al., "The IVS4 + 4A to T mutation of the Fanconi anemia gene FANCC is not associated with a severe phenotype in Japanese patients," *Blood*, vol. 95, no. 4, pp. 1493–1498, 2000.

[21] M. A. Whitney, H. Saito, P. M. Jakobs, R. A. Gibson, R. E. Moses, and M. Grompe, "A common mutation in the FACC gene causes Fanconi anaemia in Ashkenazi Jews," *Nature Genetics*, vol. 4, no. 2, pp. 202–205, 1993.

[22] D. Kutler and A. Auerbach, "Fanconi anemia in Ashkenazi Jews," *Familial Cancer*, vol. 3, no. 3-4, pp. 241–248, 2004.

[23] L. Faivre, P. Guardiola, C. Lewis et al., "Association of complementation group and mutation type with clinical outcome in Fanconi anemia," *Blood*, vol. 96, no. 13, pp. 4064–4070, 2000.

[24] T. Yamashita, N. Wu, G. Kupfer et al., "Clinical variability of Fanconi anemia (type C) results from expression of an amino terminal truncated Fanconi anemia complementation group C polypeptide with partial activity," *Blood*, vol. 87, no. 10, pp. 4424–4432, 1996.

[25] H. Joenje, "Fanconi anaemia complementation groups in Germany and the Netherlands," *Human Genetics*, vol. 97, no. 3, pp. 280–282, 1996.

[26] R. Kalb, K. Neveling, H. Hoehn et al., "Hypomorphic mutations in the gene encoding a key Fanconi anemia protein, FANCD2, sustain a significant group of FA-D2 patients with severe phenotype," *American Journal of Human Genetics*, vol. 80, no. 5, pp. 895–910, 2007.

[27] I. Demuth, M. Wlodarski, A. J. Tipping et al., "Spectrum of mutations in the Fanconi anaemia group G gene, FANCG/XRCC9," *European Journal of Human Genetics*, vol. 8, no. 11, pp. 861–868, 2000.

[28] A. D. Auerbach, J. Greenbaum, K. Pujara et al., "Spectrum of sequence variation in the FANCG gene: an International Fanconi Anemia Registry (IFAR) study," *Human Mutation*, vol. 21, no. 2, pp. 158–168, 2003.

[29] H. Yagasaki, T. Oda, D. Adachi et al., "Two common founder mutations of the fanconi anemia group G gene FANCG/XRCC9 in the Japanese population," *Human mutation*, vol. 21, no. 5, p. 555, 2003.

[30] N. V. Morgan, F. Essop, I. Demuth et al., "A common Fanconi anemia mutation in black populations of sub-Saharan Africa," *Blood*, vol. 105, no. 9, pp. 3542–3544, 2005.

[31] J. Rosendorff and R. Bernstein, "Fanconi's anemia—chromosome breakage studies in homozygotes and heterozygotes," *Cancer Genetics and Cytogenetics*, vol. 33, no. 2, pp. 175–183, 1988.

[32] B. P. Alter, "Diagnostic evaluation of FA," in *Fanconi Anemia: Guidelines for Diagnosis and Management*, M. E. Eiler et al., Ed., pp. 33–48, Fanconi Anemia Research Fund, Eugene, Ore, USA, 2008.

[33] M. Castella, R. Pujol, E. Callen et al., "Origin, functional role, and clinical impact of Fanconi anemia FANCA mutations," *Blood*, vol. 117, no. 14, pp. 3759–3769, 2011.

[34] N. Ameziane, A. Errami, F. Léveillé et al., "Genetic subtyping of Fanconi anemia by comprehensive mutation screening," *Human Mutation*, vol. 29, no. 1, pp. 159–166, 2008.

[35] J. R. Lo Ten Foe, M. T. Barel, P. Thuß, M. Digweed, F. Arwert, and H. Joenje, "Sequence variations in the Fanconi anaemia gene, FAC: pathogenicity of 1806insA and R548X and recognition of D195V as a polymorphic variant," *Human Genetics*, vol. 98, no. 5, pp. 522–523, 1996.

[36] H. Hanenberg, S. D. Batish, K. E. Pollok et al., "Phenotypic correction of primary Fanconi anemia T cells with retroviral vectors as a diagnostic tool," *Experimental Hematology*, vol. 30, no. 5, pp. 410–420, 2002.

[37] S. Chandra, O. Levran, I. Jurickova et al., "A rapid method for retrovirus-mediated identification of complementation groups in Fanconi anemia patients," *Molecular Therapy*, vol. 12, no. 5, pp. 976–984, 2005.

[38] T. N. Kaiser, A. Lojewski, C. Dougherty, L. Juergens, E. Sahar, and S. A. Latt, "Flow cytometric characterization of the response of Fanconi's anemia cells to mitomycin C treatment," *Cytometry*, vol. 2, no. 5, pp. 291–297, 1982.

[39] F. O. Pinto, T. Leblanc, D. Chamousset et al., "Diagnosis of Fanconi anemia in patients with bone marrow failure," *Haematologica*, vol. 94, no. 4, pp. 487–495, 2009.

[40] B. Hirsch, A. Shimamura, L. Moreau et al., "Association of biallelic BRCA2/FANCD1 mutations with spontaneous chromosomal instability and solid tumors of childhood," *Blood*, vol. 103, no. 7, pp. 2554–2559, 2004.

[41] J. E. Wagner, J. Tolar, O. Levran et al., "Germline mutations in BRCA2: shared genetic susceptibility to breast cancer, early onset leukemia, and Fanconi anemia," *Blood*, vol. 103, no. 8, pp. 3226–3229, 2004.

[42] K. Offit, O. Levran, B. Mullaney et al., "Shared genetic susceptibility to breast cancer, brain tumors, and Fanconi anemia," *Journal of the National Cancer Institute*, vol. 95, no. 20, pp. 1548–1551, 2003.

[43] S. Reid, D. Schindler, H. Hanenberg et al., "Biallelic mutations in PALB2 cause Fanconi anemia subtype FA-N and predispose to childhood cancer," *Nature Genetics*, vol. 39, no. 2, pp. 162–164, 2007.

[44] B. Xia, J. C. Dorsman, N. Ameziane et al., "Fanconi anemia is associated with a defect in the BRCA2 partner PALB2," *Nature Genetics*, vol. 39, no. 2, pp. 159–161, 2007.

[45] K. Somyajit, S. Subramanya, and G. Nagaraju, "RAD51C: a novel cancer susceptibility gene is linked to Fanconi anemia and breast cancer," *Carcinogenesis*, vol. 31, no. 12, pp. 2031–2038, 2010.

[46] J. P. Schouten, C. J. McElgunn, R. Waaijer, D. Zwijnenburg, F. Diepvens, and G. Pals, "Relative quantification of 40 nucleic acid sequences by multiplex ligation-dependent probe amplification," *Nucleic acids research*, vol. 30, no. 12, p. e57, 2002.

[47] A. R. Gennery, M. A. Slatter, A. Bhattacharya et al., "The clinical and biological overlap between Nijmegen Breakage syndrome and Fanconi anemia," *Clinical Immunology*, vol. 113, no. 2, pp. 214–219, 2004.

[48] P. van der Lelij, A. B. Oostra, M. A. Rooimans, H. Joenje, and J. P. de Winter, "Diagnostic overlap between Fanconi anemia and the cohesinopathies: roberts syndrome and Warsaw Breakage syndrome," *Anemia*, vol. 2010, Article ID 565268, 7 pages, 2010.

[49] J. R. Lo Ten Foe, M. L. Kwee, M. A. Rooimans et al., "Somatic mosaicism in Fanconi anemia: molecular basis and clinical significance," *European Journal of Human Genetics*, vol. 5, no. 3, pp. 137–148, 1997.

Diagnosis of Fanconi Anemia: Mutation Analysis by Multiplex Ligation-Dependent Probe Amplification...

75

[50] Q. Waisfisz, N. V. Morgan, M. Savino et al., "Spontaneous functional correction of homozygous Fanconi anaemia alleles reveals novel mechanistic basis for reverse mosaicism," *Nature Genetics*, vol. 22, no. 4, pp. 379–383, 1999.

[51] B. P. Alter, H. Joenje, A. B. Oostra, and G. Pals, "Fanconi anemia: adult head and neck cancer and hematopoietic mosaicism," *Archives of Otolaryngology*, vol. 131, no. 7, pp. 635–639, 2005.

[52] A. L. Medhurst, E. H. Laghmani, J. Steltenpool et al., "Evidence for subcomplexes in the Fanconi anemia pathway," *Blood*, vol. 108, no. 6, pp. 2072–2080, 2006.

[53] B. P. Alter, C. L. Frissora, D. S. Halperin et al., "Fanconi's anaemia and pregnancy," *British Journal of Haematology*, vol. 77, no. 3, pp. 410–418, 1991.

[54] P. S. Rosenberg, H. Tamary, and B. P. Alter, "How high are carrier frequencies of rare recessive syndromes? Contemporary estimates for Fanconi anemia in the United States and Israel," *American Journal of Medical Genetics A*, vol. 155, no. 8, pp. 1877–1883, 2011.

[55] A. D. Auerbach, "Fanconi anemia," in *Diagnosis and Treatment of the Unborn Child*, M. I. New, Ed., pp. 27–35, Idelson-Gnocchi, Naples, Italy, 1999.

[56] A. Bechtold, R. Kalb, K. Neveling et al., "Prenatal diagnosis of Fanconi anemia: functional and molecular testing," in *Fanconi Anemia. A Paradigmatic Disease for the Understanding of Cancer and Aging*, D. Schindler and H. Hoehn, Eds., Monographs in Human Genetics, pp. 131–148, Karger, Basel, Switzerland, 2007.

[57] A. Merrill, L. Rosenblum-Vos, D. A. Driscoll, K. Daley, and K. Treat, "Prenatal diagnosis of Fanconi anemia (Group C) subsequent to abnormal sonographic findings," *Prenatal Diagnosis*, vol. 25, no. 1, pp. 20–22, 2005.

[58] D. I. Kutler, B. Singh, J. Satagopan et al., "A 20-year perspective on the International Fanconi Anemia Registry (IFAR)," *Blood*, vol. 101, no. 4, pp. 1249–1256, 2003.

[59] P. C. Verlander, A. Kaporis, Q. Liu, Q. Zhang, U. Seligsohn, and A. D. Auerbach, "Carrier frequency of the IVS4 + 4 A—> T mutation of the Fanconi anemia gene FAC in the Ashkenazi Jewish population," *Blood*, vol. 86, no. 11, pp. 4034–4038, 1995.

[60] M. Berwick, J. M. Satagopan, L. Ben-Porat et al., "Genetic heterogeneity among Fanconi anemia heterozygotes and risk of cancer," *Cancer Research*, vol. 67, no. 19, pp. 9591–9596, 2007.

[61] M. Tischkowitz, D. F. Easton, J. Ball, S. V. Hodgson, and C. G. Mathew, "Cancer incidence in relatives of British Fanconi anaemia patients," *BMC Cancer*, vol. 8, article 257, 2008.

[62] N. G. Howlett, T. Taniguchi, S. Olson et al., "Biallelic inactivation of BRCA2 in Fanconi anemia," *Science*, vol. 297, no. 5581, pp. 606–609, 2002.

[63] E. Levy-Lahad and E. Friedman, "Cancer risks among BRCA1 and BRCA2 mutation carriers," *British Journal of Cancer*, vol. 96, no. 1, pp. 11–15, 2007.

[64] N. Rahman, S. Seal, D. Thompson et al., "PALB2, which encodes a BRCA2-interacting protein, is a breast cancer susceptibility gene," *Nature Genetics*, vol. 39, no. 2, pp. 165–167, 2007.

[65] M. J. Garcia, V. Fernandez, A. Osorio et al., "Analysis of FANCB and FANCN/PALB2 Fanconi anemia genes in BRCA1/2-negative Spanish breast cancer families," *Breast Cancer Research and Treatment*, vol. 113, no. 3, pp. 545–551, 2009.

[66] A. Meindl, H. Hellebrand, C. Wiek et al., "Germline mutations in breast and ovarian cancer pedigrees establish RAD51C as a human cancer susceptibility gene," *Nature Genetics*, vol. 42, no. 5, pp. 410–414, 2010.

[67] A. R. Meetei, M. Levitus, Y. Xue et al., "X-linked inheritance of Fanconi anemia complementation group B," *Nature Genetics*, vol. 36, no. 11, pp. 1219–1224, 2004.

10

A DOG's View of Fanconi Anemia: Insights from *C. elegans*

Martin Jones and Ann Rose

Department of Medical Genetics, University of British Columbia, Vancouver, BC, Canada V6T 1Z4

Correspondence should be addressed to Ann Rose, annroseubc@gmail.com

Academic Editor: Laura Hays

C. elegans provides an excellent model system for the study of the Fanconi Anemia (FA), one of the hallmarks of which is sensitivity to interstrand crosslinking agents. Central to our understanding of FA has been the investigation of DOG-1, the functional ortholog of the deadbox helicase *FANCJ*. Here we review the current understanding of the unique role of DOG-1 in maintaining stability of G-rich DNA in *C. elegans* and explore the question of why DOG-1 animals are crosslink sensitive. We propose a dynamic model in which noncovalently linked G-rich structures form and un-form in the presence of DOG-1. When DOG-1 is absent but crosslinking agents are present the G-rich structures are readily covalently crosslinked, resulting in increased crosslinks formation and thus giving increased crosslink sensitivity. In this interpretation DOG-1 is neither upstream nor downstream in the FA pathway, but works alongside it to limit the availability of crosslink substrates. This model reconciles the crosslink sensitivity observed in the absence of DOG-1 function with its unique role in maintaining G-Rich DNA and will help to formulate experiments to test this hypothesis.

1. Introduction

The helicase, FANCJ, is required for the Fanconi Anemia (FA) pathway to function properly and thus maintain genome integrity. In humans, *FANCJ* mutations have been identified in early-onset breast cancer patients [1, 2] and FA complementation group J patients [3–5]. However, the role of FANCJ in the FA pathway of DNA repair is not fully understood. Some insights have been gained from research on DOG-1 (Deletions Of G-rich DNA), the *Caenorhabditis elegans* functional ortholog of FANCJ [6–9]. However, even in this relatively simple model system, important questions remain. An outstanding issue is the relationship between the relatively well-known function of DOG-1/FANCJ in preventing replication blocks at unresolved secondary structures and its function in resistance to interstrand crosslinks (ICLs). Previous work from our group has shown that DOG-1 acts upstream of, or parallel to, FCD-2 in the maintenance of G-tracts [7] but is dispensable for FCD-2 focus formation in response to ICL generating agents [8]. One possibility is that DOG-1 takes on two different functions, one in G4 DNA resolution and one in FA crosslink repair. On the other hand, it is possible that its ability to unwind G-rich secondary structure may be sufficient to explain its role in both situations.

Here we summarize the current understanding of DOG-1/FANCJ function and hypothesize how to reconcile the two known roles for this protein with its helicase function.

2. DOG-1 Is Required for Maintenance of G-Tracts

DOG-1 was discovered as being essential for the maintenance of G-rich DNA [6] and was subsequently shown to be the functional ortholog of FANCJ [8]. The value of *C. elegans* as a model for Fanconi Anemia and ICL repair has been thoroughly reviewed in Youds et al. [9]. An understanding of DOG-1's role in replication and repair began with the observation that it is a mutator. This was immediately recognizable in *C. elegans* because of the appearance of spontaneous morphological mutants (described in Cheung et al. [6]) and further explored by the capture and characterization of mutational changes in genes essential for survival (lethal mutations) maintained using a genetic balancer [10]. In *dog-1* mutants, the manifestation of the morphological *Vab* (Variable ABnormal) phenotype was linked to the gene *vab-1*. An examination of the molecular nature of the *vab-1* mutations revealed small deletions that were detectable by PCR. These deletions initiated at the 5′ end of poly-C or

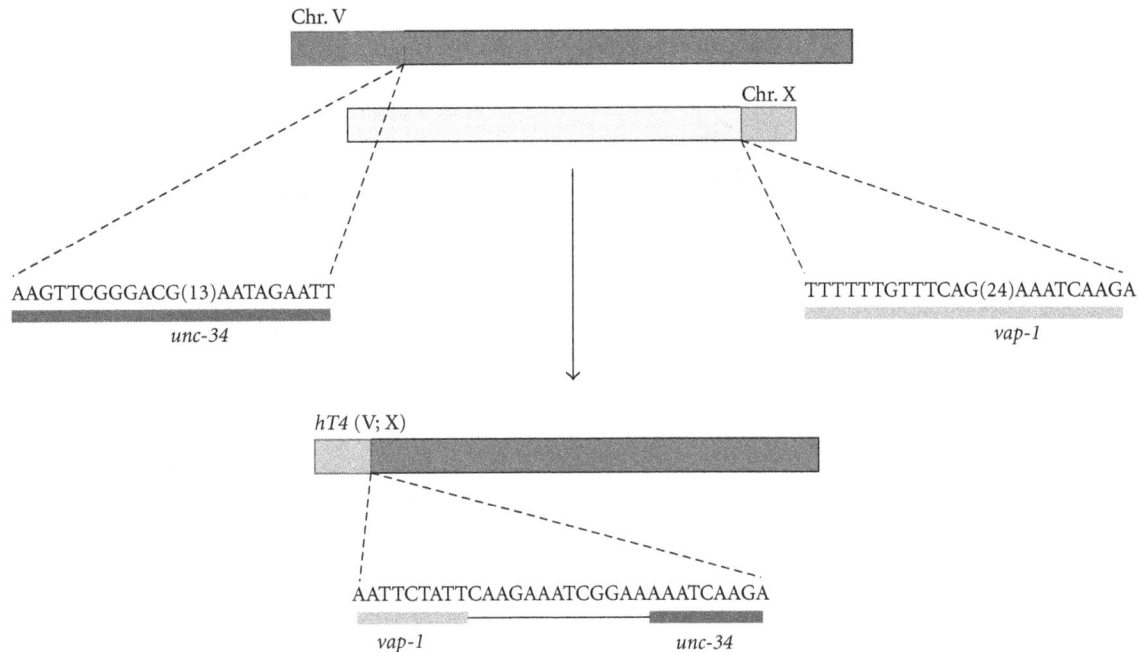

FIGURE 1: Schematic of the *dog-1*-derived translocation, *hT4* (V; X). Sequences near the left end of chromosome V were deleted (red box), whereas the right end of chromosome X was duplicated (blue box). PCR primers were designed and used to determine the DNA sequence across the junction of V and X in *hT4* (described in [10]).

the 3′ end of poly-G stretches of DNA and extended for variable distances. These observations led to the proposal that the deletions were occurring as a result of structural blocks to lagging-strand synthesis [6]. In this model, poly-G stretches present in the *C. elegans* genome form secondary structures. These secondary structures require the helicase function of DOG-1 to resolve them, allowing fork progression. In the absence of the helicase function, deletions are formed between the stalled fork and the upstream Okazaki fragment initiation. Another research group subsequently confirmed the prediction that Okazaki-sized deletions occurred on the lagging strand by using unbiased array comparative hybridization (aCGH) of DOG-1-minus genomes [11]. In this study, it was shown that deletions occurred exclusively at sequences that could form quadruplex structures (G4) at a frequency of 4% per site per animal generation. In the human genome, there are estimated to be >300,000 G4 forming sites [12], and these have potentially mutagenic properties implicated in development of cancer susceptibility in the absence of FANCJ function.

Further work from our laboratory revealed that in the absence of DOG-1 large chromosomal rearrangements occurred [10]. The rearrangements included larger deletions, duplications of chromosomal fragments, and translocations between chromosomes, in addition to the small deletions detectable by PCR. These large rearrangements were identified because they acquired lethal mutations, which could be isolated and characterized with the use of a balancer chromosome that provided a rescuing wild-type allele in a stable genetic construct (reviewed in [13]). The analysis showed that 1% of the chromosomes acquired lethal lesions [10], giving a forward mutation frequency greater than tenfold of

the spontaneous frequency. The frequency is equivalent to that for 500 Rads of ionizing radiation [14]. Rearrangements derived from *dog-1* mutant that were examined by aCGH revealed that in most (but not all) cases the breakpoints occurred in G-rich DNA. In one example, a translocation between chromosome V and the X-chromosome was formed. In this case, the right end of the X-chromosome was duplicated and attached to the left breakpoint of a deletion at left end of chromosome V (Figure 1). The breakpoint on chromosome V is in a 24 bp G/C tract, while the breakpoint on the X is in a "short" 13 bp G-rich sequence. In vertebrates, large rearrangements have also been observed in the absence of FANCJ function. In avian DT40 cell lines, large-scale genomic deletions occurred at the rearranged immunoglobulin heavy chain locus (IgH) in the absence of *FANCJ*, but not other FA genes [15]. These researchers found that in *FANCJ* mutant cells cultured for two months, G4 sequences detected by aCGH were found at the breakpoints of one deletion. However, not all breaks occurred in G-rich DNA, suggesting that other sequences are also susceptible to breakage in the absence of FANCJ.

3. Homologous Recombination and Translesion Synthesis Compensate for the Absence of DOG-1

Repair pathways that compensate for the absence of DOG-1 in *C. elegans* have been identified. These include homologous recombination (HR) repair and translesion synthesis (TLS), but not nonhomologous end joining (NHEJ) [7]. In human cell lines, monoubiquitylation of FANCD2 is followed by HR repair. Our genetic analysis has shown that DOG-1 mutants

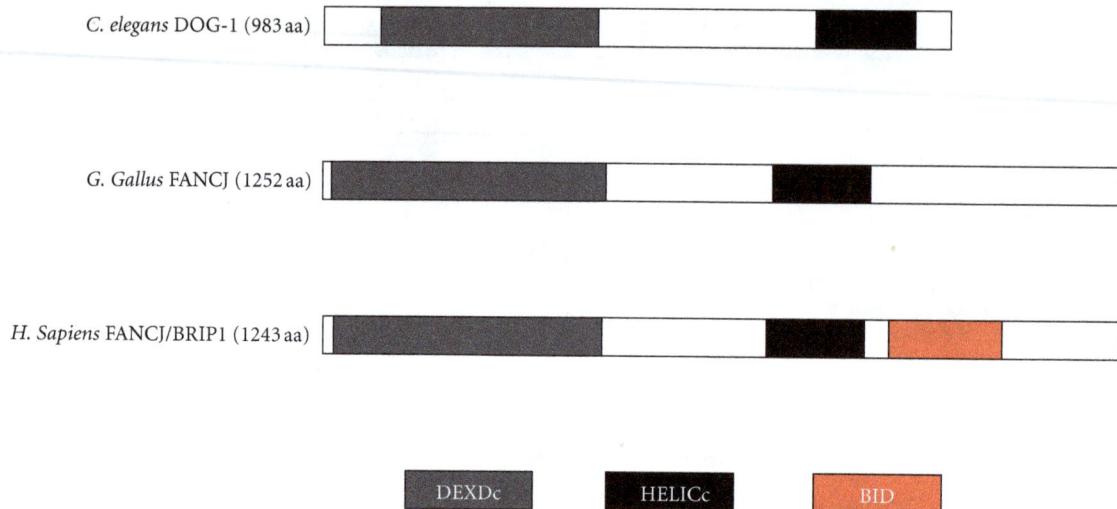

FIGURE 2: Protein schematic of FANCJ orthologs. *C. elegans* DOG-1, 983 aa, chicken FANCJ, 1252 aa and human, 1243 aa FANCJ proteins illustrating the position of the conserved DEAD Box (DEXDc) and helicase (HELICc) domains. The BRCA-1 interaction domain of human FANCJ is illustrated (BID). A full protein sequence alignment of DOG-1 and human FANCJ is shown in [8].

that are also mutant for FCD-2 (FANCD2) exacerbate G-tract deletions [8], as are the HR repair components, BRD-1 (BARD1), RAD-51 (RAD51), and XPF-1 (XPF). Similarly, DOG-1 mutants lacking the TLS polymerases, POL eta and POL kappa have significantly more PCR-detectable G-tract deletions than DOG-1 by itself. That the FA pathway and its downstream repair mechanisms are capable of resolving some G-tract-associated secondary structures in the absence of DOG-1 function indicates that the FA pathway is parallel to DOG-1, at least with respect to the maintenance of G-tracts.

A recent study in DT40 cells has expanded the endogenous role of FANCJ. Recently, Sarkies et al. have shown that FANCJ coordinates two independent mechanisms to maintain epigenetic stability near G4 DNA motifs [16]. These mechanisms are dependent on the function of the Y-family polymerase REV1 and the helicases WRNs and BLMs. Similar epigenetic studies have not been performed in *C. elegans*. However, G-tract instability is significantly increased in DOG-1 mutants animals deficient in the BLM ortholog HIM-6 [7]. Mutants in the *C. elegans* WRNs ortholog WRN-1 do not exacerbate G-tract deletions, indicting that if a function in G-tract resolution is conserved in *C. elegans*, it is dependent on the presence of DOG-1. The *C. elegans* REV1 ortholog REV-1 has not been studied with respect to G-tract stability.

4. DOG-1 Functions to Reduce ICL-Induced Damage

A diagnostic feature of FA defects is the cross-link sensitivity of cultured cells. The presence of ICLs can result in error-prone repair leading to chromosomal instability (CIN) and cell death. In *C. elegans*, the absence of DOG-1 also results in sensitivity to ICL-inducing agents such as UVA-activated trimethylpsoralen, nitrogen mustard, and cisplatin, but not

to X-rays or UVC [8]. Treatment of DOG-1-deficient animals with ICL agents can result in checkpoint-induced cell cycle arrest and apoptosis of germ cells, as well as chromatin bridges and breaks [8]. In response to ICL treatments, animal's doubly mutant for DOG-1 and FCD-2 are as equally sensitive as each of the single mutants, potentially placing the helicase function of DOG-1 in the same pathway as FCD-2 [8]. Furthermore, DOG-1 is not required for RAD-51 or FCD-2 foci formation after replication stress or ICL induction, possibly placing DOG-1 downstream of FCD-2. This data correlates with that reported by Bridge et al. [17] who demonstrated that *FANCJ* mutant DT40 cells are also not defective for FANCD2 focus formation.

In human cell lines, monoubiquitinlation of FANCD2 is followed by HR repair. During S phase, ICLs can block replication; consequently, HR and TLS are required to stabilize the fork and restart replication (reviewed in [18]). In *C. elegans*, HR repair alleviates the loss of DOG-1. DOG-1 does not function directly in DSB repair, however, as it is not sensitive to radiation-induced DSBs [8]. Bridge et al. determined that FANCJs role in ICL repair is independent of BRCA1 function by demonstrating rescue of *FANCJ* phenotypes in DT40 cells with the expression of human FANCJ/BRIP1 lacking its BRCA1-interaction domain [17]. Since DOG-1, like the avian FANCJ, does not contain the BRCA-1 interaction domain found in human FANCJ (Figure 2), we infer that the helicase function of DOG-1 is not required for HR-mediated DSB repair following replication block or ICL induction.

The type of repair pathway recruited following replication block is important in maintaining genome stability. In *C. elegans* [8] and in human and chicken cells [19], FA proteins regulate the decision to repair double strand breaks (DSBs) resulting from replication blocks or ICLs using error-free HR repair rather than error-prone nonhomologous end joining (NHEJ). In the Adamo et al. study [20], it was shown that FA-deficient human cell lines and *C. elegans* mutants had chromosomal abnormalities similar to those found in cell lines from cancer and FA patients. However, when the NHEJ component LIG-4 (LIG4) is lacking, the abnormalities do not occur. HR-mediated repair is proposed to be favored due to single-stranded DNA produced by FANCD2 [19]. In *C. elegans*, this result provides a potential inroad to further dissection of the role of FA in DNA repair and the maintenance of genome stability.

The relationship between TLS and HR repair in *C. elegans* has been teased apart somewhat by the characterization of two genes, *polq-1* (*POLQ*) and *hel-308* (*HELQ*) [21]. POLQ-1 has a helicase domain at the N-terminus and a polymerase domain at the C-terminus and has been implicated in recombination-independent and TLS-dependent ICL repair (reviewed in [22]). The helicase HEL-308, on the other hand, is proposed to function in HR along with the FA pathway in ICL repair. In *C. elegans*, there are two genetically distinct pathways, a BRC-1-POLQ-1 pathway and an FA (FCD-2, DOG-1)-HR-HEL-308 pathway. At least one of these pathways must be functional for animals survival as mutants in *hel-308* results in synthetic lethality when combined with *brc-1* mutants (reviewed in [9]). These results separate the helicase function of DOG-1 from the BRC-1/BRCA-1 repair pathway and further distinguish the role of DOG-1 as independent of HR repair. Initially these results may appear paradoxical. FCD-2 is not required for G-tract stability and the double mutant *dog-1*; *fcd-2* increased G-tract deletions 3-fold [8], placing DOG-1 upstream of the FA pathway. However, in the case of ICL sensitivity, the double mutant is not more sensitive. One interpretation of these data is that DOG-1 is epistatic to the FA pathway. Both findings are consistent with DOG-1 attempting unsuccessfully to remove the cross-linked structure.

How does this inform our understanding of DOG-1's helicase function and the relationship between G-rich secondary structures and ICLs? There is ample evidence that DOG-1 is unique in its role to maintain G-rich DNA that can form G4-like secondary structures [7, 8, 11]. Additionally, it has been demonstrated that purified FANCJ efficiently unwinds a variety of G4 structures dependent upon intrinsic FANCJ ATP hydrolysis and the availability of a 5′ ssDNA tail [22]. None of the other helicases that are able to unwind G4 structures can compensate for the loss of DOG-1. This is supported by the fact that in *C. elegans* DOG-1 has a unique phenotype and that in other systems only FANCJ has been shown to prevent breaks in G-rich DNA. These structures are, however, not covalently linked. There is no evidence that the DOG-1/FANCJ helicase can resolve covalently linked ICLs. So what is the connection?

We propose the following model as a resolution of this apparent paradox (Figure 3). G4 structures are known to form in a variety of circumstances as proposed by Wu et al. [22], which could include within a single strand of DNA, between DNA strands and between strands on separate chromosomes. The latter resulting in chromosomal translocations if not repaired correctly. In the absence of crosslinking agents, these secondary structures can form and unform depending upon the availability of DOG-1. In the *C. elegans* genome, there are nearly 400 poly-G regions distributed

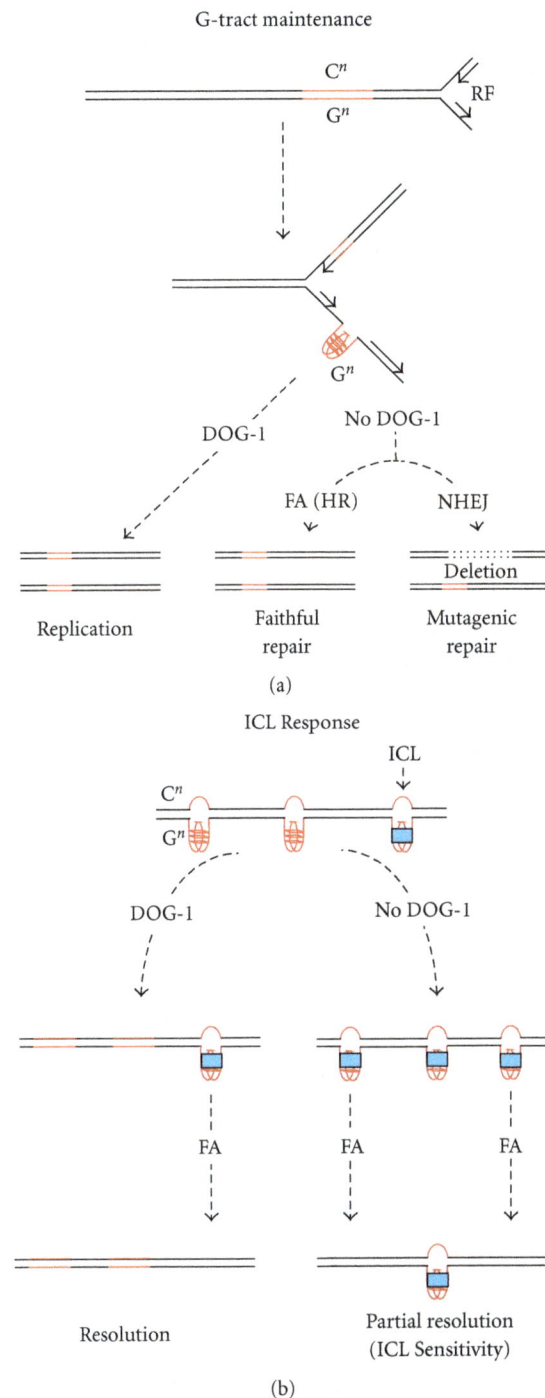

FIGURE 3: A model for DOG-1 function in genome stability and ICL response. The left panel illustrates DOG-1's role in G-tract maintenance. G4 formation on the lagging strand is resolved by the helicase function of DOG-1 and replication proceeds efficiently. In the absence of DOG-1 HR mediated by the FA pathway resolves a subset of stalled forks. Repair utilizing the mutagenic NHEJ repair mechanism results in deletions. The right panel describes a possible model for DOG-1 ICL sensitivity. In the presence of DOG-1, G4 structures may be resolved and not available as substrate for ICL stabilization. In the absence of DOG-1 G4 structures are available as substrate for ICL stabilization leading to an in increase in fork stalling, which is interpreted as an ICL sensitivity phenotype.

along each of the chromosomes and this pattern of distribution is conserved in a related nematode [23] providing a rich source of substrate for DOG-1. In the presence of a crosslinking agent, many of which have affinity for G's, secondary structures formed by these G-rich regions might be targets for covalent crosslinking. Here we suggest that once the secondary structures are detected by FA pathway components the first responder is DOG-1. The pathway detector may not distinguish between a noncovalent secondary structure and a crosslink. If the structure is not covalently linked, DOG-1 resolves it. If it is covalently linked, and not resolved by DOG-1, FA pathway-directed TLS and HR repair the lesion. In the absence of DOG-1, there is likely to be an increase in stabilized G-rich structures that may be beyond the ability of the FA pathway to respond to, giving the appearance of a crosslink sensitive phenotype. Further experiments will be needed to move towards a more complete understanding of the crosstalk among FA proteins.

Acknowledgments

The authors wish to thank Dr. David Baillie for inspiring conversations. Research has been funded by a CIHR grant to A. Rose and a CIHR Fanconi Anemia Canada Fellowship to M. Jones.

References

[1] S. B. Cantor, D. W. Bell, S. Ganesan et al., "BACH1, a novel helicase-like protein, interacts directly with BRCA1 and contributes to its DNA repair function," *Cell*, vol. 105, no. 1, pp. 149–160, 2001.

[2] S. Seal, D. Thompson, A. Renwick et al., "Truncating mutations in the Fanconi anemia J gene BRIP1 are low-penetrance breast cancer susceptibility alleles," *Nature Genetics*, vol. 38, no. 11, pp. 1239–1241, 2006.

[3] M. Levitus, Q. Waisfisz, B. C. Godthelp et al., "The DNA helicase BRIP1 is defective in Fanconi anemia complementation group J," *Nature Genetics*, vol. 37, no. 9, pp. 934–935, 2005.

[4] O. Levran, C. Attwooll, R. T. Henry et al., "The BRCA1-interacting helicase BRIP1 is deficient in Fanconi anemia," *Nature Genetics*, vol. 37, no. 9, pp. 931–933, 2005.

[5] R. Litman, M. Peng, Z. Jin et al., "BACH1 is critical for homologous recombination and appears to be the Fanconi anemia gene product FANCJ," *Cancer Cell*, vol. 8, no. 3, pp. 255–265, 2005.

[6] I. Cheung, M. Schertzer, A. Rose, and P. M. Lansdorp, "Disruption of dog-1 in *Caenorhabditis elegans* triggers deletions upstream of guanine-rich DNA," *Nature Genetics*, vol. 31, no. 4, pp. 405–409, 2002.

[7] J. L. Youds, N. J. O'Neil, and A. M. Rose, "Homologous recombination is required for genome stability in the absence of DOG-1 in *Caenorhabditis elegans*," *Genetics*, vol. 173, no. 2, pp. 697–708, 2006.

[8] J. L. Youds, L. J. Barber, J. D. Ward et al., "DOG-1 is the *Caenorhabditis elegans* BRIP1/FANCJ homologue and functions in interstrand cross-link repair," *Molecular and Cellular Biology*, vol. 28, no. 5, pp. 1470–1479, 2008.

[9] J. L. Youds, L. J. Barber, and S. J. Boulton, "*C. elegans*: a model of Fanconi anemia and ICL repair," *Mutation Research*, vol. 668, no. 1-2, pp. 103–116, 2009.

[10] Y. Zhao, M. Tarailo-Graovac, N. J. O'Neil, and A. M. Rose, "Spectrum of mutational events in the absence of DOG-1/FANCJ in *Caenorhabditis elegans*," *DNA Repair*, vol. 7, no. 11, pp. 1846–1854, 2008.

[11] E. Kruisselbrink, V. Guryev, K. Brouwer, D. B. Pontier, E. Cuppen, and M. Tijsterman, "Mutagenic capacity of endogenous G4 DNA underlies genome instability in FANCJ-defective *C. elegans*," *Current Biology*, vol. 18, no. 12, pp. 900–905, 2008.

[12] J. Eddy and N. Maizels, "Selection for the G4 DNA Motif at the 5' end of human genes," *Molecular Carcinogenesis*, vol. 48, no. 4, pp. 319–325, 2009.

[13] M. R. Jones, Z. Lohn, and A. M. Rose, "Specialized chromosomes and their uses in *Caenorhabditis elegans*," *Methods in Cell Biology*, vol. 106, pp. 23–64, 2011.

[14] R. E. Rosenbluth, C. Cuddeford, and D. L. Baillie, "Mutagenesis in *Caenorhabditis elegans*. II. A spectrum of mutational events induced with 1500 r of gamma-radiation," *Genetics*, vol. 109, no. 3, pp. 493–511, 1985.

[15] H. Kitao, S. Hirano, and M. Takata, "Evaluation of homologous recombinational repair in chicken B lymphoma cell line, DT40," *Methods in Cell Biology*, vol. 745, pp. 293–309, 2011.

[16] P. Sarkies et al., "FANCJ coordinates two pathways that maintain epigenetic stability at G-quadruplex DNA," *Nucleic Acids Research*, vol. 40, no. 4, pp. 1485–1498, 2012.

[17] W. L. Bridge, C. J. Vandenberg, R. J. Franklin, and K. Hiom, "The BRIP1 helicase functions independently of BRCA1 in the Fanconi anemia pathway for DNA crosslink repair," *Nature Genetics*, vol. 37, no. 9, pp. 953–957, 2005.

[18] A. J. Deans and S. C. West, "DNA interstrand crosslink repair and cancer," *Nature Reviews Cancer*, vol. 11, no. 7, pp. 467–480, 2011.

[19] P. Pace, G. Mosedale, M. R. Hodskinson, I. V. Rosado, M. Sivasubramaniam, and K. J. Patel, "Ku70 corrupts DNA repair in the absence of the fanconi anemia pathway," *Science*, vol. 329, no. 5988, pp. 219–223, 2010.

[20] A. Adamo, S. J. Collis, C. A. Adelman et al., "Preventing nonhomologous end joining suppresses DNA repair defects of fanconi anemia," *Molecular Cell*, vol. 39, no. 1, pp. 25–35, 2010.

[21] D. M. Muzzini, P. Plevani, S. J. Boulton, G. Cassata, and F. Marini, "*Caenorhabditis elegans* POLQ-1 and HEL-308 function in two distinct DNA interstrand cross-link repair pathways," *DNA Repair*, vol. 7, no. 6, pp. 941–950, 2008.

[22] Y. Wu, S. Y. Kazuo, and R. M. Brosh Jr., "FANCJ helicase defective in Fanconia anemia and breast cancer unwinds G-quadruplex DNA to defend genomic stability," *Molecular and Cellular Biology*, vol. 28, no. 12, pp. 4116–4128, 2008.

[23] Y. Zhao, N. J. O'Neil, and A. M. Rose, "Poly-G/poly-C tracts in the genomes of Caenorhabditis," *BMC Genomics*, vol. 8, article 403, 2007.

11

Assessment of Serum Zinc Levels of Patients with Thalassemia Compared to their Siblings

Mohamed El Missiry,[1] **Mohamed Hamed Hussein,**[1] **Sadaf Khalid,**[1] **Naila Yaqub,**[2]
Sarah Khan,[2] **Fatima Itrat,**[2] **Cornelio Uderzo,**[1] **and Lawrence Faulkner**[1]

[1] *Cure2Children Foundation, Via Marconi 30, 50131 Florence, Italy*
[2] *Children's Hospital Pakistan Institute of Medical Sciences, Islamabad, Pakistan*

Correspondence should be addressed to Mohamed El Missiry; mohamed.elmissiry@cure2children.org

Academic Editor: Aurelio Maggio

Zinc (Zn) is essential for appropriate growth and proper immune function, both of which may be impaired in thalassemia children. Factors that can affect serum Zn levels in these patients may be related to their disease or treatment or nutritional causes. We assessed the serum Zn levels of children with thalassemia paired with a sibling. Zn levels were obtained from 30 children in Islamabad, Pakistan. Serum Zn levels and anthropometric data measures were compared among siblings. Thalassemia patients' median age was 4.5 years (range 1–10.6 years) and siblings was 7.8 years (range 1.1–17 years). The median serum Zn levels for both groups were within normal range: 100 μg/dL (10 μg/dL–297 μg/dL) for patients and 92 μg/dL (13 μg/dL–212 μg/dL) for siblings. There was no significant difference between the two groups. Patients' serum Zn values correlated positively with their corresponding siblings (r = 0.635, P < 0.001). There were no correlations between patients' Zn levels, height for age Z-scores, serum ferritin levels, chelation, or blood counts (including both total leukocyte and absolute lymphocyte counts). Patients' serum Zn values correlated with their siblings' values. In this study, patients with thalassemia do not seem to have disease-related Zn deficiency.

1. Introduction

Zinc (Zn) is an essential element for cell growth, differentiation, and survival. It is a structural element of many proteins [1]. Zinc affects growth in children. It is known that adequate zinc levels in the body are essential for maintaining suitable levels of growth hormone and insulin-like growth factor in the body [2]. Impairment of zinc levels will consequently lead to growth hormone decrease. Zinc supplement is given to children on growth hormone replacement therapy. In addition, zinc is important for nucleic acid synthesis, cell division, and metabolism of lipids, proteins and carbohydrates. It is also essential in bone homeostasis and bone growth as well as in the maintenance of connective tissues. Decreased Zn may compromise growth and immune functions [2, 3].

Zn is known to be important for the integrity of the immune system, although its role and mechanism of action are not fully understood [1, 4–6]. Zn deficiency affects the adaptive immune system and results in thymus atrophy, lymphopenia, and impaired lymphocyte function [4, 7, 8].

Zinc deficiency is prevalent in children of developing countries where food is often vegetable-based and rarely includes animal products. Zinc is easily absorbed with animal proteins, while excess plant meals lead to decreased zinc absorption due to its binding to phytates [9, 10]. In such countries, Zn deficiency results in growth retardation, hypogonadism, and increased mortality and morbidly from infection-related diarrhea and pneumonia due to compromised immune function [4, 9].

Despite deficits of several specific micronutrients reported in children with thalassemia major, Zn studies yielded conflicting results [7, 11, 12]. Several factors contribute to zinc deficiency in thalassemia. One of these most important factors is chelation therapy. Chelators, namely, deferoxamine and deferiprone, may contribute to Zn deficiency in thalassemia as they tend to eliminate positive divalent ions, like iron and Zn, into urine [7, 13, 14]. On the other side, some studies showed no significant correlation between zinc level and short stature, serum ferritin level, desferrioxamine dose, age at first blood transfusion, and chelation therapy [7]. Zinc can be normal in some patients especially those who are on regular blood transfusions [7, 11, 12]. What is notable that these studies were performed on adequately treated patients subjects which is not the case in many thalassemia affected areas where access to treatment is not always possible.

In the present study, we aimed to assess serum Zn levels in patients with thalassemia and their siblings in a lower middle income country, namely, Pakistan (http://data.worldbank.org/country/pakistan), to determine whether Zn deficiency is present and, if so, if it is related to the disease per se, the use of chelation or to nutritional factors.

2. Patients and Methods

The present study was performed at the Children's Hospital of the Pakistan Institute of Medical Sciences (PIMS), Islamabad, Pakistan, between June 2009 and February 2012. A total of 30 patients with β-thalassemia major and 30 siblings were included. Parental informed consent was obtained. The following data were obtained from the patients' clinical file records: blood transfusion history, last ferritin measurement, onset of chelation therapy and type of chelation used, and infection profile. In addition to serum Zn levels, anthropometric measures such as height, weight, and body mass index (BMI) (BMI = weight (kg)/height^2 (m^2) were obtained).

Sampling and processing: Three mL of peripheral venous blood was withdrawn from each patient and sibling in the early morning, three hours before having breakfast. The samples were left for 20 minutes to clot at room temperature and then centrifuged at 2000 ×g for 10 minutes, and sera were separated and put into aliquots which were stored at −70°C till they were analyzed by atomic absorption spectrometer (AAS; AA300). Zn normal values were estimated to lie between 65 and 120 μg/dL [15].

Statistical analyses were performed by parametric single and paired t-test (after the run of normality test to check that data is normally distributed) and Pearson's correlation coefficient test. A P value ≤ 0.05 was considered to be statistically significant.

3. Results

Median patient age was 4.5 years (ranging from 1 to 10.6 years) and median sibling age was 7.3 years (ranging from 1.1 to 17 years). Patients' serum Zn ranged from 10 μg/dL to 297 μg/dL (median 100 μg/dL), while siblings' serum Zn ranged from 13 μg/dL to 212 μg/dL (median 92 μg/dL) (Figure 1). There were no significant differences in Zn levels between the patients and their corresponding siblings ($P = 0.19$) on matched pair analysis (Table 1). However, it was found that Zn levels were significantly correlated between patients with their corresponding siblings (r correlation coefficient = 0.63, $P < 0.0001$) (Figure 2).

After measuring the height for age Z-scores for the 30 patients with thalassemia, it was found that heights ranged between −4.2 at minimum and 1.09 at maximum (median = −1.5). Height for age Z-scores and Zn levels did not correlate ($r = 0.05$).

For siblings, the median height for age Z-scores was −1.2 and ranged from −3.78 to 2.6 (median = −1.2). A comparison of patient height for age Z-scores with corresponding values for siblings revealed that patients' Z-scores levels were significantly lower than corresponding siblings ($P = 0.02$). Correlation between the two groups was weakly positive ($r = 0.4$), and pairing between the two groups was statistically significant ($P = 0.01$).

The median patient serum ferritin level was 2065 ng/mL (range: 5475 ng/mL–81.15 ng/mL) and showed no correlation with patients' Zn level ($P = 0.7$).

Regular chelation therapy was used by 14 patients: 7 cases were on deferasirox and 7 cases on desferrioxamine, while 16 cases received no chelation therapy. No significant difference in Zn levels was found between chelated and nonchelated groups (median zinc levels were 103.5 μg/dL and 96 μg/dL for chelated and nonchelated patients, respectively, $P = 0.63$). There was also no significant difference in zinc values between patients on desferrioxamine and those on deferasirox (median zinc levels were 96 μg/dL and 102 μg/dL for patients with desferrioxamine and deferasirox, respectively, $P = 0.37$).

Absolute lymphocytic count (ALC) ranged between 817 and 9040 microL, with a median of 3882 microL. No correlation was found between patients' Zn values and ALC ($r = 0.36$).

4. Discussion

Zinc is an essential element for growth and immunity. In this study we aimed to compare serum Zn levels between thalassemia patients and their healthy siblings as to assess whether a possible deficiency is influenced by the disease itself or by nutritional and familial/environmental causes.

Patients' and siblings' Zn median values were within the normal range (median values were 100 μg/dL and 92 μg/dL for patients and siblings, resp.) with no significant difference (patients' serum Zn median value was 100 μg/dL versus 92 μg/dL for siblings) (Figure 1). This finding is in agreement with studies by Rea et al. (1984) [12] and Donma et al. (1990) [11] who noted that the serum Zn levels of patients with thalassemia can be higher than normal [11, 12]. Among the 30 siblings in this study, 18 were carriers for beta thalassemia and 12 were not with no significant differences between the two groups, suggesting that Zn status is not related to thalassemia—the disease itself or trait. The patients' Zn values in this study correlated significantly with corresponding siblings (r correlation coefficient = 0.63, $P < 0.0001$) (Figure 2) suggesting that Zn level was not influenced by thalassemia or its treatment [7], but rather seems more likely related to familial factors either genetic or nutritional/environmental [7].

No correlation between Zn values and growth (height for age Z-scores) was observed in our patients. Similar results

TABLE 1: (a) A collective table for the data of the patients: zinc level in μg/dL, sex (m: male, f: female), age (in years), height (in cm), height-age z-score, ferritin level (in ng/mL), chelation type, and ALC (in microL). (b) A collective table for the data of the patients: zinc level in μg/dL, sex (m: male, f: female), age (in years), height (in cm), and height-age z-score.

(a)

Patient number	Zinc level (μg/dL)	Sex	Age (years)	Height (cm)	Height-age z-score	Ferritin (ng/mL)	Chelation	ALC (microL)
1	94	m	2.6	84	−1.33	694	None	6325
2	58	m	2.9	92	−0.97	2527	None	6200
3	68	f	5.3	100	−2.29	3004	Deferasirox	3903
4	297	m	2.5	92	−0.04	785	None	3891
5	130	m	1	72	−2	641	None	7956
6	66	m	5.5	106	−1.51	2129	Deferoxamine	2156
7	102	f	2.5	91	−1	2000	Deferasirox	8024
8	80	f	8.8	122	−1.57	3513	Deferoxamine	2340
9	109	m	3.8	88	−4	1551	None	7526
10	157	m	4.4	106	−1	2425	Deferoxamine	3872
11	120	m	8.2	115	−2.31	1502	Deferoxamine	3008
12	74	m	2.5	89	−1.17	616	None	4884
13	127	m	5.4	105	−1.48	3810	None	3570
14	75	f	4	95	−1.79	1150	None	1700
15	117	f	4.6	111	0.92	1804	Deferasirox	1218
16	295	m	1.9	81	−1.6	850	None	9040
17	88	m	10.6	131	−1.5	5475	Deferasirox	1160
18	116	f	4	95	−2	2836	None	2813
19	17	m	4.7	113	1.09	658	None	2592
20	111	m	5.6	109	−1.18	2411	Deferoxamine	5002
21	112	m	7.1	114	−1.53	1951	None	1353
22	10	m	1.6	72	−4.2	81.15	None	817
23	79	m	2.2	83	−1.9	2621	None	5490
24	15	f	5	110	0.14	5036	Deferoxamine	1980
25	97	f	10	124	−2.32	706	Deferasirox	4312
26	96	f	10.4	139	−0.32	4487	Deferoxamine	3062
27	120	m	4.5	106	−0.33	5054	None	3180
28	105	f	7.4	117	−1.41	1760	Deferasirox	4260
29	98	m	1.3	75	−1.9	3812	None	5535
30	260	m	4.4	98	−2.01	4100	Deferasirox	3944

(b)

Sibling number	Zinc level (μg/dL)	Sex	Age (years)	Height (cm)	Height-age z-score	Sibling carrier status
Sibling of 1	25	f	12.0	143	−1.23	Not a carrier
Sibling of 2	75	m	5.9	128	2.62	Carrier
Sibling of 3	28	f	9.4	127	−1.31	Not a carrier
Sibling of 4	203	m	6.2	108	−1.85	Not a carrier
Sibling of 5	68	f	11.5	136	−1.8	Carrier
Sibling of 6	35	m	2.4	89	−0.48	Carrier
Sibling of 7	151	f	1.1	77	0.74	Not a carrier
Sibling of 8	89	m	4.1	108	0.95	Carrier
Sibling of 9	212	f	8.7	117	−2.24	Carrier
Sibling of 10	194	f	12.4	150	−0.53	Carrier

(b) Continued.

Sibling number	Zinc level (μg/dL)	Sex	Age (years)	Height (cm)	Height-age z-score	Sibling carrier status
Sibling of 11	138	m	6.9	110	−2.16	Not a carrier
Sibling of 12	72	m	6.9	119	−0.41	Carrier
Sibling of 13	81	m	1.5	75	−2.5	Not a carrier
Sibling of 14	82	m	12.0	140	−1.26	Carrier
Sibling of 15	98	f	2.6	144	−1.51	Not a carrier
Sibling of 16	90	f	5.3	104	−1.39	Carrier
Sibling of 17	79	f	17.0	149	−2.07	Carrier
Sibling of 18	98	m	14.1	150	−1.8	Not a carrier
Sibling of 19	42	f	9.0	137	0.74	Not a carrier
Sibling of 20	94	f	7.5	118	−1.03	Not a carrier
Sibling of 21	107	f	11.9	132	−2.7	Carrier
Sibling of 22	13	m	3.2	89	−2.18	Carrier
Sibling of 23	96	m	11.2	134	1.5	Carrier
Sibling of 24	13	f	7.2	124	0.39	Carrier
Sibling of 25	113	m	8.0	106	−3.78	Carrier
Sibling of 26	87	f	2.4	90	−0.01	Carrier
Sibling of 27	123	f	7.2	130	1.45	Carrier
Sibling of 28	114	f	1.2	73	−1.1	Carrier
Sibling of 29	103	f	9.2	140	0.98	Not a carrier
Sibling of 30	180	f	12.0	138	−1.94	Not a carrier

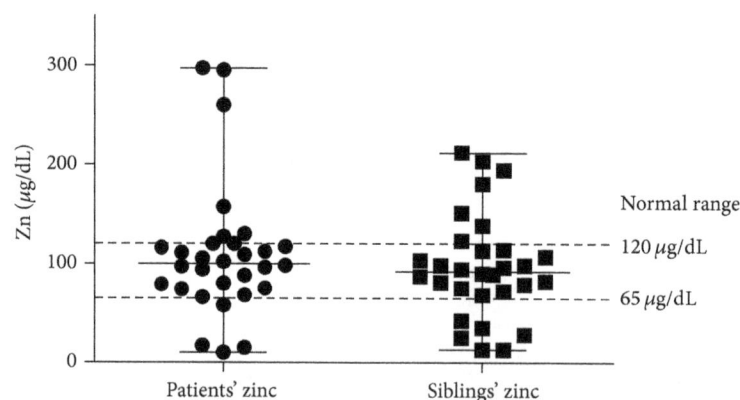

FIGURE 1: Comparison between serum Zn levels for patients and their corresponding siblings. Median levels were within normal range: 100 μg/dL (10 μg/dL–297 μg/dL) for patients and 92 μg/dL (13 μg/dL–212 μg/dL) for siblings.

have been found in several other studies; thus, it is assumed that a Zn deficiency is not related to short stature [7, 16]. However, in a study by Kyriakou and Skordis (2009) [17], the authors proposed that Zn deficiency could be a concomitant factor for growth failure among patients with thalassemia [17]. As patients were found to have significant lower height-for-age compared to their siblings, however there are other concomitant variables such as chronic anemia, iron overload-related endocrine problems, and impaired bone growth which play an important role [18–20]. In our study zinc levels did not seem to differ among siblings suggesting that Zn deficiency may not play a significant role in growth

differences often observed between thalassemic children and their brothers or sisters.

It appears that elevated ferritin levels are inversely related to Zn levels so that as ferritin increases, Zn decreases. However, in this study, the correlation was not statically significant. Decreased zinc levels or increased ferritin values have been previously reported [7, 21] and might be explained by inadequacy of clinical care and proper management affecting independently both ferritin and nutritional Zn levels.

With the limitation of a small sample size, in our study chelation therapy did not seem to affect zinc levels. Deferoxamine and deferiprone have been reported to also chelate and

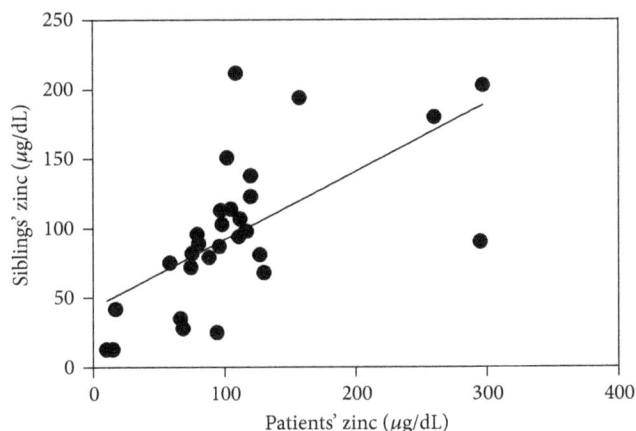

FIGURE 2: Correlation between patients' serum Zn values. Levels correlated positively with corresponding ($r = 0.635$, $P < 0.001$).

eliminate zinc into urine, while for deferasirox, which has a lower affinity for divalent zinc, this seems not to be the case [7, 13, 14].

Several studies have assumed that Zn is important to maintain intact lymphocytic function and counts [4, 7]. Fraker and King (2004) [8] found that a Zn deficiency led to lymphopenia [8]. In conclusion, this study showed that patients with thalassemia do not seem to be prone to Zn deficiency. Patients' serum Zn values correlated with their sibling suggesting that serum Zn levels are possibly more influenced by familial and environmental factors rather than by thalassemia per se or its treatment.

Abbreviations

ALC: Absolute lymphocytic count
BMI: Body mass index
CMV: Cytomegalovirus
IL-2: Interleukin 2
IL-10: Interleukin 10
Treg: T regulatory cells
Zn: Zinc.

Conflict of Interests

The authors declare that there is no conflict of interests regarding the publication of this paper.

Acknowledgments

The authors would like to thank the patients and their families for showing cooperativeness and they acknowledge the support of Cure2Children foundation (C2C), Florence, Italy, and Pakistani-Italian Debt-for-Development Swap Agreement (PIDSA), Islamabad, Pakistan, for the support of the study. Special thanks are due to Assistant Adjunct Professor of Nursing, Julia Challinor, RN, Ph.D., University of California, San Francisco, USA, for revising this paper.

References

[1] T. Hirano, M. Murakami, T. Fukada, K. Nishida, S. Yamasaki, and T. Suzuki, "Roles of zinc and zinc signaling in immunity: zinc as an intracellular signaling molecule," *Advances in Immunology*, vol. 97, pp. 149–176, 2008.

[2] R. S. MacDonald, "The role of zinc in growth and cell proliferation," *Journal of Nutrition*, vol. 130, pp. 1500S–1508S, 2000.

[3] J. Brandão-Neto, V. Stefan, B. B. Mendonça, W. Bloise, and A. V. B. Castro, "The essential role of zinc in growth," *Nutrition Research*, vol. 15, pp. 335–358, 1995.

[4] M. Yu, W.-W. Lee, D. Tomar et al., "Regulation of T cell receptor signaling by activation-induced zinc influx," *The Journal of Experimental Medicine*, vol. 208, no. 4, pp. 775–785, 2011.

[5] J. L. Kadrmas and M. C. Beckerle, "The LIM domain: from the cytoskeleton to the nucleus," *Nature Reviews Molecular Cell Biology*, vol. 5, no. 11, pp. 920–931, 2004.

[6] G. Moshtaghi-Kashanian, A. Gholamhoseinian, A. Hoseinimoghadam, and S. Rajabalian, "Splenectomy changes the pattern of cytokine production in β-thalassemic patients," *Cytokine*, vol. 35, no. 5-6, pp. 253–257, 2006.

[7] M. Mehdizadeh, G. Zamani, and S. Tabatabaee, "Zinc status in patients with major β-thalassemia," *Pediatric Hematology and Oncology*, vol. 25, no. 1, pp. 49–54, 2008.

[8] P. J. Fraker and L. E. King, "Reprogramming of the immune system during zinc deficiency," *Annual Review of Nutrition*, vol. 24, pp. 277–298, 2004.

[9] M. Y. Yakoob, E. Theodoratou, A. Jabeen et al., "Preventive zinc supplementation in developing countries: impact on mortality and morbidity due to diarrhea, pneumonia and malaria," *BMC Public Health*, vol. 11, no. 3, article S23, 2011.

[10] R. S. Gibson and E. L. Ferguson, "Nutrition intervention strategies to combat zinc deficiency in developing countries," *Nutrition Research Reviews*, vol. 11, no. 1, pp. 115–131, 1998.

[11] O. Donma, S. Gunbey, and M. A. M. tas Donma, "Zinc, copper, and magnesium concentrations in hair of children from southeastern Turkey," *Biological Trace Element Research*, vol. 24, no. 1, pp. 39–47, 1990.

[12] F. Rea, L. Perrone, A. Mastrobuono, G. Toscano, and M. D'Amico, "Zinc levels of serum, hair and urine in homozygous beta-thalassemic subjects under hypertransfusional treatment," *Acta Haematologica*, vol. 71, no. 2, pp. 139–142, 1984.

[13] R. Galanello, "Deferiprone in the treatment of transfusion-dependent thalassemia: a review and perspective," *Therapeutics and Clinical Risk Management*, vol. 3, no. 5, pp. 795–805, 2007.

[14] M. D. Cappellini, "Exjade (deferasirox, ICL670) in the treatment of chronic iron overload associated with blood transfusion," *Therapeutics and Clinical Risk Management*, vol. 3, no. 2, pp. 291–299, 2007.

[15] M. Hambidge, "Human zinc deficiency," *Journal of Nutrition*, vol. 130, no. 5, pp. 1344S–1349S, 2000.

[16] G. J. Fuchs, P. Tienboon, S. Linpisarn et al., "Nutritional factors and thalassaemia major," *Archives of Disease in Childhood*, vol. 74, no. 3, pp. 224–227, 1996.

[17] A. Kyriakou and N. Skordis, "Thalassaemia and aberrations of growth and puberty," *Mediterranean Journal of Hematology and Infectious Diseases*, vol. 1, no. 1, 2009.

[18] V. de Sanctis, A. Eleftheriou, and C. Malaventura, "Prevalence of endocrine complications and short stature in patients with thalassaemia major: a multicenter study by the Thalassaemia International Federation (TIF)," *Pediatric Endocrinology Reviews*, vol. 2, supplement 2, pp. 249–255, 2004.

[19] C. Theodoridis, V. Ladis, A. Papatheodorou et al., "Growth and management of short stature in thalassaemia major," *Journal of Pediatric Endocrinology and Metabolism*, vol. 11, no. 3, pp. 835–844, 1998.

[20] Guidelines for the clinical management of thalassemia, 2008.

[21] A. Mahyar, P. Ayazi, A. A. Pahlevan, H. Mojabi, M. R. Sehhat, and A. Javadi, "Zinc & copper status in children with Beta-thalassemia major," *Iranian Journal of Pediatrics*, vol. 20, pp. 297–302, 2010.

12

Loss of Ercc1 Results in a Time- and Dose-Dependent Reduction of Proliferating Early Hematopoietic Progenitors

Judith H. E. Verhagen-Oldenampsen,[1] Jurgen R. Haanstra,[1] Paulina M. H. van Strien,[1] Marijke Valkhof,[1] Ivo P. Touw,[1] and Marieke von Lindern[1,2]

[1] Department of Hematology, Erasmus Medical Center, Dr Molewaterplein 50, 3015 GE Rotterdam, The Netherlands
[2] Department of Hematopoiesis, Sanquin Research and Landsteiner Laboratory, AMC/UvA, Plesmanlaan 125, 1066 CX Amsterdam, The Netherlands

Correspondence should be addressed to Marieke von Lindern, m.vonlindern@sanquin.nl

Academic Editor: Laura Hays

The endonuclease complex Ercc1/Xpf is involved in interstrand crosslink repair and functions downstream of the Fanconi pathway. Loss of Ercc1 causes hematopoietic defects similar to those seen in Fanconi Anemia. $Ercc1^{-/-}$ mice die 3-4 weeks after birth, which prevents long-term follow up of the hematopoietic compartment. We used alternative Ercc1 mouse models to examine the effect of low or absent Ercc1 activity on hematopoiesis. Tie2-Cre-driven deletion of a floxed $Ercc1$ allele was efficient (>80%) in fetal liver hematopoietic cells. Hematopoietic stem and progenitor cells (HSPCs) with a deleted allele were maintained in mice up to 1 year of age when harboring a wt allele, but were progressively outcompeted when the deleted allele was combined with a knockout allele. Mice with a minimal Ercc1 activity expressed by 1 or 2 hypomorphic $Ercc1$ alleles have an extended life expectancy, which allows analysis of HSPCs at 10 and 20 weeks of age. The HSPC compartment was affected in all Ercc1-deficient models. Actively proliferating multipotent progenitors were most affected as were myeloid and erythroid clonogenic progenitors. In conclusion, lack of Ercc1 results in a severe competitive disadvantage of HSPCs and is most deleterious in proliferating progenitor cells.

1. Introduction

The Ercc1/Xpf complex is an endonuclease involved in nucleotide excision repair (NER) and in repair of interstrand crosslinks (ICL) [1, 2]. Mice lacking Ercc1 ($Ercc1^{-/-}$) suffer from severe premature aging, which shows as small size, ruffled fur, liver polyploidy, and loss of hematopoietic progenitors from bone marrow (BM), resulting in death at 3-4 weeks of age [3–6]. Hypomorphic $Ercc1$ ($Ercc1^{d/d}$ or Ercc1*292) mice that harbor 2 C-terminally truncated alleles are also small but they survive longer (~6 months), probably as a result of their residual DNA repair capacity (~4%) [1, 2]. The hypomorphic allele has a 7 amino acid deletion at the C-terminus, which impairs dimerization with Xpf [1].

The short life span and severe aging phenotype of $Ercc1^{-/-}$ is shared with other models of defective NER such as the $Xpa^{-/-}$ $Csb^{m/m}$ mice that die at 3 weeks of age [7–9]. The hematopoietic defect of $Ercc1^{-/-}$ mice, however, is specifically linked to defective ICL repair ([5]; Verhagen-Oldenampsen et al., unpublished). The correlation of specific phenotypes with either NER or ICL repair is likely due to the activation of distinct tumor suppressor mechanisms that impact differently on specific tissues. For instance, persistent DNA damage due to defective NER results in deregulation of the growth axis and is independent of p53 and p16^{INK4a} [8]. Hematopoiesis, on the other hand, is particularly sensitive to activation of p53 (Haanstra, Verhagen-Oldenampsen in preparation).

Both fibroblasts and hematopoietic cells of $Ercc1^{-/-}$ mice and mice lacking Fanconi proteins are hypersensitive to the DNA crosslinker mitomycin C (MMC) [1, 5, 10]. Importantly, the endonuclease complex Ercc1/Xpf participates in the same ICL repair pathway as the Fanconi Anemia (FA) proteins [11, 12]. It associates with FancP/Sxl4 and is required for FancD2 focus formation [13, 14]. Mice lacking for instance the $Fancc$ gene only develop hematopoietic defects when challenged with MMC, or when hematopoietic cells are cultured at atmospheric oxygen prior to transplantation [10, 15]. Mice lacking Ercc1 develop hypoplasia of the BM compartment without applying an external challenge similar to FA patients [16] and Fancp/Slx4-deficient mice [14].

The Ercc1 mice are a useful model to study BM failure in FA, which is, however, limited by the short life span of $Ercc1^{-/-}$ mice. The BM of $Ercc1^{-/-}$ mice contains fewer progenitors, and the remaining myeloid and erythroid progenitors fail to proliferate *in vitro* [5]. The aim of this study was to characterize progression of BM failure in Ercc1 models with an extended life span, and to examine how low levels of Ercc1 activity impact on hematopoiesis. We used mice with a single floxed Ercc1 allele and a Tie2-driven Cre recombinase. Tie2 is expressed in the early hematopoietic stem cell (HSC) when they dissociate from the hemogenic endothelium, and in quiescent adult HSC [17, 18]. We show that the Ercc1 allele recombines efficiently in fetal liver. In presence of an intact Ercc1 allele, the recombination frequency remained stable, while the frequency of cells lacking Ercc1 rapidly decreased in BM when the second Ercc1 allele was lacking. This indicated that Ercc1-deficient hematopoietic cells have a severe competitive disadvantage. To investigate how low levels of Ercc1 affect hematopoietic stem and progenitor cells, we compared hematopoiesis in mice harboring one or two hypomorph alleles ($Ercc1^{-/d}$ and $Ercc1^{d/d}$, encoding proteins with impaired Xpf dimerisation capacity) at 3, 10, and 20 weeks of age. At week 3, we included $Ercc1^{-/-}$ in this comparison. This analysis showed that proliferating stem and progenitor cells decreased, whereas the most immature cells within the LSK fraction were less affected once these cells became quiescent after 3 weeks of age. The decrease of multipotent progenitors preceded the decrease of committed progenitors indicating that the earliest proliferating progenitors are most sensitive to defective ICL repair.

2. Materials and Methods

2.1. Animals. $Ercc1^{+/d}$, $Ercc1^{+/-}$ [1], $Ercc1^{+/f}$ (obtained from Dr. L. Niedernhofer, University of Pittsburgh School of Medicine, Pittsburgh, PA), *Tie2-Cre* [19], and wt littermates were kept in a pure background of both C57/Bl6 and FVB/n at the Animal Resource Center (Erasmus MC). Experimental animals were generated as F1 in a mixed background of C57/Bl6 and FVB/n. $Ercc1^{+/-}$ and $Ercc1^{+/d}$ mice displayed a wild-type phenotype and were used as controls. All animal studies were approved by an independent Animal Ethical Committee. Mice were sacrificed by CO_2 inhalation between postnatal weeks 3 and 20. Neonatal mice and embryo's were sacrificed by decapitation on ice. Femurs, tibia, and sternum were isolated and BM cell suspensions were obtained by crushing the bones in HBSS supplemented with 5% (v/v) foetal calf serum, 100 units/mL penicillin, and 100 μg/mL streptomycin. Fetal livers and neonatal spleens were resuspended by pipetting in the same medium.

2.2. Colony-Forming Unit Assays. Bone marrow cell suspensions were plated in methyl cellulose medium (Methocult M3234, StemCell Technologies SARL, Grenoble, France) containing huGCSF (0.1 μg/mL), muGM-CSF (0.1 μg/mL), or Epo (4 mU/mL) plus transferrin (0.3 mM), hemin (0.2 mM), and muSCF (0.1 μg/mL). Colonies containing 30 cells or more were scored after 7-8 days of culture.

2.3. Flow Cytometry. Single-bone-marrow cell suspensions were analyzed by flow cytometry using a BD LSR II Flow Cytometer System with FCS Express Diva software (BD Biosciences, San Jose, CA). FCS files were analyzed using FlowJo (Tree Star, Inc., Ashland, OR). Cells were labelled with the following antibodies; mouse biotinylated lineage depletion kit, CD16/CD32-PE, CD117-APC, CD135-PE and streptavidin-APC-Cy7 (BD Pharmingen), Sca1-PE-Cy7, CD34-pacific blue and CD127-pacific blue (Ebioscience), and 7'AAD (Invitrogen).

2.4. Genotyping PCR and Q-PCR. Genomic DNA was isolated from tail segments or from blood (NucleoSpin Tissue XS, MACHEREY-NAGEL GmbH & Co). Genotypes were determined by PCR. Genomic Q-PCR used an Applied Biosystems 7900 instrument (Applied Biosystems, Weiterstadt, Germany) and SYBR Green PCR Master Mix (Applied Biosystems). Primers used were HPRT—forward: AGCCTAAGATGAGCGCAAGT, reverse: ATGGCCACAGGACTAGAACA; Recombined Ercc1 allele—forward: TGCAGCATGCTCTAGACTCG, reverse: CCATGAATTCCGGGATCTCTCGAC; nonrecombined Ercc1 allele—forward: TCCACTTCGCATATTAAGGTGA, reverse: AACCTGCGTGCAATCCAT; Ercc1 knock out locus—forward: TCCTCGTGCTTTACGGTATC, reverse: CAGGATCAGGAGGTACAGGA.

2.5. Histology. Livers were embedded in Tissue-Tek O.C.T (Sakura Finetek, Zoeterwoude, Netherlands). 4 μm sections were made using a cryostat (Leica) and stained with hematoxylin and eosin. Slides were imaged on a Leica DMLB light microscope equipped with Leica application suite 2.7.1 (Leica Microsystems, Switzerland).

3. Results

3.1. Ercc1-Deficient Hematopoietic Stem and Progenitor Cells Have a Competitive Disadvantage. $Ercc1^{-/-}$ mice have an average lifespan of 3 weeks. Because we aimed to study long-term effects of Ercc1-deficiency on hematopoietic stem cell function, we used a Cre-lox conditional mouse model expressing Cre-recombinase from the Tie2 promoter (*Tie2-Cre*). Tie2 is expressed on vascular endothelial cells and HSCs [17, 18]. Mice with a single floxed Ercc1 allele ($Ercc1^{+/f}$) were crossed with $Ercc1^{+/-}$ *Tie2-Cre* mice. We compared $Ercc1^{-/f}$ and $Ercc1^{+/f}$ mice with and without expression of Tie2-Cre. Because the recombination efficiency in Cre-lox mouse models is never 100% [20], deletion of the floxed allele was analyzed both pre- and postnatal in the most active hematopoietic organ, that is, fetal liver in the embryo, spleen in newborn animals, and BM in adult animals. The presence of the floxed allele was analyzed by real-time genomic PCR on DNA isolated from the various tissues. The fraction of cells with a deleted floxed allele was calculated by comparing the relative signals in tissues with or without Cre. *Tie2-Cre/Ercc1*$^{+/f}$ mice showed stable deletion of the floxed allele in 50% or more of the hematopoietic cells (Figure 1). In *Tie2-Cre/Ercc1*$^{-/f}$ mice, the Ercc1 allele was deleted in 80% of fetal liver cells at prenatal days E12.5 and E15.5. In newborn *Tie2-Cre/Ercc1*$^{-/f}$ animals (postnatal day 1), ~50% of spleen cells carried a deleted floxed allele. At ten weeks of age, the recombined allele was undetectable or present in a low percentage of cells. In *Tie2-Cre/Ercc1*$^{-/f}$ animals of 1 year old, the BM contained hardly any cells with a recombined allele (Figure 1). Accordingly, blood cell parameters and colony-forming progenitors in BM were similar in *Ercc1*$^{-/f}$ mice with or without *Tie2-Cre* expression at 10 weeks and 1 year of age (data not shown). This indicates that Ercc1-deleted cells are outcompeted by cells in which the floxed allele was not recombined. The presence of one *Ercc1* allele is sufficient to maintain the hematopoietic cell compartment at a similar level as in nondeleted animals.

3.2. The Composition of the Hematopoietic Stem Cell Pool Is Affected by the Level of Ercc1 Activity.

To find a window of Ercc1 expression that allows for the analysis of hematopoiesis for several weeks, we compared hematopoiesis in bone marrow of *Ercc1*$^{-/-}$ mice with mice harboring one C-terminally truncated Ercc1 allele and a knock out allele (*Ercc1*$^{-/d}$), or two C-terminally truncated Ercc1 alleles (*Ercc1*$^{d/d}$). The truncated allele has been described as *293 [1] or as *delta* [21], we adopted *delta*, indicated as "*d*", that should not to be confused with a recombined floxed allele. Three-week-old mice with low or absent Ercc1 activity had a dose-dependent decrease in body size (Figure 2(a)). *Ercc1*$^{-/-}$ mice died between weeks 3 and 4. The *Ercc1*$^{d/d}$ and *Ercc1*$^{-/d}$ mice survived longer, but their low body weight persisted at 10 and 20 weeks of age (Figures 2(b) and 2(c)). A comparison of liver morphology of the various Ercc1-deficient mice at 3 weeks of age indicated that livers from both *Ercc1*$^{-/-}$, *Ercc1*$^{-/d}$, and *Ercc1*$^{d/d}$ mice contained cells with enlarged nuclei, compared to wt livers (larger than 8 μm; Figures 2(d) and 2(e)) as previously described [21].

To analyze the effect of low levels of Ercc1 on hematopoiesis, we first examined the stem and progenitor cell compartment using flow cytometry. Hematopoietic stem cells and progenitor cells (HSPCs) were defined as negative for lineage markers (Lin−) and positive for the surface markers Sca (Sca1+) and the SCF receptor cKit (cKit+), indicated as the LSK fraction. The stem cell compartment was further subdivided into long-term HSC (LT-HSC, CD34−, CD135−), short-term HSC (ST-HSC, CD34+ CD135−), and multipotent progenitors (MPP, CD34+ CD135+) [22].

Because BM cellularity corrected for body weight was comparable between the different genotypes at 3, 10, and 20 weeks of age, a comparison of the subset ratios was permitted between Ercc1-deficient mice and their wt littermates. The

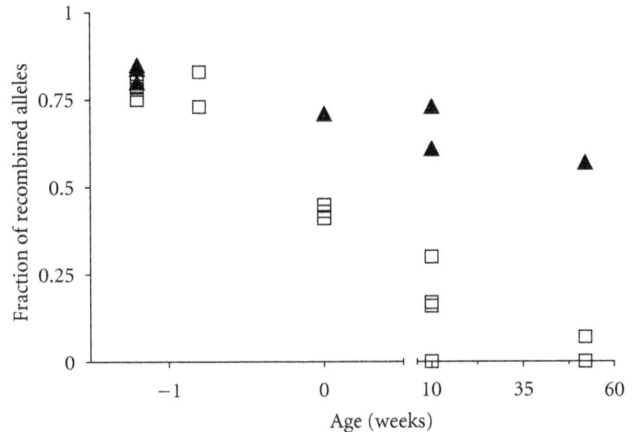

FIGURE 1: Recombination in Ercc1-flox Tie2-Cre model. The fraction of recombined alleles in the presence of Tie2-Cre was calculated after measuring the nondeleted floxed allele by real-time genomic PCR and comparing it to the presence of the floxed allele in absence of Cre. HPRT was measured to control for total DNA. DNA was isolated from fetal livers at embryonic days E12.5 and E15.5, from the spleen of neonatal mice, and from bone marrow of 10- and 52-week-old mice. Closed triangles: *Tie2-Cre; Ercc1*$^{+/f}$, open boxes: *Tie2-Cre; Ercc1*$^{-/f}$. Each symbol is an independent measurement.

percentage of LSK cells in the total bone marrow of 3-week-old mice was decreased to 17% of wt for *Ercc1*$^{-/-}$, 28% of wt for *Ercc1*$^{-/d}$, and 27% of wt in *Ercc1*$^{d/d}$ mice (Figure 3(a)). At 10 weeks of age, the percentage of LSK cells present in the BM further decreased in *Ercc1*$^{-/d}$ mice to 10% of wt but stabilized to 50% of wt for *Ercc1*$^{d/d}$ mice (Figure 3(b)). At 20 weeks, the percentage of LSK was 26% of wt for *Ercc1*$^{-/d}$ and 31% of wt for *Ercc1*$^{d/d}$ (Figure 3(c)). Thus, the size of the stem cell compartment correlates with Ercc1 activity but fluctuates over time.

We next investigated how distinct subpopulations within the LSK compartment depend on Ercc1 protein activity. The distribution of LT-HSC, ST-HSC, and MPP displayed relatively minor changes at week 3 (Figure 3(d)). At 10 weeks of age, the fraction of actively dividing MPP was more than 3-fold decreased in both hypomorphic models (Figure 3(e)). The *Ercc1*$^{-/d}$ BM contained predominantly quiescent LT-HSC, while proliferating ST-HSC was the most abundant fraction in *Ercc1*$^{d/d}$ BM (Figure 3(e)). The enrichment of quiescent LT-HSC is in accordance with the further reduction of LSK in *Ercc1*$^{-/d}$ BM. In contrast, the LSK fraction in *Ercc1*$^{d/d}$ BM partly recovered at week 10, which is in accordance to the increase in ST-HSC fraction. At 20 weeks of age, the distribution of quiescent and dividing subfractions within the population of LSK cells remained similar to the distribution at 10 weeks for both *Ercc1*$^{-/d}$ and *Ercc1*$^{d/d}$ mice (Figure 3(f)).

To specify the distribution of progenitors that arise from the LSK fraction in relation to the remaining Ercc1 activity, we analyzed the following lineage committed progenitor subsets: common myeloid progenitors (CMP, Lin− cKit+ CD34+ CD16/CD32int), granulocyte-monocyte progenitors (GMP, Lin− cKit+ CD34+ CD16/CD32hi),

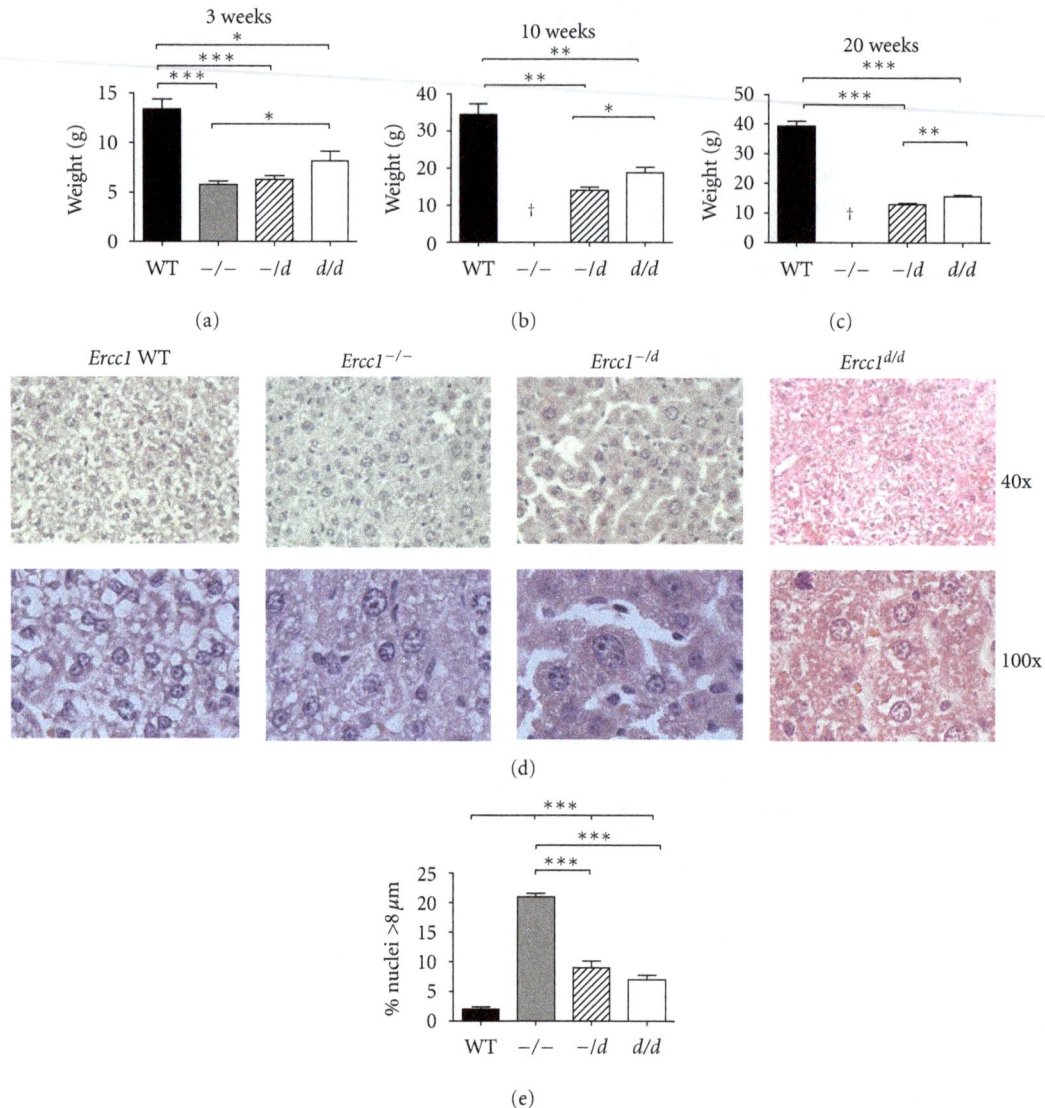

FIGURE 2: Weight and liver cell morphology of mice with distinct levels of Ercc1 activity. ((a)–(c)) Mean body weight of (a) 3-week-old $Ercc1^{-/-}$ ($n = 6$), $Ercc1^{-/d}$ ($n = 7$), $Ercc1^{d/d}$ ($n = 4$), and wt ($n = 13$) mice. (b) 10-week-old $Ercc1^{d/d}$ ($n = 3$), $Ercc1^{-/d}$ ($n = 3$), and wt ($n = 6$) mice. (c) 20-week-old $Ercc1^{-/d}$ ($n = 8$), $Ercc1^{d/d}$ ($n = 5$), and wt ($n = 12$) mice. (d) Hematoxylin- and eosin-stained sections of liver from 3-week-old wt, $Ercc1^{-/-}$, $Ercc1^{-/d}$, and $Ercc1^{d/d}$ mice. (e) Quantification of enlarged nuclei ($>8\,\mu m$). Error bars indicate standard deviation. *indicates $P \leq 0.05$, **indicates $P \leq 0.01$, and ***indicates $P \leq 0.001$.

megakaryocyte-erythroid progenitors (MEP, Lin− cKit+ CD34− CD16/CD32low), and common lymphoid progenitors (CLP, Lin− CD127+ Sca1/cKit+ int). At 3 weeks of age, the CMP fraction of $Ercc1^{-/-}$ mice decreased to 46% of wt, the GMP fraction to 16% of wt, the MEP fraction to 45% of wt, and the CLP fraction to 48% of wt levels (Figure 3(g)). In $Ercc1^{-/d}$ mice, the progenitor subsets decreased to, respectively, 39%, 54%, and 88% of wt levels and no change in CLP levels (Figure 3(g)). For $Ercc1^{d/d}$ mice, these percentages were 23%, 38%, and 41% of wt levels and no difference in CLP levels (Figure 3(g)). For all myeloid subsets, except the CMP compartment, the numbers increased in $Ercc1^{-/d}$ mice as compared to $Ercc1^{-/-}$ mice.

At 10 weeks of age, BM of $Ercc1^{-/d}$ mice contained 20% of wt CMP levels, 29% of wt GMP levels, 49% of wt MEP levels, and 87% of wt CLP levels (Figure 3(h)). In $Ercc1^{d/d}$

mice, these subsets contained 32%, 27%, 39%, and 74% of wt levels, respectively (Figure 3(h)). At 20 weeks of age, $Ercc1^{-/d}$ BM contained 35% of wt CMP levels, 77% of wt GMP levels, 53% of wt MEP levels, and 67% of wt CLP levels (Figure 3(i)). In $Ercc1^{d/d}$ mice, these subsets contained 13%, 23%, 31%, and 69% of wt levels, respectively (Figure 3(i)).

In conclusion, decreased Ercc1 levels reduce all compartments of actively proliferating stem and progenitor cells except for the CLP fraction that is only moderately affected. Despite reduced numbers of progenitors in BM, we observed normal cell numbers in peripheral blood (data not shown). The presence of a hypomorphic Ercc1 allele extends the life span of the mice and marginally improves hematopoiesis in the mice. Also in $Ercc1^{d/d}$ mice, the number of HSPCs remains severely compromised.

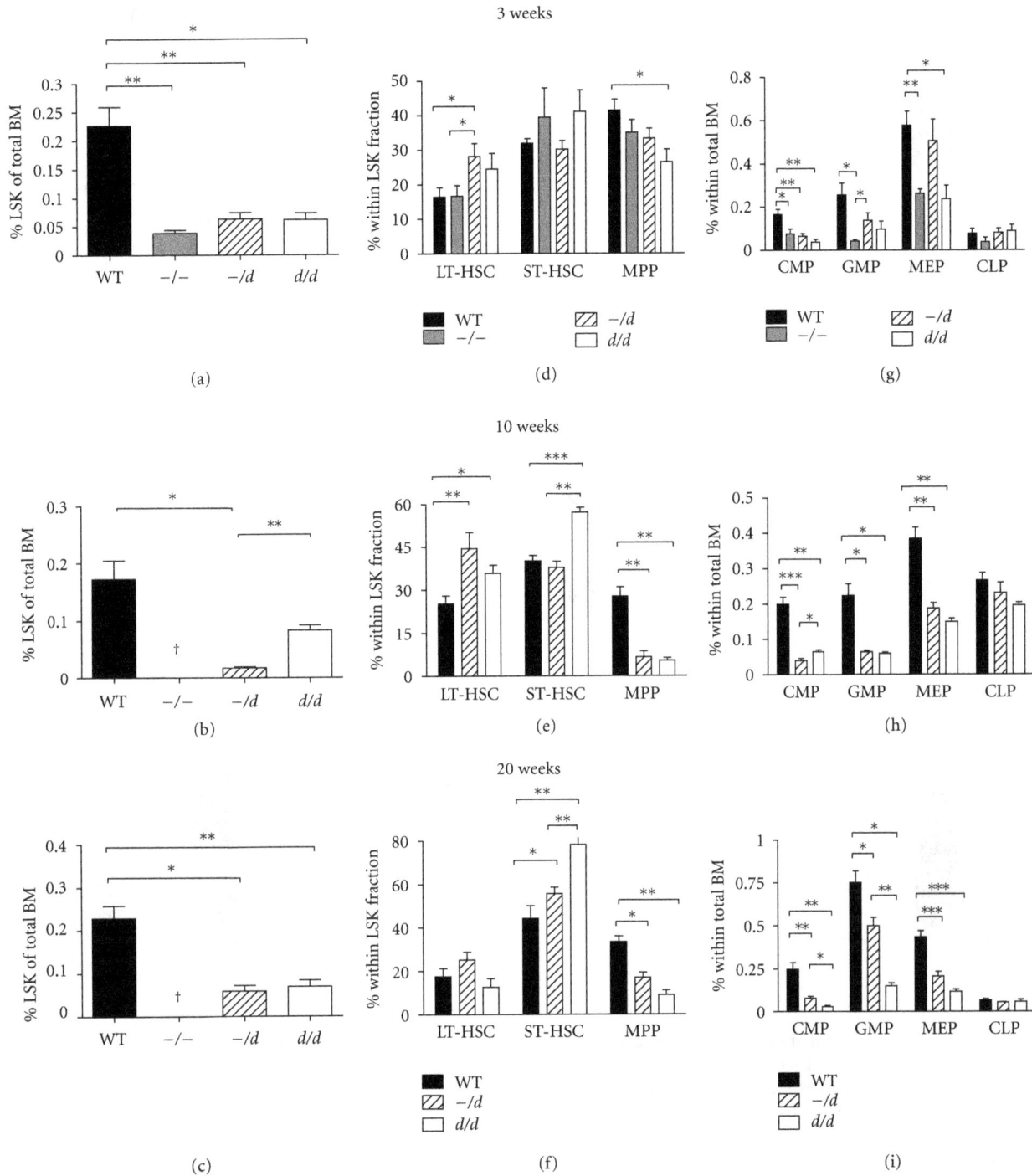

3 weeks

(a)

(d)

(g)

10 weeks

(b)

(e)

(h)

20 weeks

(c)

(f)

(i)

FIGURE 3: Ercc1 levels influence the composition of the stem and progenitor cell pool. Whole BM suspensions were stained with surface antigen specific antibodies for hematopoietic stem cells. ((a)–(c)) LSK (Lin− Sca1+ cKit+) cells as percentage of total bone marrow cells. ((d)–(f)) Distribution of stem cells within the LSK fraction (LT HSC(CD34− CD135−), ST-HSC (CD34+ CD135−) and MPP (CD34+ CD135+)). ((g)–(i)) Distribution of progenitor cells within total bone marrow (CMP (Lin− cKit+ CD34+ CD16/CD32intermediate), GMP (Lin− cKit+ CD34+ CD16/CD32high), MEP (Lin− cKit+ CD34− CD16/CD32low) and CLP (Lin− CD127+ Sca1/cKit intermediate)). Mean percentages are plotted; error bars indicate standard deviation. *indicates $P \leq 0.05$, **indicates $P \leq 0.01$ and ***indicates $P \leq 0.001$.

3.3. Ercc1 Deficiency Impairs Colony Formation by Hematopoietic Progenitors. To assess the colony-forming potential of hematopoietic progenitors, bone marrow suspensions were plated in semisolid medium supplemented with lineage-specific cytokines. At 3 weeks of age, the number of erythroid (BFU-E, Figure 4(a)), granulocytic (CFU-G, Figure 4(b)),

and granulocytic-macrophage colony-forming cells (CFU-GM, Figure 4(c)) were significantly reduced in all Ercc1-deficient models relative to wt (Figures 4(a)–4(c)).

Similar results were obtained in BM of 10- and 20-week-old mice; Ercc1−/d BM formed no BFU-E colonies (Figures 4(d) and 4(g)), no CFU-G colonies (Figures 4(e) and 4(h))

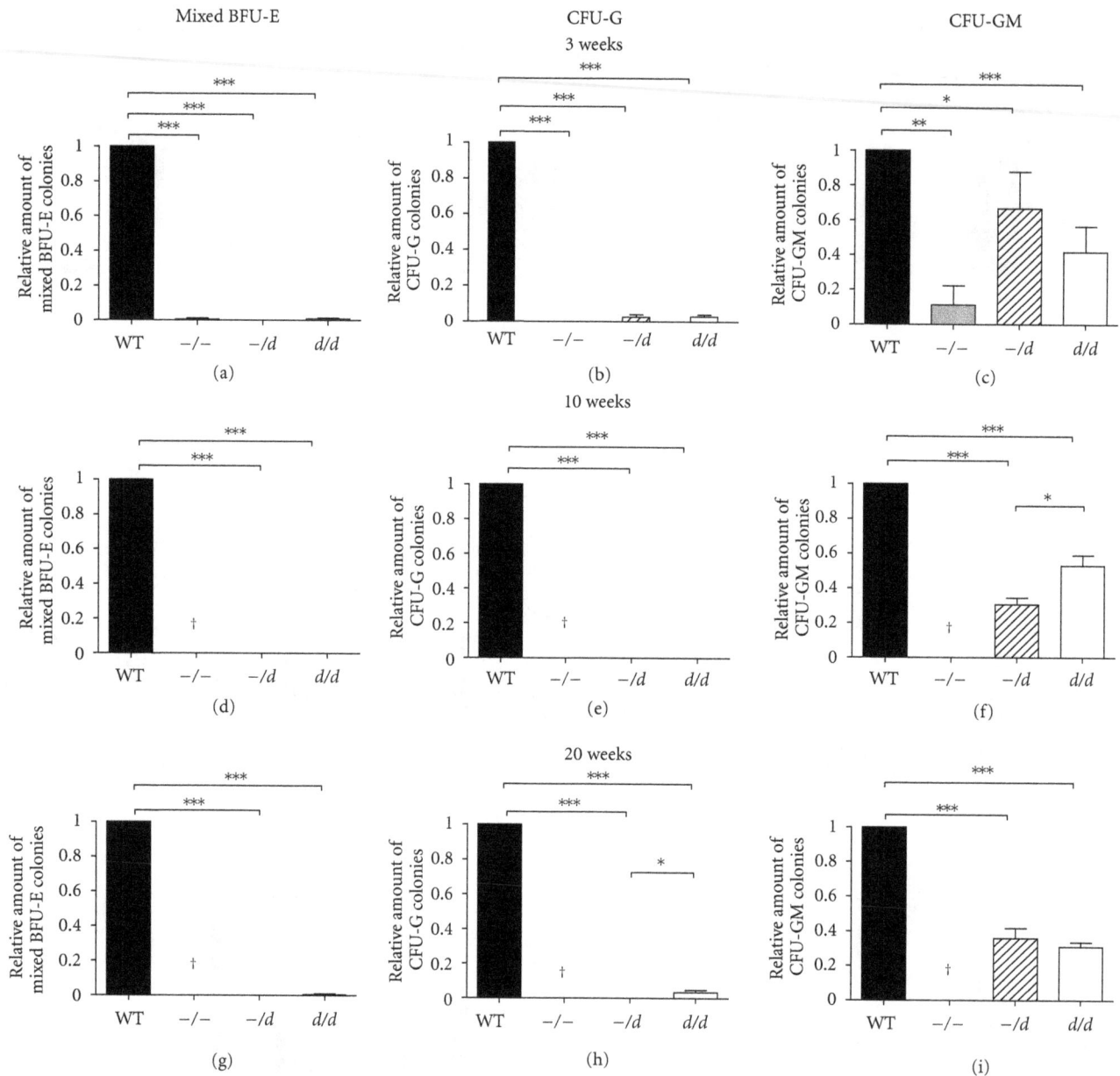

Figure 4: Colony-forming potential of bone marrow progenitors is affected in hypomorphic models or Ercc1. BFU-E, CFU-G, and CFU-GM colonies per 5×10^4 bone marrow cells derived from ((a)–(c)) 3-week-old $Ercc1^{-/-}$ ($n = 6$), $Ercc1^{-/d}$ ($n = 7$), $Ercc1^{d/d}$ ($n = 4$), and wt mice ($n = 7$) ((d)–(f)) 10-week-old $Ercc1^{-/d}$ ($n = 3$), $Ercc1^{d/d}$ ($n = 3$), and wt mice ($n = 3$), ((g)–(i)) 20-week-old $Ercc1^{-/d}$ ($n = 3$), $Ercc1^{d/d}$ ($n = 6$), and wt mice ($n = 8$). Error bars indicate standard deviation. *indicates $P \leq 0.05$, **indicates $P \leq 0.01$, and ***indicates $P \leq 0.001$.

and only 31% of CFU-GM colonies compared to wt (Figures 4(f) and 4(i)). In $Ercc1^{d/d}$ BM, the percentages were 0%, 0%, and 35% of wt, respectively. These results imply that the residual Ercc1 activity in $Ercc1^{-/d}$ and $Ercc1^{d/d}$ mice is not sufficient to support BFU-E or CFU-G colony formation, whereas CFU-GM colony outgrowth is only partly restored.

4. Discussion

The Ercc1/Xpf endonuclease complex acts downstream of the Fanconi pathway in ICL repair [1, 2, 12]. The hematopoietic defects in Ercc1-deficient mice are reminiscent of the

hematopoietic defect of FA patients [23]. It mostly takes several years before FA patients develop anemia. In most FA mouse models, loss of HSC is only seen when the mice are challenged with Mitomycin C [24, 25]. The fact that most mouse models lacking Fanconi genes fail to display overt BM failure may reflect the time it takes to develop anemia. An important factor in the onset of BM failure and leukemia development may be the level of residual DNA repair activity. We employed Ercc1-deficient mouse models to show progressive loss of the number of hematopoietic stem and progenitor cells dependent on Ercc1 activity. Remaining progenitors were compromised in their *in vitro* proliferation capacity, which was similarly severe in $Erccl^{-/-}$, $Erccl^{-/d}$, and $Erccl^{d/d}$ mice.

4.1. Reduced Competitiveness of Erccl-Deficient Hematopoietic Cells.

The conditional knock out model showed that a small percentage of hematopoietic stem and progenitor cells in which the floxed Erccl allele did not recombine outcompeted the Erccl-deficient cells in which Cre-driven deletion had occurred. This progressive loss of Erccl-deficient hematopoietic cells resembles what has been found in a small fraction of FA patients. In some FA patients, a mutation was reverted because two mutated alleles were recombined and yielded an unaffected allele. Such a naturally corrected hematopoietic stem cell is able to out-compete the hematopoietic cells with two defective alleles resulting in the restoration of BM cellularity. In these patients, the fibroblasts retained two mutated alleles [26]. The conditional knock out mice that we used here underscore that defective ICL repair mainly affects continuously regenerating tissues such as the hematopoietic system. It is also in the continuously proliferating bone marrow compartment that few cells with an intact allele can out-compete cells that lack a functional FA pathway.

4.2. Reduced Hematopoietic Reserves with Normal Peripheral Blood Levels.

The hematopoietic defect in Erccl-deficient mice, and in FA, is specifically associated with DNA crosslinks that stall the replication fork. The inability to repair spontaneous DNA damage limits stress-hematopoiesis by diminishing the ability of HSCs to proliferate and self-renew. During embryo development and in young mice (<3 weeks), the HSC compartment is continuously expanded, whereas HSC become largely quiescent in adult mice [27, 28]. These quiescent HSCs are less sensitive to replication-coupled DNA damage repair defects. Progenitor cells have a higher proliferation rate compared to HSC and are, therefore, more prone to DNA damage both during development and in adult mice. Accordingly, we found that LSK numbers are 3- to 5-fold decreased compared to their wt littermates in Erccl-deficient mice. At 3 weeks of age, the distribution within the LSK compartment hardly shows a tendency towards more primitive cells, most likely because all compartments contained proliferative cells. At 10 and 20 weeks of age, when the mice are adult, there is a significant shift towards the more primitive cells in the LSK compartment in the $Erccl^{-/d}$ and $Erccl^{d/d}$ compared to their wt littermates, indicating that maintenance of the LT-HSC fraction is less sensitive to DNA interstrand cross links than the maintenance of the proliferative MPP fraction [29].

However, the mice did not develop overt anemia, and peripheral blood contained near normal amounts of red and white blood cells. This is most likely due to compensatory mechanisms controlled by a network of cytokines and hormones: only small and transient alterations in local-and/or systemic concentrations will be needed to maintain or restore homeostasis. Notably, Epo serum concentrations were normal in Erccl-deficient mice (data not shown), but this result was expected given that the mice were not anemic and Epo production in the kidney is activated by hypoxia.

Because cell numbers in peripheral blood are hardly affected, the hematopoietic defect in $Erccl^{-/d}$ mice does not represent overt BM failure but can be regarded as a situation prone to such overt BM failure. Also in FA patients, reduced stem cell numbers precede overt BM failure and leukemia development [30, 31]. When challenged for regeneration following insult, the Erccl-deficient stem and progenitor cells lack the robustness to do so. Analysis of BM and leukemogenesis in FA and in FA mouse models shows that hypoplasia precedes leukemic transformation [32, 33]. Hypoplastic compartments are most at risk for leukemic transformation [34]. FA patients mainly develop acute myeloid leukemia (AML) and only very rarely acute lymphoid leukemia (ALL) [35]. In the Erccl models, we also found that the myeloid compartment is affected by Erccl deficiency while the CLP compartment is hardly affected. Therefore, the hypomorphic Erccl mice may be a very useful model to study BM failure mechanisms and subsequent leukemogenic transformation in FA.

4.3. Comparison of the Hematopoietic Phenotype of $Erccl^{-/-}$, $Erccl^{-/d}$, and $Erccl^{d/d}$ Mice.

In myeloid and erythroid colony-forming assays, Erccl-deficient progenitors show a 50% (on GM-CSF) to a 100% (on EPO/SCF or G-CSF) decrease in colony numbers. In $Erccl^{-/d}$, and $Erccl^{d/d}$ mice, the decrease in colony numbers was not significantly different from those in $Erccl^{-/-}$ mice. This implies that low levels of functional protein cannot repair the damage inflicted by the rapid proliferation that occurs in these assays. Flow cytometry measurements indicated that the decrease in myeloid and erythroid colony-forming cell numbers was only moderate in the Erccl-deficient models at 3 weeks of age. Thus, the progenitors are present, and they are able to generate progeny in vivo, but not in vitro. In vitro conditions challenge the proliferation capacity more than the in vivo condition and may be more mutagenic such as higher oxygen levels.

Conflict of Interests

The authors have no conflict of interests.

Authors' Contributions

J. H. E. Verhagen-Oldenampsen and J. R. Haanstra contributed equally to this paper. I. P. Touw and M. von Lindern share equal responsibility of this paper.

Acknowledgments

This paper was supported by the Dutch Cancer Society (Koningin Wilhelmina Fonds, Grants 2005-3314 and 2007-3754). The authors would like to thank Jan Hoeijmakers and his staff at the Department of Cell Biology and Genetics at Erasmus MC for the Erccl mouse models and the EDC staff for taking care of their animals.

References

[1] G. Weeda, I. Donker, J. de Wit et al., "Disruption of mouse *Errc1* results in a novel repair syndrome with growth failure, nuclear abnormalities and senescence," *Current Biology*, vol. 7, no. 6, pp. 427–439, 1997.

[2] S. Q. Gregg, A. R. Robinson, and L. J. Niedernhofer, "Physiological consequences of defects in *Errc1*-XPF DNA repair endonuclease," *DNA Repair*, vol. 10, no. 7, pp. 781–791, 2011.

[3] J. Doig, C. Anderson, N. J. Lawrence, J. Selfridge, D. G. Brownstein, and D. W. Melton, "Mice with skin-specific DNA repair gene (*Errc1*) inactivation are hypersensitive to ultraviolet irradiation-induced skin cancer and show more rapid actinic progression," *Oncogene*, vol. 25, no. 47, pp. 6229–6238, 2006.

[4] J. McWhir, J. Selfridge, D. J. Harrison, S. Squires, and D. W. Melton, "Mice with DNA repair gene (ERCC-1) deficiency have elevated levels of p53, liver nuclear abnormalities and die before weaning," *Nature Genetics*, vol. 5, no. 3, pp. 217–224, 1993.

[5] J. M. Prasher, A. S. Lalai, C. Heijmans-Antonissen et al., "Reduced hematopoietic reserves in DNA interstrand crosslink repair-deficient *Errc1* $^{-/-}$ mice," *EMBO Journal*, vol. 24, no. 4, pp. 861–871, 2005.

[6] L. J. Niedernhofer, J. Essers, G. Weeda et al., "The structure-specific endonuclease *Errc1*-Xpf is required for targeted gene replacement in embryonic stem cells," *EMBO Journal*, vol. 20, no. 22, pp. 6540–6549, 2001.

[7] M. Murai, Y. Enokido, N. Inamura et al., "Early postnatal ataxia and abnormal cerebellar development in mice lacking Xeroderma pigmentosum group A and Cockayne syndrome group B DNA repair genes," *Proceedings of the National Academy of Sciences of the United States of America*, vol. 98, no. 23, pp. 13379–13384, 2001.

[8] G. A. Garinis, L. M. Uittenboogaard, H. Stachelscheid et al., "Persistent transcription-blocking DNA lesions trigger somatic growth attenuation associated with longevity," *Nature Cell Biology*, vol. 11, no. 5, pp. 604–615, 2009.

[9] I. van der Pluijm, G. A. Garinis, R. M. C. Brandt et al., "Impaired genome maintenance suppresses the growth hormone-insulin-like growth factor 1 axis in mice with cockayne syndrome," *PLoS Biology*, vol. 5, no. 1, article e2, 2007.

[10] T. Otsuki, J. Wang, I. Demuth, M. Digweed, and J. M. Liu, "Assessment of mitomycin C sensitivity in Fanconi anemia complementation group C gene (Fac) knock-out mouse cells," *International Journal of Hematology*, vol. 67, no. 3, pp. 243–248, 1998.

[11] N. Bhagwat, A. L. Olsen, A. T. Wang et al., "XPF-*Errc1* participates in the Fanconi anemia pathway of cross-link repair," *Molecular and Cellular Biology*, vol. 29, no. 24, pp. 6427–6437, 2009.

[12] G. P. Crossan and K. J. Patel, "The Fanconi anaemia pathway orchestrates incisions at sites of crosslinked DNA," *The Journal of Pathology*, vol. 226, no. 2, pp. 326–337, 2012.

[13] K. M. McCabe, A. Hemphill, Y. Akkari et al., "*Errc1* is required for FANCD2 focus formation," *Molecular Genetics and Metabolism*, vol. 95, no. 1-2, pp. 66–73, 2008.

[14] G. P. Crossan, L. van der Weyden, I. V. Rosado et al., "Disruption of mouse Slx4, a regulator of structure-specific nucleases, phenocopies Fanconi anemia," *Nature Genetics*, vol. 43, no. 2, pp. 147–152, 2011.

[15] X. Li, M. M. Le Beau, S. Ciccone et al., "Ex vivo culture of Fancc$^{-/-}$ stem/progenitor cells predisposes cells to undergo apoptosis, and surviving stem/progenitor cells display cytogenetic abnormalities and an increased risk of malignancy," *Blood*, vol. 105, no. 9, pp. 3465–3471, 2005.

[16] A. D. Auerbach, "Fanconi anemia and its diagnosis," *Mutation Research*, vol. 668, no. 1-2, pp. 4–10, 2009.

[17] A. Iwama, I. Hamaguchi, M. Hashiyama, Y. Murayama, K. Yasunaga, and T. Suda, "Molecular cloning and characterization of mouse TIE and TEK receptor tyrosine kinase genes and their expression in hematopoietic stem cells," *Biochemical and Biophysical Research Communications*, vol. 195, no. 1, pp. 301–309, 1993.

[18] A. Sato, A. Iwama, N. Takakura, H. Nishio, G. D. Yancopoulos, and T. Suda, "Characterization of TEK receptor tyrosine kinase and its ligands, Angiopoietins, in human hematopoietic progenitor cells," *International Immunology*, vol. 10, no. 8, pp. 1217–1227, 1998.

[19] P. A. Koni, S. K. Joshi, U. A. Temann, D. Olson, L. Burkly, and R. A. Flavell, "Conditional vascular cell adhesion molecule 1 deletion in mice: impaired lymphocyte migration to bone marrow," *Journal of Experimental Medicine*, vol. 193, no. 6, pp. 741–754, 2001.

[20] D. Hameyer, A. Loonstra, L. Eshkind et al., "Toxicity of ligand-dependent Cre recombinases and generation of a conditional Cre deleter mouse allowing mosaic recombination in peripheral tissues," *Physiological Genomics*, vol. 31, no. 1, pp. 32–41, 2007.

[21] S. Q. Gregg, V. Gutierrez, A. R. Robinson et al., "A mouse model of accelerated liver aging due to a defect in DNA repair," *Hepatology*, vol. 55, no. 2, pp. 609–621, 2012.

[22] A. Wölfler, A. A. Danen-van Oorschot, J. R. Haanstra et al., "Lineage-instructive function of C/EBPα in multipotent hematopoietic cells and early thymic progenitors," *Blood*, vol. 116, no. 20, pp. 4116–4125, 2010.

[23] K. Neveling, D. Endt, H. Hoehn, and D. Schindler, "Genotype-phenotype correlations in Fanconi anemia," *Mutation Research*, vol. 668, no. 1-2, pp. 73–91, 2009.

[24] M. Carreau, O. I. Gan, L. Liu, M. Doedens, J. E. Dick, and M. Buchwald, "Hematopoietic compartment of Fanconi anemia group C null mice contains fewer lineage-negative CD34$^+$ primitive hematopoietic cells and shows reduced reconstitution ability," *Experimental Hematology*, vol. 27, no. 11, pp. 1667–1674, 1999.

[25] M. Carreau, O. I. Gan, L. Liu et al., "Bone marrow failure in the Fanconi anemia group C mouse model after DNA damage," *Blood*, vol. 91, no. 8, pp. 2737–2744, 1998.

[26] J. Soulier, T. Leblanc, J. Larghero et al., "Detection of somatic mosaicism and classification of Fanconi anemia patients by analysis of the FA/BRCA pathway," *Blood*, vol. 105, no. 3, pp. 1329–1336, 2005.

[27] D. J. Rossi, D. Bryder, J. Seita, A. Nussenzweig, J. Hoeijmakers, and I. L. Weissman, "Deficiencies in DNA damage repair limit the function of haematopoietic stem cells with age," *Nature*, vol. 447, no. 7145, pp. 725–729, 2007.

[28] D. J. Rossi, D. Bryder, and I. L. Weissman, "Hematopoietic stem cell aging: mechanism and consequence," *Experimental Gerontology*, vol. 42, no. 5, pp. 385–390, 2007.

[29] K. Naka and A. Hirao, "Maintenance of genomic integrity in hematopoietic stem cells," *International Journal of Hematology*, vol. 93, no. 4, pp. 434–439, 2011.

[30] A. D. Auerbach, Q. Liu, R. Ghosh, M. S. Pollack, G. W. Douglas, and H. E. Broxmeyer, "Prenatal identification of potential donors for umbilical cord blood transplantation for Fanconi anemia," *Transfusion*, vol. 30, no. 8, pp. 682–687, 1990.

[31] P. F. Kelly, S. Radtke, C. von Kalle et al., "Stem cell collection and gene transfer in Fanconi anemia," *Molecular Therapy*, vol. 15, no. 1, pp. 211–219, 2007.

[32] A. M. Green and G. M. Kupfer, "Fanconi Anemia," *Hematology/Oncology Clinics of North America*, vol. 23, no. 2, pp. 193–214, 2009.

[33] K. Parmar, A. D'Andrea, and L. J. Niedernhofer, "Mouse models of Fanconi anemia," *Mutation Research*, vol. 668, no. 1-2, pp. 133–140, 2009.

[34] G. C. Bagby and G. Meyers, "Myelodysplasia and acute leukemia as late complications of marrow failure: future prospects for leukemia prevention," *Hematology/Oncology Clinics of North America*, vol. 23, no. 2, pp. 361–376, 2009.

[35] D. I. Kutler, B. Singh, J. Satagopan et al., "A 20-year perspective on the International Fanconi Anemia Registry (IFAR)," *Blood*, vol. 101, no. 4, pp. 1249–1256, 2003.

13

Diagnosis of Severe Fetal Anemia Based on Perinatal Outcomes: A Comparative Analysis of the Current Reference Values

Zilma Silveira Nogueira Reis,[1,2] **Gabriel Costa Osanan,**[1] **Tiago Lanfernini Ricardo Coelho,**[3] **Cezar Alencar De Lima Rezende,**[1] **Henrique Vitor Leite,**[1] **and Antônio Carlos Vieira Cabral**[1]

[1] *Department of Gynecology and Obstetrics, Federal University of Minas Gerais, Brazil*
[2] *Obstetrics and Gynaecology Department, Universidade Federal de Minas Gerais (UFMG), Avenida Professor Alfredo Balena, 190, Funcionários, Belo Horizonte, 30.130.100 Minas Gerais, Brazil*
[3] *Federal University of Minas Gerais, Brazil*

Correspondence should be addressed to Zilma Silveira Nogueira Reis; Zilma@medicina.ufmg.br

Academic Editor: Bruno Annibale

Objectives. To compare current criteria for severe fetal anemia diagnosis. *Methodology*. A cohort study analyzed 105 alloimmunized fetuses that underwent cordocentesis due to risk of anemia. Concordance among the diagnostic criteria for severe fetal anemia, hemoglobin deficit >7 g/dL, hemoglobin deficit ≥5 g/dL, and hemoglobin concentration <0.55 MoM, was analyzed using Cohen's Kappa index. Perinatal mortality, fetal hydrops, and fetal acidosis were used to discuss discordances. *Results*. There was fair concordance among the three criteria analyzed: 0.80 (Kappa index, IC 95%: 0.67 to 0.93) when comparing hemoglobin deficit >7.0 g/dL and hemoglobin concentration <0.55 MoM criteria, 0.63 (Kappa index, IC 95%: 0.47 to 0.69) when comparing hemoglobin deficit ≥5.0 g/dL and hemoglobin deficit >7.0 g/dL reference, and 0.77 (Kappa index, IC 95%: 0.64 to 0.90) when comparing hemoglobin deficit≥5.0 g/dL and hemoglobin concentration <0.55 MoM standards. Eighteen cases were classified differently depending on the criteria used. The cut-off point of hemoglobin deficit ≥5 g/dL was the best criterion to discriminate fetuses with poor perinatal outcome in our study. *Conclusions*. Relevant discordances in classification of severe fetal anemia were pointed out. Some criteria may underestimate the real gravity of fetal anemia.

1. Introduction

Maternal alloimmunization still affects a large number of pregnancies, particularly in developing countries [1, 2]. These pregnancies need specific follow-up at tertiary referral centers to carry out proper monitoring, in the view of a high risk of perinatal morbidity and mortality [3, 4]. When severe fetal anemia is suspected by a noninvasive method, cordocentesis is necessary to assess fetal hemoglobin concentration and then to determine the need of an intrauterine transfusion (IUT) [5, 6]. In this context, perinatal outcome also will depend on timely diagnosis and treatment of fetal anemia. For severely anemic fetuses the transfusion therapy is a life-saving procedure [7–9]. However, IUT carries risks for both mother and fetuses. In this way, it is important to determine which fetus is anemic and so it will need an IUT [7–9].

In this high-risk context, assessment of the degree of fetal anemia is an essential strategy for managing these pregnancies [10]. There are three main references for diagnosis and classification of fetal anemia. The first one was proposed by Nicolaides et al., published in 1998 [11]. These criteria use fetal hemoglobin deviation or deficit (mean hemoglobin for gestational age minus measured hemoglobin) as parameter for determining the severity of anemia. The authors consider as severely anemic fetuses those at high risk of hydrops that would generally occur when the hemoglobin deficit was >7 g/dL.

The second criterion was proposed by Bahado-Singh et al., published in 1998 [12]. These authors also use the concept of hemoglobin deficit as a parameter to classify the severity of anemia. They define severe anemia as a hemoglobin deficit ≥5 g/dL, since the risk of fetal hydrops is often below this below this value [13].

And finally, the third criterion was described by Mari et al., published in 2000. This author uses a different parameter for diagnosis and classification of fetal anemia, the multiples of median (MoM) of hemoglobin levels (calculated by dividing the measured hemoglobin value by the expected value for gestational age). Mari et al. define, as severely anemic fetuses, the presence of fetal hemoglobin concentration of less than 0.55 MoM at a blood cord sample [10]. This cut-off point was also based on the risk of fetal hydrops.

In this manner the purpose of this study was to make a comparative analysis of these three criteria used to diagnose and classify fetal anemia, based on perinatal outcome of fetuses followed and treated at a university referral center for Rh alloimmunization in Brazil.

2. Patients and Methods

A cohort study analyzed 151 fetuses that underwent cordocentesis due to suspected anemia. Fetal blood was sampled from January 1999 to December 2009, at the Fetal Medicine Center at the Clinical Hospital of the Federal University of Minas Gerais, a tertiary referral center for alloimmunized pregnancies in Brazil. Clinical records were retrospectively accessed. The study was approved by UFMG Research Ethics Committee.

Eligibility criteria for inclusion in the study were fetuses submitted to cordocentesis due to the risk of anemia, access to information in medical records such as fetal hemoglobin levels before first cordocentesis; and reliable gestational age, confirmed by the latest reliable menstruation date and by an ultrasound examination performed at 20 weeks of gestation.

During this 11-year period, 329 pregnancies were referred to our Fetal Medicine Center due to rhesus alloimmunization (Figure 1). From this total, 151 (45.9%) needed cordocentesis to confirm fetal anemia and to evaluate the need of IUT. From these 151 cases, 46 were excluded from this analysis due to unclear or insufficient clinical records (40 cases had unreliable gestational age at first cordocentesis and six medical records had no information about hemoglobin values at the first IUT).

Cordocentesis was indicated, between 19 and 34 weeks of gestation, based on previous obstetric history, indirect Coombs test titer, presence of fetal hydrops, or altered cardiofemoral index (CFI) and peak systolic velocity middle cerebral artery (MCA-PSV) [13, 14]. Fetal hemoglobin concentration was measured using the HemoCue, a photometric technique on drops of blood taken immediately before the transfusion. In addition, the blood was sent for confirmation of the hemoglobin concentration measured using conventional techniques and for determination of fetal gasometry. The hemoglobin deficit was calculated based on the difference between the hemoglobin expected for the gestational age and that found in the puncture. IUT was performed when the fetal hemoglobin concentration deficit was ≥5 g/dL [12].

Finally we analyzed concordance among the criteria proposed by Nicolaides et al. [11], Bahado-Singh et al. [12],

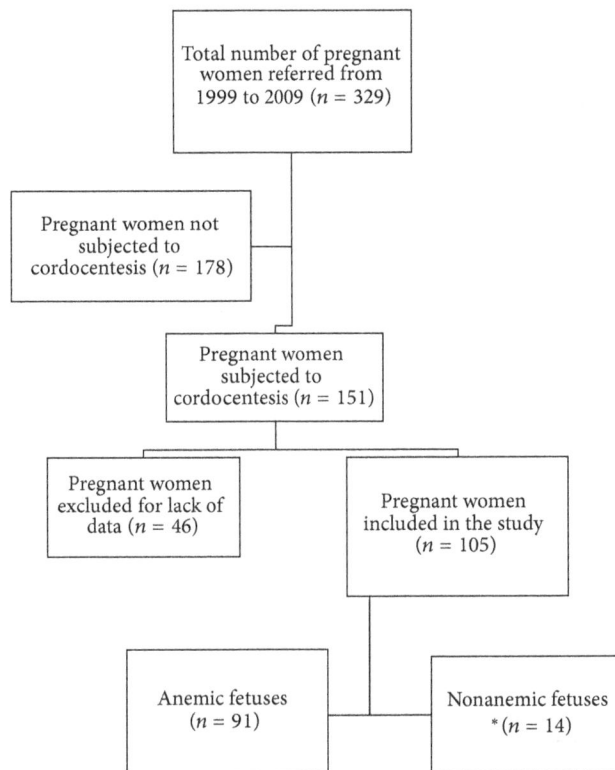

FIGURE 1: Flow diagram of enrolled fetuses at risk of fetal anemia from Rh.

and Mari et al. [10] (Table 3), by means of diagnosis of severe anemia and prediction of perinatal outcome.

For the statistical descriptive analysis, variables were presented using central tendency and dispersion measures, according to the nature of their frequency distribution and absolute and relative frequencies.

In order to provide better understanding of the concordances and discordances among the diagnostic criteria of anemia, the fetal hemoglobin levels were plotted on a graph superimposed on the reference criteria curves. The Interrater agreement among the three criteria (for diagnosis of severe anemia) was obtained by Cohen's Kappa index, with respective confidence intervals of 95%. For this purpose references for fetal severe anemia diagnosis were compared.

Perinatal outcome parameters such as pH value and hydrops [15] at first cordocentesis, perinatal mortality, and 5th minute APGAR index were compared to the criteria. After comparing the current standards, the cases were distributed into three categories of agreement: concordant severe anaemia cases, concordant nonsevere anaemia cases, and discordant severe anaemia cases.

To detect differences in perinatal outcome among the groups the nonparametrical Kruskal-Wallis and Pearson's Chi-square test were utilized. Statistical significance was defined as $P < 0.05$. Statistical analysis calculations were performed using MINITAB Release 14.12.0 1972–2004 Minitab Inc. software.

TABLE 1: Characteristics of alloimmunized pregnancies included in the study.

Gestational and perinatal characteristics	n	Values	Variation or %
Maternal age, years (mean ± SD)	105	29.7 ± 5.3	19 to 43
Parity (median, range)	105	4	1 to 11
Anti-D antibodies (alone), n(%)	99	54	54.5%
Anti-D + anti-C antibodies, n(%)	99	32	32.5%
GA, weeks, at first cordocentesis (mean ± SD)	105	27.9 ± 3.9	19 to 34
Fetal hemoglobin (g/dL), at first cordocentesis (mean ± SD)	105	9.4 ± 3.4	2.2 to 16.4
Fetal severe anemia (>7.0 g/dL hemoglobin deficit)*, n(%)	105	24	22.9%
Fetal severe anemia (≥5.0 g/dL hemoglobin deficit)**, n(%)	105	41	39.1%
Fetal severe anemia (hemoglobin < 0.55 MoM***, n(%)	105	30	28.6%
Fetal pH, at first cordocentesis (median, range)	101	7.35	7.07–7.49
Fetal hydrops at first cordocentesis, n(%)	105	26	24.8%
Perinatal mortality, n(%)	105	20	19.1%
Apgar 5 (median, range)	89	9	2 to 10

*Nicolaides et al. [11], **Bahado-Singh et al. [12], and ***Mari et al. [10]; SD: standard deviation, GA: gestational age.

3. Results

Most of the pregnant women (64.8%, n = 68) arrived at this university center during third trimester of gestation. The hydrops incidence at first cordocentesis was 24.8% (n = 26). In these cases, 80.6% (n = 122) of pregnant women showed an indirect Coombs test titre ≥1 : 64. The characterization of the pregnancies evaluated in the study was presented in Table 1. The lack of a specific Rh immunoprophylaxis, at birth and at miscarriage, was the major cause of maternal sensitization (89.9%, n = 95). The most prevalent erythrocyte antibody found in this study was the anti-D (87%, n = 86/99) (Table 1). The perinatal mortality rate found was 19.1% (n = 20). Severe fetal anemia frequency ranged from 22.9% to 39.1%, depending on the diagnosis criterion adopted (Table 1).

The fetal hemoglobin concentration values, according to the respective gestational age, were plotted on a graph with the reference standards (the three criteria) for fetal anemia (Figure 2). Eighteen fetuses could be classified as nonseverely or severely anemic, depending on the criterion employed (hollow triangles).

Concordance on the diagnosis of severe anaemia was 0.80 (Kappa index, IC 95%: 0.67–0.93) when comparing the criteria of Nicolaides et al. (hemoglobin deficits >7.0 g/dL) and Mari et al. (hemoglobin concentration <0.55 MoM) [11, 12], even though seven diagnoses were discordant.

Moderate concordance (0.63, Kappa index, IC 95%: 0.47–0.69) was observed when comparing Bahado-Singh et al. (hemoglobin deficit ≥5.0 g/dL) [12] and Nicolaides et al. (hemoglobin deficit >7.0 g/dL) [11] criteria for severe anemia. However, 18 diagnoses were discordant.

Finally, fair concordance was observed: 0.77 (Kappa index, IC 95%: 0.64–0.90) comparing Bahado-Singh et al. (hemoglobin deficit ≥5.0 g/dL) and Mari et al. (hemoglobin concentration <0.55 MoM) criteria. All the 30 cases considered severely anemic by Bahado-Singh et al. (hemoglobin deficit ≥5.0 g/dL) [12] criteria were also classified as severely anemic by Mari et al. (hemoglobin concentration

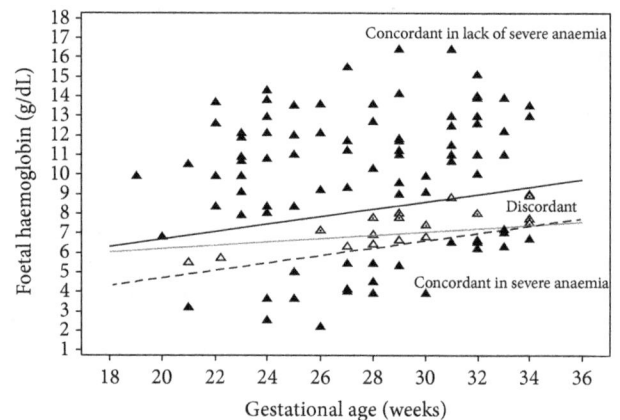

FIGURE 2: Fetal hemoglobin concentration values assessed at first cordocentesis, plotted under the severe anemia diagnosis threshold, according to the anemia different criteria. Solid triangles: concordant cases. Hollow triangles: discordant cases.

<0.55 MoM) [10]. Once more, 11 cases showed discordant classification.

Perinatal results were presented in Table 2. The outcome was characterized by high mortality (20%) and high incidence of hydrops (33.3%). Weight at birth ranged from 390 to 3180 g (median 2180 g). Only the hemoglobin deficit ≥5.0 g/dL criterion for severe anemia [12] could identify all cases with poor perinatal outcome.

As mentioned before, when comparing the current criteria for the diagnosis of severe anemia (two at each time), the cases could be distributed into three categories: the concordant severe anemia cases, the concordant nonsevere anemia cases, and the discordant severe anemia cases (Table 2). The APGAR score and the pH values at cord blood sample (at first cordocentesis) were similar among these groups (Table 2). However, the presence of hydrops and perinatal death were statistically higher in the group of concordant severe anemia

TABLE 2: Perinatal outcome, according to concordance in classifying anemia severity using the several criteria analyzed.

	N	Concordant nonsevere anemia cases	Discordant severe anemia cases	Concordant severe anemia cases	P
hb ≥ 5.0 g/dL deficit [12] versus hb < 0.55 MoM [10]		(n = 64)	(n = 11)	(n = 30)	
Fetal pH[#]	101	7.39 (7.10–7.49)	7.33 (7.19–7.43)	7.35 (7.07–7.45)	0.076[*]
Fetal hydrops[+]	105	8 (12.5%)	2 (20%)	16 (51.6%)	<0.001[**]
Perinatal death	105	5 (7.8%)	3 (30%)	12 (38.7%)	0.001[**]
Apgar 5	89	9 (2–10)	9 (9-9)	9 (2–10)	0.603[*]
hb > 7.0 g/dL deficit [11] versus hb ≥ 5.0 g/dL deficit [12]		(n = 64)	(n = 18)	(n = 23)	
Fetal pH[#]	101	7.39 (7.10–7.49)	7.34 (7.19–7.46)	7.34 (7.07–7.45)	0.069[*]
Fetal hydrops[+]	105	8 (12.5%)	6 (33.3%)	12 (52.2%)	0.001[**]
Perinatal death	105	5 (7.8%)	5 (27.8%)	10 (43.5%)	0.001[**]
Apgar 5	89	9 (2–10)	9 (9-9)	9 (2–10)	0.318[*]
hb > 7.0 g/dL deficit [11] versus hb < 0.55 MoM [10]		(n = 74)	(n = 8)	(n = 23)	
Fetal pH[#]	101	7.38 (7.10–7.49)	7.37 (7.30–7.43)	7.34 (7.07–7.45)	0.172[*]
Fetal hydrops[+]	105	10 (13.5%)	4 (50%)	12 (52.2%)	<0.001[**]
Perinatal death	105	8 (10.8%)	2 (25%)	10 (43.5%)	0.002[**]
Apgar 5	89	9 (2–10)	9 (9-9)	9 (2–10)	0.539[*]

Note: [#]1st cordocentesis, [*] Kruskal-Wallis test, [**] Chi-square test, hb: foetal hemoglobin value at first cordocentesis.

TABLE 3: Criteria for diagnosis and classification of fetal anemia.

	Mild anemia	Moderate anemia	Severe anemia
Nicolaides et al. [11]	Hemoglobin deficit <2 g/dL	Hemoglobin deficit ≥2 g/dL to 7 g/dL	Hemoglobin deficit >7 g/dL
Bahado-Singh et al. [12]	Hemoglobin deficit ≥2 g/dL to less than 5 g/dL	—	Hemoglobin deficit ≥5 g/dL
Mari et al. [10]	Hemoglobin concentration from 0.84 to 0.65 MoM	Hemoglobin concentration from less than 0.65 to 0.55 MoM	Hemoglobin concentration less than 0.55 MoM

cases than in the group of concordant nonsevere anemia (Table 2).

In this study, the standard that uses a cut-off point of hemoglobin deficit ≥5 g/dL [12] to define severe fetal anemia was the only criterion available to classify as severely anemic fetuses, all the cases that had poor perinatal outcome.

4. Discussion

The absence of previous studies that compare current criteria for the diagnoses of severe fetal anemia coexists with an uncritical clinical use of them. This study provides a retrospective analysis that compares these three standards to the perinatal outcome of pregnancies complicated by maternal alloimmunization at our service. We also highlight the potential discrepancies among these three criteria when classifying fetuses as severely anemic. It is important to emphasize that this study was not addressed to evaluate recommendations to indicate cordocentesis or to compare the noninvasive methods to predict fetal anemia or even to analyze current protocols to manage Rh-alloimmunized pregnancies [2, 14].

By pointing out concordances and discordances in classifying the severe anaemia, this study may help to define

protocol standards for the management of pregnancies complicated by maternal alloimmunization. It is important to note that such a comparative approach was possible, just because it took place at a referral center for the care of alloimmunized pregnancies. However, as all retrospective studies, some peculiar limitations were present in this analysis. An important one referred to the changes (worldwide) in the protocol for handling these pregnancies, especially when the MCA-PSV [10] substituted the amniocentesis in the prediction of fetal anemia. This fact reduced drastically the utilization of invasive procedures for diagnosing fetal anemia. The MCA-PSV measurement by ultrasound turned safer prediction of fetal anemia in these pregnancies and then reduced the risk (including fetal death) related to unnecessary cordocentesis. Furthermore, the experience of our service with another noninvasive method, the CFI [8, 9, 16], added a new and important parameter to be used in association with the MCA-PSV to predict important fetal anemia. Finally the present study faced another limitation related to the incompleteness of data (due to information not inserted into the records) or even the loss of cases, leading to exclusions.

The first study to propose a classification for fetal anemia in a group of alloimmunized pregnancies was performed by Nicolaides et al. [11]. To achieve it, the authors determined a normal reference range of fetal hemoglobin, based on 210 samples of umbilical cord blood from conceptuses without anemia, undergoing prenatal diagnosis. Subsequently, they compared the normal range of hemoglobin concentration to the levels found in umbilical cord from alloimmunized fetuses, in a way that they could evaluate severity of anemia. Thus the authors defined severe anemia as the presence of hemoglobin deficit >7 g/dL, since hydropic fetuses in their study had a hemoglobin concentration 7 to 10 g/dL below the normal mean for gestational age. This criterion is probably the most traditional reference to define and classify fetal anemia nowadays. However, in our study, some fetuses with markers of poor perinatal outcome were not classified as severely anemic by this reference.

The second criterion studied was the one created by Bahado-Singh et al. [12]. These authors, based on the references established by Nicolaides et al. [11], decided to reduce the cut-off for the diagnosis of severe anemia to a hemoglobin deficit ≥5 g/dL, in the attempt to increase sensitivity to detect severely anemic cases, and so to ensure that the anemic fetuses would be treated before development of hydrops. Moreover, he classifies severity of anemia in only two groups: mild and severe anemic fetuses. In the present study, all conceptuses that showed hydrops or died during the perinatal period were classified as severely anemic by this criterion.

The third and last criterion evaluated was defined by Mari et al. [10]. This author, as Nicolaides et al. [11], determined the normal range of hemoglobin concentration from his own population of fetuses [10, 14] and classified fetal anemia into mild, moderate, and severe anemia. Differently from Nicolaides et al. [11], Mari et al. [10] found that hemoglobin concentration increases exponentially with advancing gestation and so they decided to classify severity of anemia by means of MoM (multiples of median) for haemoglobin concentration (in order to adjust for the effect of gestational age on the measurement). With this approach, the authors demonstrated that fetuses with severe anemia had a hemoglobin value <0.55 MoM for a given gestational age [10,14]. In our analyses, unfortunately this definition of severe fetal anemia also did not include all fetuses with significant markers of poor perinatal outcome.

Evaluating the different criteria of severe anemia diagnosis, we found that there are important divergences capable of modifying perinatal outcome, especially regarding the occurrence of fetal hydrops and perinatal mortality. On comparing Bahado-Singh et al. [12] and Mari et al. [10] criteria, it was possible to observe 11 divergent cases. Out of these, three cases (30%) were classified as having a severe form of anemia by Bahado-Singh et al. [12] but not by Mari et al. [10], progressed to perinatal death. The same discordance happened with the other two cases (20%) that were hydropic at the first cordocentesis and were not considered severely anemic by Mari standards [10]. Also on comparing Bahado-Singh et al. [12] and Nicolaides et al. [11] standards, 18 fetuses were divergent in severe anemia classification were observed. At this time, five cases (27.8%) were classified as having a severe form of anemia by Bahado-Singh et al. [12] but not by Nicolaides et al. [11], progressed to perinatal death. Moreover other six (33%) that were hydropic would not

considered severely anemic by Nicolaides et al. [11] cut-off point.

Among the three recommendations, we believe that defining severe anemia in the presence of hemoglobin deficit ≥5 g/dL [12] could offer more safety intervention by allowing earlier and more timely treatment for these conceptuses, despite its risk. It is necessary for other prospective clinical trials to confirm our findings. In any event, we hope that this study may contribute to a better management of pregnancies complicated by maternal alloimmunization.

Conflict of Interests

There is no conflict of interests with any trademark or software.

References

[1] L. M. M. Nardozza, L. Camano, A. F. Moron et al., "Perinatal mortality in Rh alloimmunized patients," *European Journal of Obstetrics Gynecology and Reproductive Biology*, vol. 132, no. 2, pp. 159–162, 2007.

[2] L. M. M. Nardozza, E. A. Junior, C. Simioni, L. Camano, and A. F. Moron, "Intervalos de referência do pico de velocidade sistólica da artéria cerebral média fetal na população brasileira," *Radiologia Brasileira*, vol. 41, no. 6, pp. 385–389, 2008.

[3] A. C. V. Cabral, T. B. D. Barcelos, I. G. M. Apocalipse, H. V. Leite, and Z. S. N. Reis, *Indice Cárdio-Femoral Para Avaliação Da Anemia De Fetos De Gestantes Isoimuniza Das*, 2005.

[4] S. Kumar and F. Regan, "Management of pregnancies with RhD alloimmunisation," *British Medical Journal*, vol. 330, no. 7502, pp. 1255–1258, 2005.

[5] J. Bowman, "The management of hemolytic disease in the fetus and newborn," *Seminars in Perinatology*, vol. 21, no. 1, pp. 39–44, 1997.

[6] M. J. Bleile, A. Rijhsinghani, D. M. Dwyre, and T. J. Raife, "Successful use of maternal blood in the management of severe hemolytic disease of the fetus and newborn due to anti-Kpb," *Transfusion and Apheresis Science*, vol. 43, no. 3, pp. 281–283, 2010.

[7] R. Welch, M. W. Rampling, A. Anwar, D. G. Talbert, and C. H. Rodeck, "Changes in hemorhcology with fetal intravascular transfusion," *American Journal of Obstetrics and Gynecology*, vol. 170, no. 3, pp. 726–732, 1994.

[8] M. D. Santiago, C. A. D. L. Rezende, A. C. V. Cabral, H. V. Leite, G. C. Osanan, and Z. S. N. Reis, "Determining the volume of blood required for the correction of foetal anaemia by intrauterine transfusion during pregnancies of Rh isoimmunised women," *Blood Transfusion*, vol. 8, no. 4, pp. 271–277, 2010.

[9] G. C. Osanan, Z. N. Silveira Reis, I. G. Apocalypse, A. P. Lopes, A. K. Pereira, O. M. da Silva Ribeiro et al., "Predictive factors of perinatal mortality in transfused fetuses due to maternal alloimmunization: what really matters?" *Journal of Maternal-Fetal and Neonatal Medicine*, vol. 25, no. 8, pp. 1333–1337, 2012.

[10] G. Mari, R. L. Deter, R. L. Carpenter et al., "Noninvasive diagnosis by Doppler ultrasonography of fetal anemia due to maternal red-cell alloimmunization," *The New England Journal of Medicine*, vol. 342, no. 1, pp. 9–14, 2000.

[11] K. H. Nicolaides, W. H. Clewell, R. S. Mibashan, P. W. Soothill, C. H. Rodeck, and S. Campbell, "Fetal haemoglobin measurement in the assessment of red cell isoimmunisation," *The Lancet*, vol. 1, no. 8594, pp. 1073–1075, 1988.

[12] R. Bahado-Singh, U. Oz, G. Mari, D. Jones, M. Paidas, and L. Onderoglu, "Fetal splenic size in anemia due to Rh-alloimmunization," *Obstetrics and Gynecology*, vol. 92, no. 5, pp. 828–832, 1998.

[13] A. C. V. Cabral, Z. S. N. Reis, H. V. Leite, E. M. Lage, A. L. P. Ferreira, and I. G. Melo, "Cardiofemoral index as an ultrasound marker of fetal anemia in isoimmunized pregnancy," *International Journal of Gynecology and Obstetrics*, vol. 100, no. 1, pp. 60–64, 2008.

[14] G. Mari, "Middle cerebral artery peak systolic velocity: is it the standard of care for the diagnosis of fetal anemia?" *Journal of Ultrasound in Medicine*, vol. 24, no. 5, pp. 697–702, 2005.

[15] I. Forouzan, "Hydrops fetalis: recent advances," *Obstetrical and Gynecological Survey*, vol. 52, no. 2, pp. 130–138, 1997.

[16] A. C. V. Cabral, Z. S. N. Reis, I. G. Apocalypse, G. C. Osanan, E. M. Lage, and H. V. Leite, "Combined use of the cardiofemoral index and middle cerebral artery Doppler velocimetry for the prediction of fetal anemia," *International Journal of Gynecology and Obstetrics*, vol. 111, no. 3, pp. 205–208, 2010.

14

Reduced PKC α Activity Induces Senescent Phenotype in Erythrocytes

Rukmini B. Govekar,[1] Poonam D. Kawle,[1] Suresh H. Advani,[2] and Surekha M. Zingde[1]

[1] Advanced Centre for Treatment, Research and Education in Cancer, Tata Memorial Centre, Kharghar, Navi Mumbai 410610, India
[2] Department of Medical Oncology, Jaslok Hospital and Research Centre, Mumbai 400026, India

Correspondence should be addressed to Rukmini B. Govekar, rgovekar@actrec.gov.in

Academic Editor: Eitan Fibach

The molecular mechanism mediating expression of senescent cell antigen-aggregated or cleaved band 3 and externalized phosphatidylserine (PS) on the surface of aged erythrocytes and their premature expression in certain anemias is not completely elucidated. The erythrocytes with these surface modifications undergo macrophage-mediated phagocytosis. In this study, the role of protein kinase C (PKC) isoforms in the expression of these surface modifications was investigated. Inhibition of PKC α by 30 μM rottlerin (R30) and 2.3 nM Gö 6976 caused expression of both the senescent cell marker-externalized PS measured by FACS analysis and aggregated band 3 detected by western blotting. In contrast to this observation, but in keeping with literature, PKC activation by phorbol-12-myristate-13-acetate (PMA) also led to the expression of senescence markers. We explain this antithesis by demonstrating that PMA-treated cells show reduction in the activity of PKC α, thereby simulating inhibition. The reduction in PKC α activity may be attributed to the known downregulation of PMA-activated PKC α, caused by its membrane translocation and proteolysis. We demonstrate membrane translocation of PKC α in PMA-treated cells to substantiate this inference. Thus loss of PKC α activity either by inhibition or downregulation can cause surface modifications which can trigger erythrophagocytosis.

1. Introduction

Human erythrocytes have a definite lifespan of 120 ± 4 days in circulation and thereafter are marked for phagocytosis by cell surface modifications, such as aggregation or cleavage of protein band 3 and exposure of PS [1–3]. Time-compressed expression of these markers leads to premature eryptosis in anemias [4, 5]. Molecular events which mediate expression of these surface markers of senescence have been partly delineated in erythrocytes mainly under oxidative conditions [6, 7]. They appear to recapitulate the cytoplasmic events in apoptosis of nucleated cells such as translocation of Fas into rafts, formation of a Fas-associated complex, and activation of caspases 8 and 3 [8]. Activation of caspase 3 in turn is associated with cleavage of band 3 [9], which generates senescent cell antigen in erythrocytes [10], as well as causes impairment of aminophospholipid flippase activity and PS externalization [11]. This similarity of molecular events in eryptosis and apoptosis prompted us to explore the role of PKC isoforms, which have distinct tissue-specific roles in both cell survival and apoptosis of nucleated cells [12], in eryptosis.

PKC is a family of serine/threonine kinases comprising of eleven isoforms which differ in their cofactor requirement for activation and are accordingly categorized into classical (Ca^{2+}/diacylglycerol (DAG) dependent: α, βI, βII, γ), novel (DAG dependent: δ, ε, η, θ), and atypical (Ca^{2+}/DAG independent: ζ, ι, related kinase μ) isoforms [13]. We have earlier shown that normal erythrocytes express PKC α, ζ, ι, μ [14]. This investigation demonstrates in vitro that reduction in the activity of PKC α causes expression of the senescent cell antigens in erythrocytes.

2. Materials and Methods

2.1. Chemicals. PMA (P 8139), 4α-phorbol 12,13-didecanoate (4αPDD) (P 8014), phenyl methyl sulfonyl fluoride (PMSF) (P 7626), anti-band 3 N-terminus monoclonal antibody (B 9277), and anti-β-actin antibody (A5316) were purchased from Sigma. Rottlerin (557370) and Gö 6976 (365250) were procured from Calbiochem. PKC activity kit (RPN 77), enhanced chemiluminescence reagent (ECL plus) (RPN 2132), and the horseradish-peroxidase (HRP) conjugated-anti-mouse IgG (NA 931) were from GE Healthcare. Polyvinylidene difluoride (PVDF) membrane (IPVH 00010) was from Millipore. Annexin V-FITC apoptosis detection kit I (556547) was from BD Pharmingen. Anti-PKC α antibody was from PKC sampler kit (S 85080) of the Transduction Laboratories. Colloidal gold total protein stain (170-6527) was from Bio-Rad laboratories. $\gamma^{32}P$ ATP was obtained from Board of Radiation and Isotope Technology, Department of Atomic Energy, India.

2.2. Biological Material.

This study was undertaken after obtaining ethics clearance from the hospital ethics committee, and informed consent form was administered prior to sample collection. Peripheral blood (5 mL) was collected by venipuncture in ethylene diamine tetra acetic acid (EDTA)-containing bulbs for separation of erythrocytes. Healthy voluntary donors (N) who reported no health problems were recruited for the study ($n = 20$). The age of volunteers ranged from 22 to 56 years. An equal number of male and female volunteers in the age ranges 20–30, 30–40, 40–50, and 50–60 years were included.

2.3. Preparation of Erythrocyte Suspension.

Erythrocytes were allowed to settle from the blood sample collected in EDTA bulbs. After removing the supernatant plasma, erythrocytes were washed three times in wash buffer (10 mM Tris pH 7.6, 150 mM NaCl) separating erythrocytes each time by centrifugation at 1500 rpm for 15 min at 4°C.

2.4. Treatment of Erythrocytes with Activators and Inhibitors of PKC.

Erythrocytes (10^8 cells/mL) were incubated at 37°C for 20 min with either dimethylsulfoxide (DMSO)—solvent for all the modifiers (final concentration 1.6% as it was the highest concentration in the inhibitor/activator treated groups), 1 μM PMA-activator of classical and novel isoforms of PKC, 1 μM 4αPDD—biologically inactive structural analogue of PMA, 30 μM rottlerin (R30)—inhibitor of PKC (inhibits classical isoforms α, β, and γ and novel isoforms δ and θ at the concentration used but not atypical isoforms PKC ζ, ι or μ). This treatment group comprising of ten samples was used for the initial assessment of the role of PKC in the aggregation of band 3 and PS externalization as well as to assess membrane translocation of PKC α. To confirm the role of PKC α in expression of markers of senescence, aggregation of band 3 and externalized PS were detected in erythrocytes from ten additional samples incubated with DMSO or 2.3 nM Gö 6976—a specific inhibitor of PKC α. After treatment with modifiers the cells were aliquoted.

2.5. Analysis of PS Externalization.

Aliquots of cells (1×10^7) treated with modifiers and untreated controls were labelled with annexinV-FITC to detect PS exposure on erythrocytes. Labelling was performed using the annexinV-FITC apoptosis detection kit according to the manufacturer's instructions.

Data acquisition was performed on a Becton Dickinson FACS Calibur flow cytometer, and analysis was done with Cell Quest software. Per sample 10,000 events were acquired. The percentage of annexin V-positive erythrocytes from the gated population was determined for each treatment group and compared with a negative (unlabeled) control, which was run for each sample.

2.6. Preparation of Erythrocyte Lysates for Western Blotting.

An aliquot of the erythrocytes treated with modifiers or DMSO was lysed in equal volume of hypotonic solution (10 mM Tris pH 7.6, 1 mM EDTA, 20 μg/mL PMSF) as described by Dodge et al. [15]. After centrifugation of the lysate at 15,000 rpm for 15 min at 4°C in SS-34 rotor of Sorvall RC-5C centrifuge, the supernatant was recovered as cytosolic fraction and the pellet which contained the membrane skeleton (referred to as "membrane") was washed thrice with wash buffer (10 mM Tris pH 7.6, 150 mM NaCl, 20 μg/mL PMSF). Membrane and cytosol fractions were aliquoted and preserved at −70°C until use. Protein was estimated using the modified Lowry's method [16].

2.7. Detection of Band 3 and Translocation of PKC α.

Erythrocyte membrane protein (60 μg) and cytosolic protein (120 μg) obtained from cells treated with DMSO and modifiers were resolved on 10% SDS-polyacrylamide gels and then transferred electrophoretically to PVDF membrane [17]. The blots with membrane proteins were probed with anti-band 3 antibody. The protein-antibody complexes were further reacted with anti-mouse IgG-HRP, and the binding of HRP-labelled antibody was detected by autography using the ECL plus western blotting detection system. A duplicate blot was used for probing with antibody to β-actin, and the recorded signals were assessed to ascertain equal loading. For the samples with quantities inadequate for duplicate blot, the blot stained with band 3 antibody was stained with colloidal gold to assess equal loading of protein. Western blots of both membrane and cytosolic proteins from cells treated with DMSO, PMA, and 4αPDD were probed with PKC α antibody to assess translocation of PKC α from cytosol to membrane. Detection of protein-antibody complex was done similar to that for band 3.

2.8. Preparation of Whole Cell Lysates for the PKC Activity Assay.

Erythrocytes ($1–3 \times 10^9$) were lysed in 1 mL cold cell lysis buffer (50 mM HEPES pH 7.6, 150 mM NaCl, 10% glycerol, 1% Triton X-100, 1.5 mM MgCl$_2$, 5 mM EGTA, 1 mM leupeptin, 2 mM PMSF, 10 μg/mL aprotinin, 10 μg/mL pepstatin, 1 mM sodium orthovanadate, and 1.5 mM sodium fluoride). The mixture was kept on ice for 15 min. and spun at 1,00,000 g for 30 min. in a Beckman TL-100 ultracentrifuge. After adding an equal volume of glycerol to the supernatant, it was stored at −70°C till use.

2.9. Estimation of Activity of PKC α.

PKC activity was determined using the PKC enzyme assay system as per manufacturer's instructions. Incorporation of γ-^{32}P-labelled ATP (45,000 ± 20,000 cpm in magnesium buffer per reaction) in

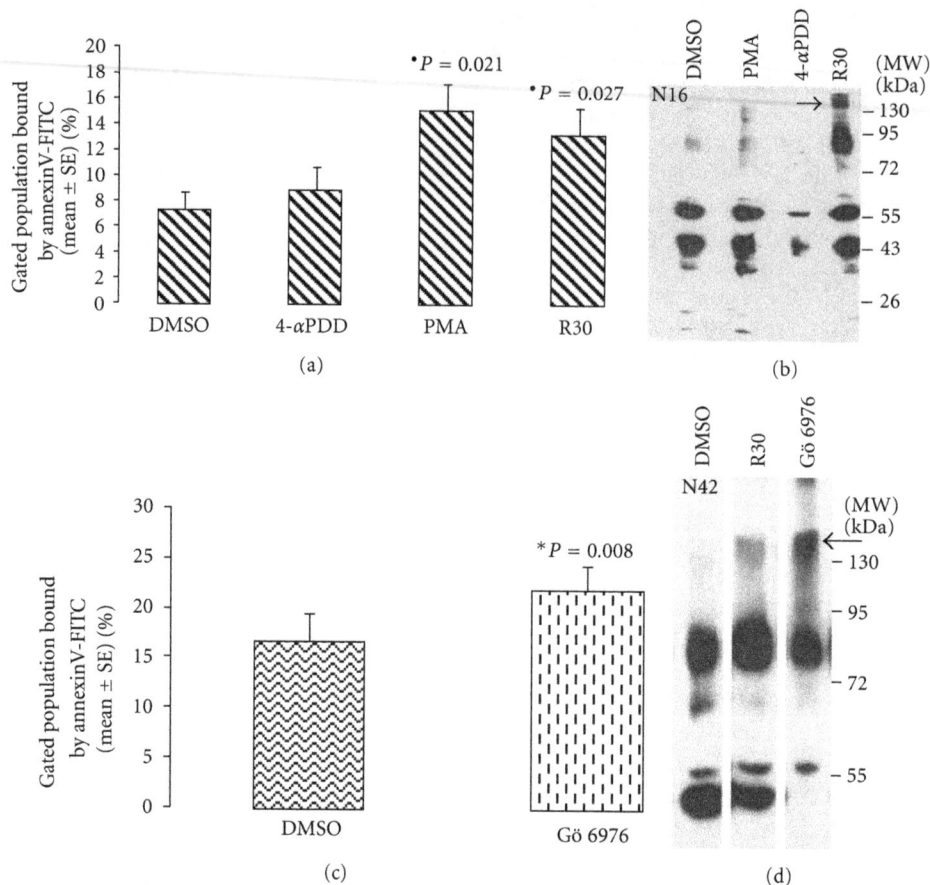

FIGURE 1: Externalization of PS and aggregation of band 3 induced by PKC α activator (PMA) and inhibitors (30 μM rottlerin-R30 and Gö 6976). Flow cytometry of annexinV-bound cells shows significant (*) increased percentage of cells with externalized PS upon treatment with (a) PMA, R30 (Wicoxon signed rank test; $n = 10$) as well as (c) with Gö 6976(paired t-test, $n = 10$). A signal for aggregated band 3 above 130 kDa (indicated by arrow) is seen in western blot of erythrocyte membrane proteins immunostained with band 3 antibody only in cells treated with (b) R30 (represented in sample $N16$) and (d) Gö 6976 (represented by $N42$).

PKC-specific substrate was measured in total lysates (25 μL) (of DMSO- and PMA-treated erythrocytes) incubated with Ca^{2+} and lipid (as a mixture of α phosphatidyl-L-serine and phorbol-12-myristate-13-acetate in the kit). Incorporation of labelled ATP in the peptide substrate was measured by liquid scintillation counting. Activity was expressed as pmol phosphate transferred/min/mg protein.

2.10. Statistical Analysis. Comparison of PS externalization observed in erythrocytes treated with different modifiers was expressed as mean ± standard error (SE) for the specified number of samples (n) and analyzed by either paired t-test or Wilcoxon signed ranks test as indicated, using SPSS software version 15.

3. Results and Discussion

We have earlier demonstrated that PKC α is the only DAG-dependent and thus PMA-activated PKC isoform expressed in erythrocytes, while PKC ζ, ι, and μ are atypical isoforms which are non-responsive to PMA [14]. Thus the significant increase ($P = 0.021$; Wilcoxon Signed Ranks Test) in cells

expressing externalized PS upon the activation of PKC with PMA (Figure 1(a)) can be attributed to PKC α. This is in keeping with the literature reports on PKC-induced PS externalization [18, 19] as well as its attribution to PKC α [20]. In cells treated with 4αPDD, a biologically inactive structural analogue of PMA, the percentage of cells expressing PS remained unchanged. The effect of PMA was less obvious on aggregation of band 3 (Figure 1(b)).

The conclusion of causative role of PKC α activation in externalization of PS was differed by our observation in the inhibition experiments. Preferential inhibition of PKC α was achieved by using 30 μM rottlerin which inhibits PKC α while the atypical isoforms ζ, ι, and μ are inhibited by 80–100 μM [21]. In erythrocyte samples ($n = 10$) treated with 30 μM rottlerin, significant PS externalization ($P = 0.027$; Wilcoxon Signed Ranks Test) (Figure 1(a)) as well as aggregation of band 3 (in 9/10 samples) was observed (represented in Figure 1(b)). The role of PKC α inhibition was confirmed by demonstrating expression of both the markers of senescence (Figures 1(c) and 1(d)) in erythrocytes treated with 2.3 nM Gö 6976, which specifically inhibits PKC

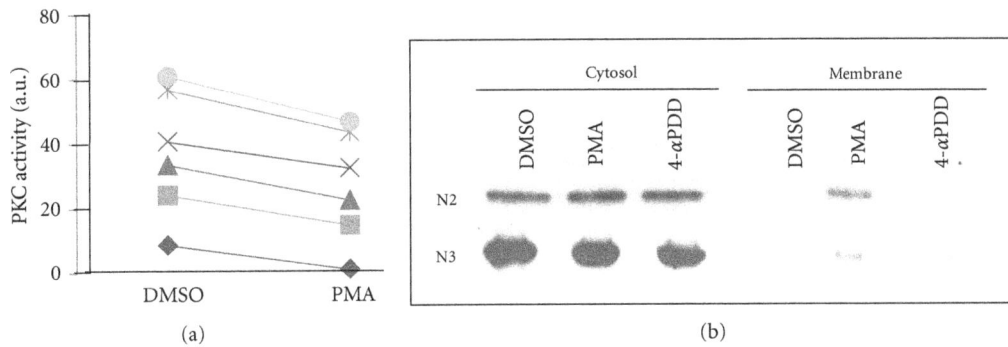

FIGURE 2: Modulation of PKC α localization and activity upon PMA treatment. (a) Activity of PKC in the presence of Ca^{2+} and lipid shows 10–30% reduction in PMA-treated group. Units of activity (a.u.) are arbitrary values assigned by the graphic tool. (b) Western blots of erythrocyte cytosolic and membrane proteins stained with anti-PKC α antibody (represented by N2 and N3) show a signal around 77 kDa in the cytosol of all treatment groups but in the membrane fractions of only the PMA-treated erythrocytes.

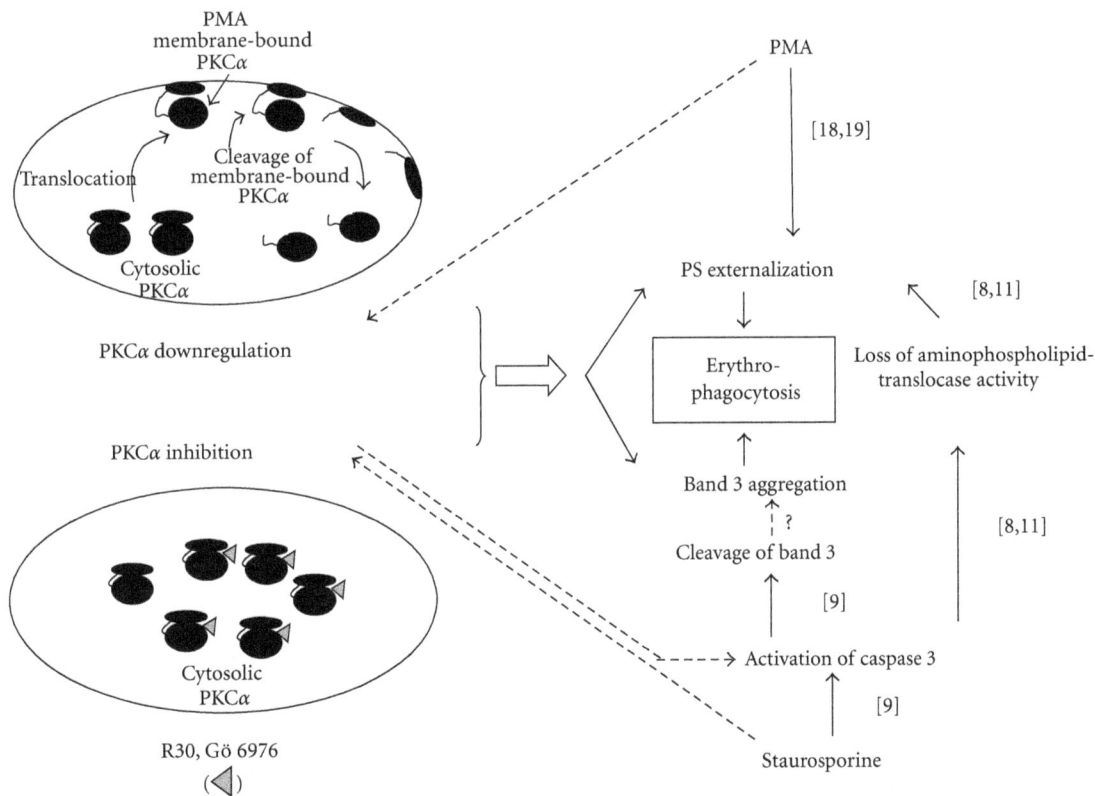

FIGURE 3: PKC α in eryptosis. Literature reports the role of activation of PKC/PKC α in the expression of externalized PS. We demonstrate that loss of PKC α activity due to inhibition or activation-linked down fregulation causes expression of not only externalized PS but also aggregated band 3. These observations along with other reports (given in brackets along the arrows) are linked to further understand the molecular mechanism of eryptosis. The molecular pathway of eryptosis emerging from the reports and the present study suggests exploration of the role of PKC α inhibition in activation of caspase 3 (indicated by dotted lines) which causes expression of both the markers of senescence.

α [22]. These observations are significant in the light of the reported [23] loss of PKC activity in senescent erythrocytes.

Generation of similar responses with agents which activate (PMA) or inhibit (rottlerin) PKC in an isoform-non-specific manner is also reported by Liu et al. [24]. We explain this antithesis by the demonstration of 10–30% reduction in PKC α activity (Figure 2(a)) in the presence of Ca^{2+} and

DAG (which activate only PKC α in erythrocyte) in PMA-treated cells as compared to control. We show translocation of activated PKC α (Figure 2(b)) in PMA-treated cells which is known to cause their downregulation by calpain-mediated proteolysis [25]. Translocation is not observed in samples treated with DMSO or 4αPDD. In erythrocytes which do not synthesize protein, downregulation would lead to permanent loss of activatable protein, thereby simulating conditions of inhibition. We therefore redefine the mechanism of PMA-mediated expression of externalized PS in erythrocytes as caused by loss of PKC α activity due to downregulation rather than activation of the molecule.

Thus we report for the first time that loss of PKC α activity due to inhibition or downregulation causes expression of both markers of erythrocyte senescence which can mediate erythrophagocytosis. Figure 3 highlights the insights provided by this finding into the aspects of PMA-mediated molecular events in erythrocyte aging reported in literature.

4. Conclusion

Thus, PKC isoforms, which have distinct tissue-specific roles in both cell survival and apoptosis of nucleated cells, can also mediate eryptosis. While literature reports the role of activation of PKC/PKC α in the expression of externalized PS, we demonstrate that loss of PKC α activity due to inhibition or activation-linked downregulation can cause expression of not only externalized PS but also aggregated band 3. The study has thus unravelled a molecular event causative of the expression of two cell surface modifications, which can trigger erythrophagocytosis.

Acknowledgments

This study received financial support from the Lady Tata Memorial Trust and additional funds from ACTREC to complete the PKC α inhibition experiments. Mrs. Namrata Gosar-Dedhia, SIES College, Mumbai worked as a trainee on this project and has participated in this work. The authors thank Miss Shyamal Vetale and Mrs. Rekha Gaur from Flow Cytometry Facility, ACTREC for their help in the flow cytometry experiments and analysis.

References

[1] P. Arese, F. Turrini, and E. Schwarzer, "Band 3/complement-mediated recognition and removal of normally senescent and pathological human erythrocytes," *Cellular Physiology and Biochemistry*, vol. 16, no. 4–6, pp. 133–146, 2005.

[2] F. E. Boas, L. Forman, and E. Beutler, "Phosphatidylserine exposure and red cell viability in red cell aging and in hemolytic anemia," *Proceedings of the National Academy of Sciences of the United States of America*, vol. 95, no. 6, pp. 3077–3081, 1998.

[3] G. J. C. G. M. Bosman, F. L. A. Willekens, and J. M. Werre, "Erythrocyte aging: a more than superficial resemblance to apoptosis?" *Cellular Physiology and Biochemistry*, vol. 16, no. 1–3, pp. 1–8, 2005.

[4] M. Kundu, J. Basu, and P. Chakrabarti, "Chronic myelogenous leukemia: alterations in red cell membrane band 3 and increased IgG binding," *Indian Journal of Biochemistry and Biophysics*, vol. 27, no. 6, pp. 456–459, 1990.

[5] J. D. Corbett and D. E. Golan, "Band 3 and glycophorin are progressively aggregated in density- fractionated sickle and normal red blood cells. Evidence from rotational and lateral mobility studies," *Journal of Clinical Investigation*, vol. 91, no. 1, pp. 208–217, 1993.

[6] P. S. Low, S. M. Waugh, K. Zinke, and D. Drenckhahn, "The role of hemoglobin denaturation and band 3 clustering in red blood cell aging," *Science*, vol. 227, no. 4686, pp. 531–533, 1985.

[7] K. Schluter and D. Drenckhahn, "Co-clustering of denatured hemoglobin with band 3: its role in binding of autoantibodies against band 3 to abnormal and aged erythrocytes," *Proceedings of the National Academy of Sciences of the United States of America*, vol. 83, no. 16, pp. 6137–6141, 1986.

[8] D. Mandal, A. Mazumder, P. Das, M. Kundu, and J. Basu, "Fas-, caspase 8-, and caspase 3-dependent signaling regulates the activity of the aminophospholipid translocase and phosphatidylserine externalization in human erythrocytes," *Journal of Biological Chemistry*, vol. 280, no. 47, pp. 39460–39467, 2005.

[9] D. Mandal, V. Baudin-Creuza, A. Bhattacharyya et al., "Caspase 3-mediated proteolysis of the N-terminal cytoplasmic domain of the human erythroid anion exchanger 1 (Band 3)," *Journal of Biological Chemistry*, vol. 278, no. 52, pp. 52551–52558, 2003.

[10] M. M. B. Kay, G. J. Bosman, S. S. Shapiro, A. Bendich, and P. S. Bassel, "Oxidation as a possible mechanism of cellular aging: vitamin E deficiency causes premature aging and IgG binding to erythrocytes," *Proceedings of the National Academy of Sciences of the United States of America*, vol. 83, no. 8, pp. 2463–2467, 1986.

[11] D. Mandal, P. K. Moitra, S. Saha, and J. Basu, "Caspase 3 regulates phosphatidylserine externalization and phagocytosis of oxidatively stressed erythrocytes," *FEBS Letters*, vol. 513, no. 2-3, pp. 184–188, 2002.

[12] M. E. Reyland, "Protein kinase C isoforms: multi-functional regulators of cell life and death," *Frontiers in Bioscience*, vol. 14, no. 6, pp. 2386–2399, 2009.

[13] P. J. Parker and J. Murray-Rust, "PKC at a glance," *Journal of Cell Science*, vol. 117, no. 2, pp. 131–132, 2004.

[14] R. B. Govekar and S. M. Zingde, "Protein kinase C isoforms in human erythrocytes," *Annals of Hematology*, vol. 80, no. 9, pp. 531–534, 2001.

[15] J. T. Dodge, C. Mitchell, and D. J. Hanahan, "The preparation and chemical characteristics of hemoglobin-free ghosts of human erythrocytes," *Archives of Biochemistry and Biophysics*, vol. 100, no. 1, pp. 119–130, 1963.

[16] G. L. Peterson, "A simplification of the protein assay method of Lowry et al. Which is more generally applicable," *Analytical Biochemistry*, vol. 83, no. 2, pp. 346–356, 1977.

[17] H. Towbin, T. Staehelin, and J. Gordon, "Electrophoretic transfer of proteins from polyacrylamide gels to nitrocellulose sheets: procedure and some applications," *Proceedings of the National Academy of Sciences of the United States of America*, vol. 76, no. 9, pp. 4350–4354, 1979.

[18] K. De Jong, M. P. Rettig, P. S. Low, and F. A. Kuypers, "Protein kinase C activation induces phosphatidylserine exposure on red blood cells," *Biochemistry*, vol. 41, no. 41, pp. 12562–12567, 2002.

[19] B. A. Klarl, P. A. Lang, D. S. Kempe et al., "Protein kinase C mediates erythrocyte "programmed cell death" following glucose depletion," *American Journal of Physiology*, vol. 290, no. 1, pp. C244–C253, 2006.

[20] D. B. Nguyen, L. Wagner-Britz, and S. Maia, "Regulation of phosphatidylserine exposure in red blood cells," *Cellular Physiology and Biochemistry*, vol. 28, pp. 847–856, 2011.

[21] M. Gschwendt, H. J. Muller, K. Kielbassa et al., "Rottlerin, a novel protein kinase inhibitor," *Biochemical and Biophysical Research Communications*, vol. 199, no. 1, pp. 93–98, 1994.

[22] G. Martiny-Baron, M. G. Kazanietz, H. Mischak et al., "Selective inhibition of protein kinase C isozymes by the indolocarbazole Gö 6976," *Journal of Biological Chemistry*, vol. 268, no. 13, pp. 9194–9197, 1993.

[23] H. K. Jindal, Z. Ai, P. Gascard, C. Horton, and C. M. Cohen, "Specific loss of protein kinase activities in senescent erythrocytes," *Blood*, vol. 88, no. 4, pp. 1479–1487, 1996.

[24] J. Liu, E. Someren, A. Mentink et al., "The effect of PKC activation and inhibition on osteogenic differentiation of human mesenchymal stem cells," *Journal of Tissue Engineering and Regenerative Medicine*, vol. 4, no. 5, pp. 329–339, 2010.

[25] P. J. Parker, L. Bosca, L. Dekker, N. T. Goode, N. Hajibagheri, and G. Hansra, "Protein kinase C (PKC)-induced PKC degradation: a model for down-regulation," *Biochemical Society Transactions*, vol. 23, no. 1, pp. 153–155, 1995.

15

Targeting the Fanconi Anemia Pathway to Identify Tailored Anticancer Therapeutics

Chelsea Jenkins, Jenny Kan, and Maureen E. Hoatlin

Department of Biochemistry and Molecular Biology, Oregon Health and Science University, 3181 SW Sam Jackson Parkway, Portland, OR 97239, USA

Correspondence should be addressed to Maureen E. Hoatlin, hoatlinm@gmail.com

Academic Editor: Henri J. Van De Vrugt

The Fanconi Anemia (FA) pathway consists of proteins involved in repairing DNA damage, including interstrand cross-links (ICLs). The pathway contains an upstream multiprotein core complex that mediates the monoubiquitylation of the FANCD2 and FANCI heterodimer, and a downstream pathway that converges with a larger network of proteins with roles in homologous recombination and other DNA repair pathways. Selective killing of cancer cells with an intact FA pathway but deficient in certain other DNA repair pathways is an emerging approach to tailored cancer therapy. Inhibiting the FA pathway becomes selectively lethal when certain repair genes are defective, such as the checkpoint kinase ATM. Inhibiting the FA pathway in ATM deficient cells can be achieved with small molecule inhibitors, suggesting that new cancer therapeutics could be developed by identifying FA pathway inhibitors to treat cancers that contain defects that are synthetic lethal with FA.

1. Introduction

Fanconi anemia is a rare genetic disease featuring characteristic developmental abnormalities, a progressive pancytopenia, genomic instability, and predisposition to cancer [1, 2]. The FA pathway contains a multiprotein core complex, including at least twelve proteins that are required for the monoubiquitylation of the FANCD2/FANCI protein complex and for other functions that are not well understood [3–6]. The core complex includes the Fanconi proteins FANCA, FANCB, FANCC, FANCE, FANCF, FANCG, FANCL, and FANCM. At least five additional proteins are associated with the FA core complex, including FAAP100, FAAP24, FAAP20, and the histone fold dimer MHF1/MHF2 [1, 4, 7–10]. The core complex proteins function together as an E3 ubiquitin ligase assembly to monoubiquitylate the heterodimeric FANCI/FANCD2 (ID) complex. The monoubiquitylation of FANCD2 is a surrogate marker for the function of the FA pathway [11]. USP1 and its binding partner UAF1 regulate the deubiquitination of FANCD2 [12]. The breast cancer susceptibility and Fanconi proteins FANCD1/BRCA2, the partner of BRCA2 (PALB2/FANCN), a helicase associated with BRCA1 (FANCJ/BACH1), and several newly identified components including FAN1, FANCO/RAD51C, and FANCP/SLX4 [13–17] participate in the pathway to respond to and repair DNA damage (for review, see [5]).

Although FA is rare, understanding the functional role of the FA proteins in context with other DNA damage response pathways will provide broader opportunities for new cancer therapeutics. Two general strategies could accomplish this, as illustrated in Figure 1: inhibiting the FA pathway in tumor cells to sensitize them to cross-linking agents, or by exploiting synthetic lethal relationships. The latter approach depends on inhibiting the FA pathway in tumor cells that are defective for a secondary pathway required for survival in the absence of the FA pathway.

2. Chemosensitizing and Resensitizing Tumor Cells

A defining characteristic of FA cells is hypersensitivity to cross-linking agents, such as the chemotherapeutic agent cisplatin [2, 5]. Cisplatin (and other platinum-based

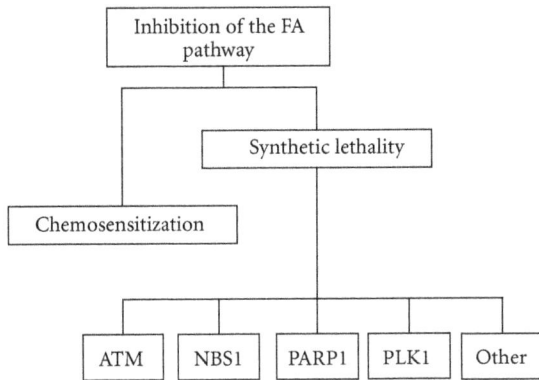

FIGURE 1: Inhibition of the FA pathway. Strategy for selectively targeting tumor cells by inhibition of the FA pathway by (a) chemo-sensitization to cross-linking agents or by (b) exploiting specific synthetic lethal interactions.

compounds) has been used as a chemotherapeutic drug for over 30 years (for review see [18]). The toxicity of platinum-based chemotherapy (nephrotoxicity, neurotoxicity, and ototoxicity) and development of cisplatin resistance are limitations of the therapy [18–20]. Once inside the cell, cisplatin enters the nucleus and forms covalent DNA inter-strand cross-links via platinum-DNA adducts. These cross-links block ongoing DNA replication, and in the absence of repair, activate apoptotic pathways [18, 19]. A functional FA pathway is required for processing damage after exposure to cisplatin and other crosslinking agents, and is at least partially responsible for resistance to cisplatin. Cell-free and cell-based assays have identified inhibitors of the FA pathway, and some of these inhibitors can resensitize platinum-resistant tumors and cell lines [19, 21, 22]. Further efforts to identify small molecule compounds that specifically inhibit the FA pathway could lead to improved resensitization from treatment-induced resistance.

3. Exploiting Synthetic Lethal Interactions

In addition to sensitization, inhibiting the FA pathway may be an effective strategy to exploit synthetic lethal interactions aimed at improving targeted killing of tumor cells. Current approaches in cancer treatment are generally not selective, affecting both cancer cells and normal cells. However, inactivation of DNA repair pathways, an event that occurs frequently during tumor development [23], can make cancer cells overdependent on a reduced set of DNA repair pathways for survival. There is new evidence that targeting the remaining functional pathways by using a synthetic lethal approach can be useful for single-agent and combination therapies in such tumors. Two genes have a synthetic lethal relationship if mutants for either gene are viable but simultaneous mutations are lethal [20]. A successful example of this approach is specific targeting of BRCA-deficient tumors with PARP (poly (ADP-ribose) polymerase) inhibitors [24].

4. Defects in Homologous Recombination and Sensitivity to PARP Inhibitors

Defects in HR repair can result in an overreliance on the protein PARP1, which is responsible for repair of DNA single strand breaks by the base excision repair pathway. Unrepaired single-strand breaks are converted to double-strand breaks during replication and must be repaired by HR [25–27]. Thus, treating cells that are defective in HR with PARP inhibitors results in a targeted killing of the defective cells, while cells with intact HR are capable of repair. Defects in breast cancer susceptibility proteins BRCA1 and BRCA2 (FANCD1) result in HR defects [28]. Clinical trials investigating the effectiveness of PARP inhibitors against recurrent ovarian cancer have been promising, but rigorous stratification of tumors for HR status or "BRCA-ness" (defects in HR) is needed to identify the patients who are likely to benefit [29–31]. Future clinical trials with PARP1 inhibitors in breast cancer may require combination therapies, evaluation of resistance, and identification of non-BRCA biomarkers [32].

PARP1 Inhibition has also been shown to be selectively toxic to ATM-defective tumor cell lines *in vitro* and to increase radiosensitivity of other ATM-proficient cell lines, including nonsmall-cell lung cancer, medulloblastoma, ependymoma, and high-grade gliomas [33–35]. In addition, cell lines lacking functional Mre11 are sensitive to PARP1 inhibitors, strengthening the case for combined use of PARP1 inhibitors with inhibitors of the FA pathway [36, 37].

PTEN (phosphatase and tensin homolog) is a tumor-suppressor gene and one of the most commonly mutated genes in human tumor cells [38, 39] (see Figure 2). PTEN deficiency results in decreased expression of RAD51, which is required for homologous recombination [38, 40]. PTEN deficient tumors are thus candidates for targeted therapy by PARP1 inhibition [36, 38]. Although approximately 470,000 (48%) of 977,628 newly diagnosed cancers each year in the US may have PTEN defects, only a subset of these cancers will have PTEN mutations that result in homologous recombination defects and sensitivity to PARP inhibitors [28, 39, 41–51]. Current studies are aimed at determining the relationship between PTEN loss, RAD51 expression, and PARP1 inhibitor sensitivity [36]. Efforts to asses HR status to establish which PTEN mutations lead to an HR defect, and determining under what circumstances RAD51 expression could be used as a biomarker, will be useful to stratify and predict PARP1 inhibitor sensitivity.

Synthetic lethal interactions with the FA pathway have been explored. An siRNA-based screen of cells deficient in the Fanconi core complex protein, FANCG, showed that ATM, PARP1, NBS1, and PLK1 were among the genes with a synthetic lethal interaction [52] (see Table 1). The FA-ATM synthetic lethal relationship is particularly interesting since ATM deficiency has been reported in a subset of patients with hematological malignancies, including mantle cell lymphoma, chronic lymphocytic leukemia, and acute lymphoblastic leukemia [53, 54], making these potential targets for treatment with FA pathway inhibitors (see Table 2).

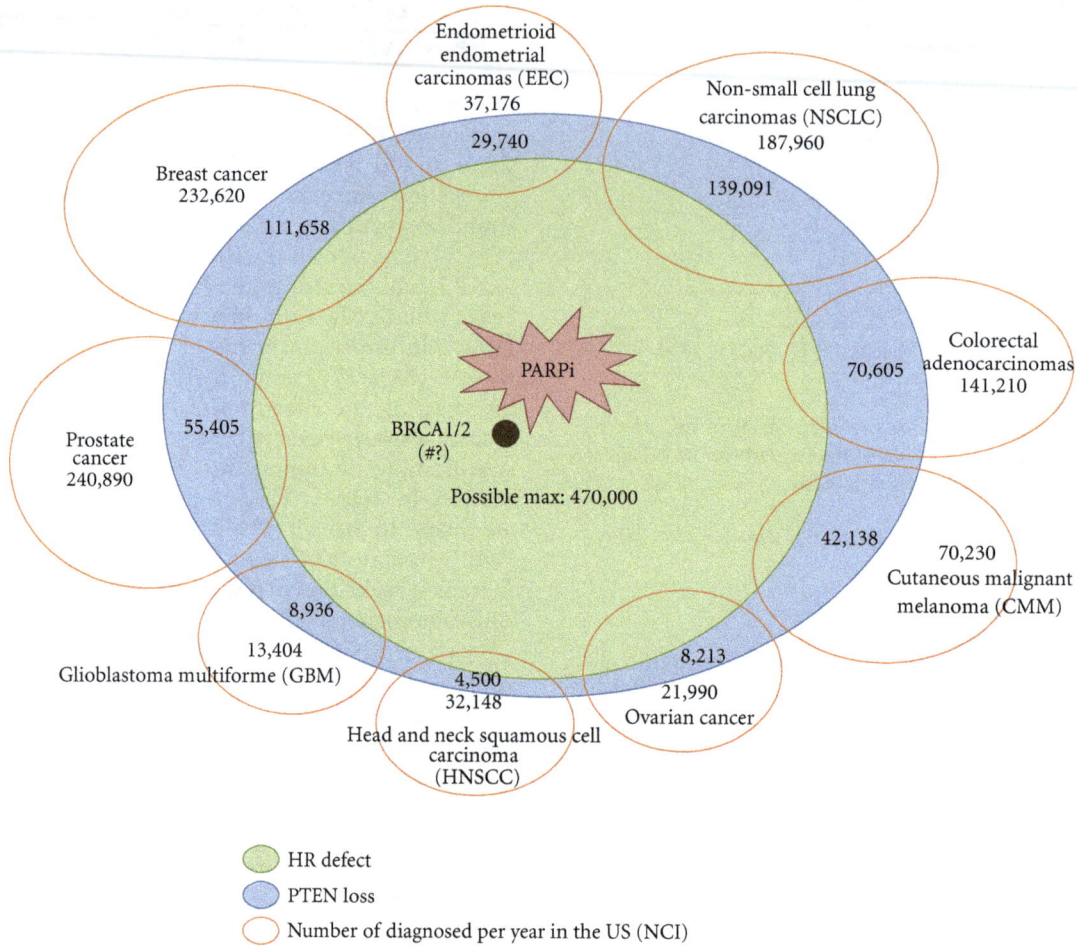

FIGURE 2: PTEN defects in cancers. Types of cancer diagnosed annually in the US (orange oval), with the estimates for PTEN deficiencies shown in each type (blue oval). An unknown percentage of tumors with PTEN deficiencies will have a defect in homologous recombination (HR) repair, predicting sensitivity to treatment with PARP1 inhibitors (green oval).

TABLE 1: Function and expression of genes synthetically lethal with FA.

Gene synthetically lethal with FA genes	Function	Expression in tumor cells
TREX2 [52]	DNA exonuclease; SAGA complex pathway	Expressed in most tumor cell lines [60]
PARP1 [52]	BER	Overexpressed in tumors, including medulloblastoma, ependymoma, HGG, melanoma, and breast cancers [35, 61–63]
PLK1 [52]	Cell-cycle progression	Over-expressed in many human tumors [64]
RAD6/HR6B [52]	Switching of DNA polymerases	Upregulated in metastatic mammary tumors [65]
CDK7 [52]	Transcription	Moderately over-expressed in tumor cell lines [66]
TP53BP1 [52]	DSB sensing; ATM activation	Underexpressed in most cases of triple negative breast cancer [67]
ATM [52]	DSB response kinase	Under-expressed in some tumors, see Figure 3
NEIL1 [52]	BER	Expression reduced in 46% of gastric cancers [68]
RAD54B [52]	HR	Known to be mutated in cancer cell lines [69, 70]
NBS1 [52]	DSB sensing; ATM activation	Over-expressed in HNSCC tumors [71]
ADH5 [6]	Formaldehyde processing	Reduced expression in melanoma cells [72]

TABLE 2: ATM-deficiency in cancer.

Malignancy	ATM-deficient cell lines/number tested
T-cell prolymphocytic leukemia [73]	17/32
Mantle cell lymphoma [53]	12/28
Rhabdomyosarcoma [74]	7/17
Chronic lymphoblastic leukemia [54, 73]	16/50, 38/111
BRCA1-negative breast cancer [75]	12/36
BRCA2 negative breast cancer [75]	12/40
Acute lymphoblastic leukemia [54]	4/15
Non-BRCA1/BRCA2 negative breast cancers [75]	118/1106
Other lymphomas [53]	10/97

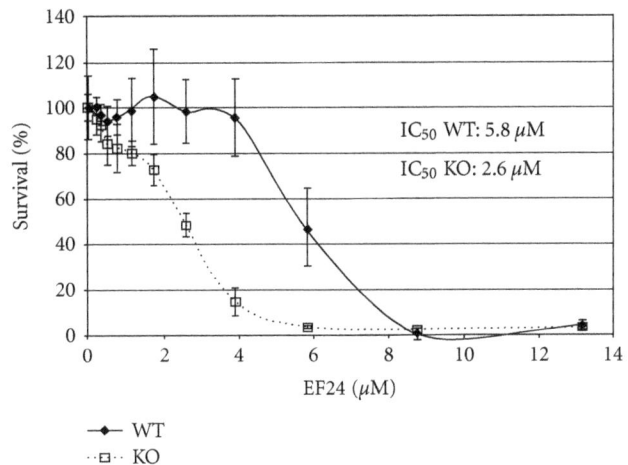

FIGURE 3: EF24 is selectively toxic to ATM-deficient cells [57]. 309ATM-deficient and 334ATM wild type cells were treated with the FA pathway inhibitor EF24. Cell viability was measured after 3 days by MTS assay. Each point represents the mean of 3 repeats. Error bars represent standard deviation.

5. Inhibiting the FA Pathway

Inhibition of the FA pathway could occur at any point in the multistep FA protein network, but a key predictive readout for FA function and resistance to ICLs is the monoubiquitylation of FANCD2 [11, 55]. Several inhibitors of FANCD2 monoubiquitylation have been identified including proteasome inhibitors bortezomib and MG132, curcumin, and the curcumin analogs EF24 and 4H-TTD [19, 22, 56, 57]. Curcumin, a natural product derived from turmeric, was identified as a weak inhibitor of FANCD2 monoubiquitylation in a cell-based screen [19]. We developed a cell-free assay in *Xenopus* egg extracts to screen small molecules for stronger and more specific inhibitors of FANCD2 monoubiquitylation. Unlike cell-based screening assays for small molecules capable of inhibiting the FA pathway, the cell-free method uncouples FANCD2 monoubiquitylation from DNA replication, thus focusing more specifically on the key biochemical steps in a soluble context enriched for nuclear proteins and capable of full genomic replication [22]. Screening in egg extracts identified 4H-TTD, a compound with structural similarity to curcumin as an inhibitor, and this inhibitory effect was verified in human cells [22, 57]. A series of curcumin analogs were also tested, including EF24, a potent monoketone analog of curcumin [58, 59]. The prediction that an FA inhibitor would selectively kill ATM-deficient cells was tested in cell-based assays for synthetic lethality in ATM-proficient and ATM-deficient cells. ATM-deficient cells treated with EF24 demonstrated an increased sensitivity compared to ATM wt cells (see Figure 3) [22, 57]. The increased lethality in ATM-deficient cells provides evidence for future synthetic lethal approaches with FA pathway inhibitors in the treatment of ATM-deficient tumors, and other tumors with deficiencies in genes that are synthetically lethal with FA (see Table 1) [6, 52].

6. Conclusion and Future Directions

Understanding how the Fanconi anemia pathway functions in concert with other DNA damage response networks is essential for understanding genomic stability and for exploiting synthetic lethality for new cancer treatments. New chemotherapeutic agents could be developed by identifying potent and specific inhibitors of the FA pathway, for example, by screening for compounds that inhibit key FA pathway steps (e.g., monoubiquitylation and deubiquitylation of FANCD2/FANCI). While a long-term defect in the function of the FA pathway would result in genomic instability, short-term inhibition could provide a treatment strategy for tumors with deficiencies in certain other DNA repair pathways. Stringent identification of additional genes with synthetic lethal relationships with the FA pathway, and identification of malignancies with deficiencies or mutations in genes that are synthetic lethal with FA will be required for these tailored therapeutic approaches.

Acknowledgments

This work was supported in part by funds from the Medical Research Fund of Oregon.

References

[1] W. Wang, "Emergence of a DNA-damage response network consisting of Fanconi anaemia and BRCA proteins," *Nature Reviews Genetics*, vol. 8, no. 10, pp. 735–748, 2007.

[2] J. P. de Winter and H. Joenje, "The genetic and molecular basis of Fanconi anemia," *Mutation Research*, vol. 668, no. 1-2, pp. 11–19, 2009.

[3] H. Takata, Y. Tanaka, and A. Matsuura, "Late S phase-specific recruitment of Mre11 complex triggers hierarchical assembly of telomere replication proteins in Saccharomyces cerevisiae," *Molecular Cell*, vol. 17, no. 4, pp. 573–583, 2005.

[4] Z. Yan, M. Delannoy, C. Ling et al., "A histone-fold complex and FANCM form a conserved DNA-remodeling complex to maintain genome stability," *Molecular Cell*, vol. 37, no. 6, pp. 865–878, 2010.

[5] H. Kitao and M. Takata, "Fanconi anemia: a disorder defective in the DNA damage response," *International Journal of Hematology*, vol. 93, no. 4, pp. 417–424, 2011.

[6] I.V. Rosado, F. Langevin, G. P. Crossan et al., "Formaldehyde catabolism is essential in cells deficient for the Fanconi anemia DNA-repair pathway," *Nature Structural & Molecular Biology*, vol. 18, no. 12, pp. 1432–1434, 2011.

[7] A. Ciccia, C. Ling, R. Coulthard et al., "Identification of FAAP24, a Fanconi Anemia core complex protein that interacts with FANCM," *Molecular Cell*, vol. 25, no. 3, pp. 331–343, 2007.

[8] C. Ling, M. Ishiai, A. M. Ali et al., "FAAP100 is essential for activation of the Fanconi anemia-associated DNA damage response pathway," *EMBO Journal*, vol. 26, no. 8, pp. 2104–2114, 2007.

[9] A. M. Ali, P. A. Singh, T. R. Singh et al., "FAAP20: a novel ubiquitin-binding FA nuclear core complex protein required for functional integrity of the FA-BRCA DNA repair pathway," *Blood*, vol. 119, no. 14, pp. 3285–3294, 2012.

[10] H. Kim, K. Yang, D. Dejsuphong, and A. D. D'Andrea, "Regulation of Rev1 by the Fanconi anemia core complex," *Nature Structural and Molecular Biology*, vol. 19, no. 2, pp. 164–170, 2012.

[11] A. Shimamura, R. M. De Oca, J. L. Svenson et al., "A novel diagnostic screen for defects in the Fanconi anemia pathway," *Blood*, vol. 100, no. 13, pp. 4649–4654, 2002.

[12] K. Yang, G. L. Moldovan, P. Vinciguerra, J. Murai, S. Takeda, and A. D. D'Andrea, "Regulation of the Fanconi anemia pathway by a SUMO-like delivery network," *Genes and Development*, vol. 25, no. 17, pp. 1847–1858, 2011.

[13] A. Smogorzewska, R. Desetty, T. T. Saito et al., "A Genetic screen identifies FAN1, a Fanconi Anemia-associated nuclease necessary for DNA interstrand crosslink repair," *Molecular Cell*, vol. 39, no. 1, pp. 36–47, 2010.

[14] C. MacKay, A. C. Déclais, C. Lundin et al., "Identification of KIAA1018/FAN1, a DNA repair nuclease recruited to DNA damage by monoubiquitinated FANCD2," *Cell*, vol. 142, no. 1, pp. 65–76, 2010.

[15] T. Liu, G. Ghosal, J. Yuan, J. Chen, and J. Huang, "FAN1 acts with FANCI-FANCD2 to promote DNA interstrand cross-link repair," *Science*, vol. 329, no. 5992, pp. 693–696, 2010.

[16] K. Kratz, B. Schöpf, S. Kaden et al., "Deficiency of FANCD2-associated nuclease KIAA1018/FAN1 sensitizes cells to interstrand crosslinking agents," *Cell*, vol. 142, no. 1, pp. 77–88, 2010.

[17] R. D. Shereda, Y. Machida, and Y. J. Machida, "Human KIAA1018/FAN1 localizes to stalled replication forks via its ubiquitin-binding domain," *Cell Cycle*, vol. 9, no. 19, pp. 3977–3983, 2010.

[18] Y. Jung and S. J. Lippard, "Direct cellular responses to platinum-induced DNA damage," *Chemical Reviews*, vol. 107, no. 5, pp. 1387–1407, 2007.

[19] D. Chirnomas, T. Taniguchi, M. De La Vega et al., "Chemosensitization to cisplatin by inhibitors of the Fanconi anemia/BRCA pathway," *Molecular Cancer Therapeutics*, vol. 5, no. 4, pp. 952–961, 2006.

[20] T. Helleday, E. Petermann, C. Lundin, B. Hodgson, and R. A. Sharma, "DNA repair pathways as targets for cancer therapy," *Nature Reviews Cancer*, vol. 8, no. 3, pp. 193–204, 2008.

[21] T. Taniguchi, M. Tischkowitz, N. Ameziane et al., "Disruption of the Fanconi anemia-BRCA pathway in cisplatin-sensitive ovarian tumors," *Nature Medicine*, vol. 9, no. 5, pp. 568–574, 2003.

[22] I. Landais, A. Sobeck, S. Stone et al., "A novel cell-free screen identifies a potent inhibitor of the fanconi anemia pathway," *International Journal of Cancer*, vol. 124, no. 4, pp. 783–792, 2009.

[23] R. Rai, G. Peng, K. Li, and S. Y. Lin, "DNA damage response: the players, the network and the role in tumor suppression," *Cancer Genomics and Proteomics*, vol. 4, no. 2, pp. 99–106, 2007.

[24] P. C. Fong, D. S. Boss, T. A. Yap et al., "Inhibition of poly(ADP-ribose) polymerase in tumors from BRCA mutation carriers," *New England Journal of Medicine*, vol. 361, no. 2, pp. 123–134, 2009.

[25] T. Helleday, H. E. Bryant, and N. Schultz, "Poly(ADP-ribose) polymerase (PARP-1) in homologous recombination and as a target for cancer therapy," *Cell Cycle*, vol. 4, no. 9, pp. 1176–1178, 2005.

[26] C. J. Lord, S. McDonald, S. Swift, N. C. Turner, and A. Ashworth, "A high-throughput RNA interference screen for DNA repair determinants of PARP inhibitor sensitivity," *DNA Repair*, vol. 7, no. 12, pp. 2010–2019, 2008.

[27] M. K. Weil and A. P. Chen, "PARP inhibitor treatment in ovarian and breast cancer," *Current Problems in Cancer*, vol. 35, no. 1, pp. 7–50, 2011.

[28] K. J. Dedes, P. M. Wilkerson, D. Wetterskog, B. Weigelt, A. Ashworth, and J. S. Reis-Filho, "Synthetic lethality of PARP inhibition in cancers lacking BRCA1 and BRCA2 mutations," *Cell Cycle*, vol. 10, no. 8, pp. 1192–1199, 2011.

[29] W. Z. Wysham, P. Mhawech-Fauceglia, H. Li et al., "BRCAness profile of sporadic ovarian cancer predicts disease recurrence," *PLoS One*, vol. 7, no. 1, article e30042, 2012.

[30] S. B. Kaye, J. Lubinski, U. Matulonis et al., "Phase II, open-label, randomized, multicenter study comparing the efficacy and safety of olaparib, a poly (ADP-ribose) polymerase inhibitor, and pegylated liposomal doxorubicin in patients with BRCA1 or BRCA2 mutations and recurrent ovarian cancer," *Journal of Clinical Oncology*, vol. 30, no. 4, pp. 372–379, 2012.

[31] C. Sessa, "Update on PARP1 inhibitors in ovarian cancer," *Annals of Oncology*, vol. 22, supplement 8, pp. viii72–viii76, 2011.

[32] M. Guha, "PARP inhibitors stumble in breast cancer," *Nature Biotechnology*, vol. 29, no. 5, pp. 373–374, 2011.

[33] V. J. Weston, C. E. Oldreive, A. Skowronska et al., "The PARP inhibitor olaparib induces significant killing of ATM-deficientlymphoid tumor cells in vitro and in vivo," *Blood*, vol. 116, no. 22, pp. 4578–4587, 2010.

[34] J. M. Senra, B. A. Telfer, K. E. Cherry et al., "Inhibition of PARP-1 by olaparib (AZD2281) increases the radiosensitivity of a lung tumor xenograft," *Molecular Cancer Therapeutics*, vol. 10, no. 10, pp. 1949–1958, 2011.

[35] D. G. van Vuurden, E. Hulleman, O. L. M. Meijer et al., "PARP inhibition sensitizes childhood high grade glioma, medulloblastoma and ependymoma to radiation," *Oncotarget*, vol. 2, no. 12, pp. 984–996, 2011.

[36] M. Fraser, H. Zhao, K. R. Luoto et al., "PTEN deletion in prostate cancer cells does not associate with loss of RAD51 function: implications for radiotherapy and chemotherapy," *Clinical Cancer Research*, vol. 18, no. 4, pp. 1015–1027, 2012.

[37] P. Pichierri, D. Averbeck, and F. Rosselli, "DNA cross-link-dependent RAD50/MRE11/NBS1 subnuclear assembly requires the Fanconi anemia C protein," *Human Molecular Genetics*, vol. 11, no. 21, pp. 2531–2546, 2002.

[38] A. M. Mendes-Pereira, S. A. Martin, R. Brough et al., "Synthetic lethal targeting of PTEN mutant cells with PARP

inhibitors," *EMBO Molecular Medicine*, vol. 1, no. 6-7, pp. 315–322, 2009.

[39] L. Salmena, A. Carracedo, and P. P. Pandolfi, "Tenets of PTEN tumor suppression," *Cell*, vol. 133, no. 3, pp. 403–414, 2008.

[40] W. H. Shen, A. S. Balajee, J. Wang et al., "Essential role for nuclear PTEN in maintaining chromosomal integrity," *Cell*, vol. 128, no. 1, pp. 157–170, 2007.

[41] G. L. Mutter, M. C. Lin, J. T. Fitzgerald et al., "Altered PTEN expression as a diagnostic marker for the earliest endometrial precancers," *Journal of the National Cancer Institute*, vol. 92, no. 11, pp. 924–931, 2000.

[42] C. J. Marsit, S. Zheng, K. Aldape et al., "PTEN expression in non-small-cell lung cancer: evaluating its relation to tumor characteristics, allelic loss, and epigenetic alteration," *Human Pathology*, vol. 36, no. 7, pp. 768–776, 2005.

[43] J. G. Paez, P. A. Jänne, J. C. Lee et al., "EGFR mutations in lung, cancer: correlation with clinical response to gefitinib therapy," *Science*, vol. 304, no. 5676, pp. 1497–1500, 2004.

[44] K. S. Jang, Y. S. Song, S. H. Jang et al., "Clinicopathological significance of nuclear PTEN expression in colorectal adenocarcinoma," *Histopathology*, vol. 56, no. 2, pp. 229–239, 2010.

[45] C. Darido, S. R. Georgy, T. Wilanowski et al., "Targeting of the tumor suppressor GRHL3 by a miR-21-dependent proto-oncogenic network results in PTEN loss and tumorigenesis," *Cancer Cell*, vol. 20, no. 5, pp. 635–648, 2011.

[46] J. M. Garcia Pedrero, D. Garcia Carracedo, C. Muñoz Pinto et al., "Frequent genetic and biochemical alterations of the PI 3-K/AKT/PTEN pathway in head and neck squamous cell carcinoma," *International Journal of Cancer*, vol. 114, no. 2, pp. 242–248, 2005.

[47] Y. Wang, G. B. Kristensen, A. Helland, J. M. Nesland, A. L. Børresen-Dale, and R. Holm, "Protein expression and prognostic value of genes in the erb-b signaling pathway in advanced ovarian carcinomas," *American Journal of Clinical Pathology*, vol. 124, no. 3, pp. 392–401, 2005.

[48] H. Tsao, M. C. Mihm, and C. Sheehan, "PTEN expression in normal skin, acquired melanocytic nevi, and cutaneous melanoma," *Journal of the American Academy of Dermatology*, vol. 49, no. 5, pp. 865–872, 2003.

[49] L. Li, A. Dutra, E. Pak et al., "EGFRvIII expression and PTEN loss synergistically induce chromosomal instability and glial tumors," *Neuro-Oncology*, vol. 11, no. 1, pp. 9–21, 2009.

[50] J. Yang, Y. Ren, L. Wang et al., "PTEN mutation spectrum in breast cancers and breast hyperplasia," *Journal of Cancer Research and Clinical Oncology*, vol. 136, no. 9, pp. 1303–1311, 2010.

[51] M. Schmitz, G. Grignard, C. Margue et al., "Complete loss of PTEN expression as a possible early prognostic marker for prostate cancer metastasis," *International Journal of Cancer*, vol. 120, no. 6, pp. 1284–1292, 2007.

[52] R. D. Kennedy, C. C. Chen, P. Stuckert et al., "Fanconi anemia pathway-deficient tumor cells are hypersensitive to inhibition of ataxia telangiectasia mutated," *Journal of Clinical Investigation*, vol. 117, no. 5, pp. 1440–1449, 2007.

[53] N. Y. Fang, T. C. Greiner, D. D. Weisenburger et al., "Oligonucleotide microarrays demonstrate the highest frequency of ATM mutations in the mantle cell subtype of lymphoma," *Proceedings of the National Academy of Sciences of the United States of America*, vol. 100, no. 9, pp. 5372–5377, 2003.

[54] M. A. Haidar, H. Kantarjian, T. Manshouri et al., "ATM gene deletion in patients with adult acute lymphoblastic leukemia," *Cancer*, vol. 88, no. 5, pp. 1057–1062, 2000.

[55] I. Garcia-Higuera, T. Taniguchi, S. Ganesan et al., "Interaction of the Fanconi anemia proteins and BRCA1 in a common pathway," *Molecular Cell*, vol. 7, no. 2, pp. 249–262, 2001.

[56] C. Jacquemont and T. Taniguchi, "Proteasome function is required for DNA damage response and fanconi anemia pathway activation," *Cancer Research*, vol. 67, no. 15, pp. 7395–7405, 2007.

[57] I. Landais, S. Hiddingh, M. McCarroll et al., "Monoketone analogs of curcumin, a new class of Fanconi anemia pathway inhibitors," *Molecular Cancer*, vol. 8, article 133, 2009.

[58] B. K. Adams, J. Cai, J. Armstrong et al., "EF24, a novel synthetic curcumin analog, induces apoptosis in cancer cells via a redox-dependent mechanism," *Anti-Cancer Drugs*, vol. 16, no. 3, pp. 263–275, 2005.

[59] B. K. Adams, E. M. Ferstl, M. C. Davis et al., "Synthesis and biological evaluation of novel curcumin analogs as anti-cancer and anti-angiogenesis agents," *Bioorganic and Medicinal Chemistry*, vol. 12, no. 14, pp. 3871–3883, 2004.

[60] M. J. Chen, L. C. Dumitrache, D. Wangsa et al., "Cisplatin depletes TREX2 and causes robertsonian translocations as seen in TREX2 knockout cells," *Cancer Research*, vol. 67, no. 19, pp. 9077–9083, 2007.

[61] J. Pizem, M. Popovic, and A. Cör, "Expression of Gli1 and PARP1 in medulloblastoma: an immunohistochemical study of 65 cases," *Journal of Neuro-Oncology*, vol. 103, no. 3, pp. 459–467, 2011.

[62] V. N. Barton, A. M. Donson, B. K. Kleinschmidt-DeMasters, L. Gore, A. K. Liu, and N. K. Foreman, "PARP1 expression in pediatric central nervous system tumors," *Pediatric Blood and Cancer*, vol. 53, no. 7, pp. 1227–1230, 2009.

[63] P. Domagala, T. Huzarski, J. Lubinski, K. Gugala, and W. Domagala, "PARP-1 expression in breast cancer including BRCA1-associated, triple negative and basal-like tumors: possible implications for PARP-1 inhibitor therapy," *Breast Cancer Research and Treatment*, vol. 127, no. 3, pp. 861–869, 2011.

[64] X. Liu, M. Lei, and R. L. Erikson, "Normal cells, but not cancer cells, survive severe Plk1 depletion," *Molecular and Cellular Biology*, vol. 26, no. 6, pp. 2093–2108, 2006.

[65] M. P. V. Shekhar, A. Lyakhovich, D. W. Visscher, H. Heng, and N. Kondrat, "Rad6 overexpression induces multinucleation, centrosome amplification, abnormal mitosis, aneuploidy, and transformation," *Cancer Research*, vol. 62, no. 7, pp. 2115–2124, 2002.

[66] J. Bartkova, M. Zemanova, and J. Bartek, "Expression of CDK7/CAK in normal and tumor cells of diverse histogenesis, cell-cycle position and differentiation," *International Journal of Cancer*, vol. 66, no. 6, pp. 732–737, 1996.

[67] P. Bouwman, A. Aly, J. M. Escandell et al., "53BP1 loss rescues BRCA1 deficiency and is associated with triple-negative and BRCA-mutated breast cancers," *Nature Structural and Molecular Biology*, vol. 17, no. 6, pp. 688–695, 2010.

[68] K. Shinmura, H. Tao, M. Goto et al., "Inactivating mutations of the human base excision repair gene NEIL1 in gastric cancer," *Carcinogenesis*, vol. 25, no. 12, pp. 2311–2317, 2004.

[69] T. Hiramoto, T. Nakanishi, T. Sumiyoshi et al., "Mutations of a novel human RAD54 homologue, RAD54B, in primary cancer," *Oncogene*, vol. 18, no. 22, pp. 3422–3426, 1999.

[70] K. J. McManus, I. J. Barrett, Y. Nouhi, and P. Hieter, "Specific synthetic lethal killing of RAD54B-deficient human colorectal cancer cells by FEN1 silencing," *Proceedings of the National Academy of Sciences of the United States of America*, vol. 106, no. 9, pp. 3276–3281, 2009.

[71] M. H. Yang, W. C. Chiang, T. Y. Chou et al., "Increased NBS1 expression is a marker of aggressive head and neck cancer and overexpression of NBS1 contributes to transformation," *Clinical Cancer Research*, vol. 12, no. 2, pp. 507–515, 2006.

[72] T. Shibata, A. Kokubu, M. Miyamoto, Y. Sasajima, and N. Yamazaki, "Mutant IDH1 confers an in vivo growth in a melanoma cell line with BRAF mutation," *American Journal of Pathology*, vol. 178, no. 3, pp. 1395–1402, 2011.

[73] T. Stankovic, G. S. Stewart, C. Fegan et al., "Ataxia telangiectasia mutated-deficient B-cell chronic lymphocytic leukemia occurs in pregerminal center cells and results in defective damage response and unrepaired chromosome damage," *Blood*, vol. 99, no. 1, pp. 300–309, 2002.

[74] P. Zhang, K. S. Bhakta, P. L. Puri, R. O. Newbury, J. R. Feramisco, and J. Y. Wang, "Association of ataxia telangiectasia mutated (ATM) gene mutation/deletion with rhabdomyosarcoma," *Cancer Biology and Therapy*, vol. 2, no. 1, article 2, pp. 87–91, 2003.

[75] J. Tommiska, J. Bartkova, M. Heinonen et al., "The DNA damage signalling kinase ATM is aberrantly reduced or lost in BRCA1/BRCA2-deficient and ER/PR/ERBB2-triple-negative breast cancer," *Oncogene*, vol. 27, no. 17, pp. 2501–2506, 2008.

16

Preoperative Hematocrit Concentration and the Risk of Stroke in Patients Undergoing Isolated Coronary-Artery Bypass Grafting

Khaled M. Musallam,[1,2] Faek R. Jamali,[3] Frits R. Rosendaal,[4] Toby Richards,[5] Donat R. Spahn,[6] Kaivan Khavandi,[7] Iskandar Barakat,[8] Benjamin Demoss,[9] Luca A. Lotta,[2] Flora Peyvandi,[2] and Pier M. Sfeir[3]

[1] Department of Internal Medicine, American University of Beirut Medical Center, P.O. Box 11-0236, Beirut 1107 2020, Lebanon
[2] Angelo Bianchi Bonomi Haemophilia and Thrombosis Center, Department of Medicine and Medical Specialties, IRCCS Ca' Granda Foundation Maggiore Policlinico Hospital, University of Milan, 20122 Milan, Italy
[3] Division of General Surgery, Department of Surgery, American University of Beirut Medical Center, P.O. Box 11-0236, Beirut 1107 2020, Lebanon
[4] Departments of Clinical Epidemiology and Thrombosis & Hemostasis, Leiden University Medical Center, 2333 ZA Leiden, The Netherlands
[5] Division of Surgery and Interventional Science, University College London Hospital, London WC1E 6AU, UK
[6] Institute of Anesthesiology, University Hospital and University of Zurich, 8006 Zurich, Switzerland
[7] King's College London British Heart Foundation Centre, The Rayne Institute, St. Thomas' Hospital, King's Health Partners AHSC, London SE1 7EH, UK
[8] Department of Medicine, Staten Island University Hospital, New York, NY 10305, USA
[9] Department of Internal Medicine, Emory University School of Medicine, Atlanta, GA 30322, USA

Correspondence should be addressed to Pier M. Sfeir; ps04@aub.edu.lb

Academic Editor: Eitan Fibach

Background. Identification and management of risk factors for stroke following isolated coronary artery bypass grafting (CABG) could potentially lower the risk of such serious morbidity. Methods. We retrieved data for 30-day stroke incidence and perioperative variables for patients undergoing isolated CABG and used multivariate logistic regression to assess the adjusted effect of preoperative hematocrit concentration on stroke incidence. Results. In 2,313 patients (mean age 65.9 years, 73.6% men), 43 (1.9%, 95% CI: 1.4–2.5) developed stroke within 30 days following CABG (74.4% within 6 days). After adjustment for a priori defined potential confounders, each 1% drop in preoperative hematocrit concentration was associated with 1.07 (95% CI: 1.01–1.13) increased odds for stroke (men, OR: 1.08, 95% CI: 1.01–1.16; women, OR: 1.02, 95% CI: 0.91–1.16). The predicted probability of stroke for descending preoperative hematocrit concentration exceeded 2% for values <37% (<37% for men (adjusted OR: 2.39, 95% CI: 1.08–5.26) and <38% for women (adjusted OR: 2.52, 95% CI: 0.53–11.98), with a steeper probability increase noted in men). The association between lower preoperative hematocrit concentration and stroke was evident irrespective of intraoperative transfusion use. Conclusion. Screening and management of patients with low preoperative hematocrit concentration may alter postoperative stroke risk in patients undergoing isolated CABG.

1. Introduction

Although mortality rates for patients undergoing isolated coronary-artery bypass grafting (CABG) continue to decline, postoperative neurologic morbidity remains a concern [1]. The short-term incidence of stroke after isolated CABG is close to 2%, although reported risks vary depending on the underlying risk factors of the population under evaluation and the adopted definition of stroke [1]. Knowledge of the mechanisms of the occurrence of stroke in patients undergoing isolated CABG is limited. It was previously assumed that strokes are attributed to the use of extracorporeal cardiopulmonary bypass. However, several studies showed similar stroke rates between patients who undergo off-pump compared with conventional on-pump surgery [2–10]. Thus, efforts to reduce the incidence of stroke now focus on identifying other perioperative and patient-related risk factors. With this background in mind, we used data from the large, multicenter database of the American College of Surgeons National Surgical Quality Improvement Program (ACS NSQIP) to determine the effects of preoperative hematocrit concentration on the incidence of stroke in patients undergoing isolated CABG.

2. Materials and Methods

2.1. Study Design and Sample. This was a cohort study using data from the ACS NSQIP database. Details of the ACS NSQIP (http://www.acsnsqip.org/) have been recently described and are summarized as follows [11].

The American College of Surgeons National Surgical Quality Improvement Program

Aim. The American College of Surgeons National Surgical Quality Improvement Program (ACS NSQIP) was set up as a rigorous data collection tool for outcome measurement. The ACS NSQIP collects data on a variety of clinical variables, including preoperative risk factors, intraoperative variables, and 30-day postoperative mortality and morbidity outcomes for patients undergoing major surgical procedures in both the inpatient and outpatient setting. Using validated statistical tools that were developed and tested in large population-based studies, the ACS NSQIP program generates an expected outcome based on the case complexity mix. The observed outcomes are then compared to the expected outcomes to obtain an O/E ratio and indicate performance of a particular medical center with regards to the national average. This data is then used to identify areas in need of quality improvement.

Participants. Contribution to the ACS NSQIP is on a voluntary basis. Nonveterans hospitals that are interested in quality assurance and outcomes measurement sign-up for inclusion into the ACS NSQIP database and enter cases prospectively into this database. There are currently 289 out of 440 participating sites that are importing data to the ACS NSQIP database, located in 42 states across the US (272 sites), three Canadian provinces (15 sites), Lebanon (1 site) and the UAE (1 site). 52% of the enrolled medical centers are classified as academic/teaching and 48% are nonteaching sites. 45% of participating medical centers have ≥500 beds, 41% have 300–499 beds, 11% have 100–299 beds, and 3% have <100 beds.

Inclusion/Exclusion of Cases. The ACS NSQIP includes all major surgeries as determined by CPT codes. The ACS NSQIP has developed a comprehensive Current Procedural

Terminology (CPT) Code Inclusion List available on the website (http://www.acsnsqip.org/). Excluded cases are the following.

(i) Patients under the age of 16 years (data collected after the year 2008 was for patients over 18 years).

(ii) Cases listed on the CPT Code Exclusion List on the website (http://www.acsnsqip.org/).

(iii) Trauma cases—specifically: a patient who is admitted to the hospital with acute trauma and has surgery(s) for that trauma will be excluded. Any operation performed after the patient has been discharged from the trauma stay will be included.

(iv) Transplant cases—specifically: a patient who is admitted to the hospital for a transplant and has a transplant procedure and any additional surgical procedure during the transplant hospitalization will be excluded. Any operation performed after the patient has been discharged from the transplant stay will be included.

(v) American Society of Anesthesiologists score 6 (brain-death organ donors).

(vi) Concurrent case—an additional operative procedure performed by a different surgical team under the same anesthetic (e.g., coronary artery bypass graft procedure on a patient who is also undergoing a carotid endarterectomy). An assessment is not required on the concurrent procedure; however, this procedure would be reported as "concurrent" in the operative section for the assessed case.

To ensure a diverse surgical case mix, also excluded (at each center) are the following.

(i) More than 3 inguinal herniorrhaphies in an 8-day period.

(ii) More than 3 breast lumpectomies in an 8-day period.

(iii) More than 3 laparoscopic cholecystectomies in an 8-day period.

(iv) If the site is collecting urology cases, more than 3 transurethral resection of the prostate and/or transurethral resection of bladder tumor in an 8-day period.

It is a validated outcomes registry designed to provide feedback to member hospitals on 30-day risk-adjusted surgical mortality and morbidity [12, 13]. The database includes deidentified data on demographics, preoperative risk factors and laboratory tests, intraoperative conditions and occurrences, and 30-day postoperative outcomes for adult patients undergoing major surgery in participating nonveteran's administration hospitals [12]. Trained surgical clinical reviewers collect patient data upon admission from the medical chart, operative log, anesthesia record, interviews with the surgical attending, and telephone interviews with the patient [12]. Data quality is ensured through comprehensive training of the nurse reviewers, an interrater reliability audit of participating sites, regular conference calls, and an annual meeting [14].

For this study, the available ACS NSQIP participant use files of the years 2008 (271,368 patients from 211 sites) and 2009 (336,190 patients from 237 sites) were retrieved for major surgeries performed within various surgical subspecialties at participating ACS NSQIP medical centers in the US, Canada, Lebanon, and UAE. We identified all isolated primary CABG cases using the Current Procedural Terminology (CPT) codes: 33510–33514, 33516–33519, 33521–33523, 33530, and 33533–33536. A total of 2313 patients were identified and included in this study. In accordance with the American University of Beirut's guidelines (which follow the US Code of Federal Regulations for the Protection of Human Subjects), institutional review board approval was not needed or sought for our analysis because data were collected as part of a quality assurance activity.

2.2. Stroke. The ACS NSQIP registers data on stroke occurrence within 30-days of the index operation, which is defined as a focal brain dysfunction lasting ≥ 24 hours from a vascular cause. This definition of stroke encompasses intracranial hemorrhage, but we considered this outcome as a surrogate of ischemic stroke because hemorrhagic strokes make up only 1% of perioperative strokes [15, 16].

2.3. Preoperative Hematocrit Concentration. Retrieved preoperative hematocrit concentration reflected the last hematocrit measurement prior to the index operation. Some 99.9% of the hematocrit levels were obtained within eight weeks of the index surgery, 99.1% were obtained within four weeks and 96.6% were obtained within two weeks.

2.4. Statistical Analysis. Descriptive statistics are presented as means (standard deviation (SD)), medians (interquartile range (IQR)), or percentages. The primary study outcome measure was stroke within 30 days of surgery. We used multivariate logistic regression analysis to retrieve effect estimates (odds ratios (OR) and 95% confidence intervals (CI)) upon adjusting the association between preoperative hematocrit concentration and the outcome of stroke for potential confounders. Models were built by adjusting (Enter method) the determinant variable (preoperative hematocrit concentration) to a priori defined potential confounders of clinical relevance (risk factors that may cause both preoperative hematocrit concentration alterations as well as stroke). Two levels of adjustment were used, Model 1 (OR_{adj-1}) with basic adjustment for the most clinically relevant variables and Model 2 (OR_{adj-2}) with extended adjustment for a larger number of clinically relevant risk factors. Data were near complete, with the exception of missing values for preoperative hematocrit concentration ($n = 18$, 0.7%) and body mass index ($n = 42$, 1.8%) which were imputed by the respective means of similar sex and age groups.

We carried out the data management and analyses using the SAS software version 9.1 (SAS Institute Inc., Cary, NC, USA).

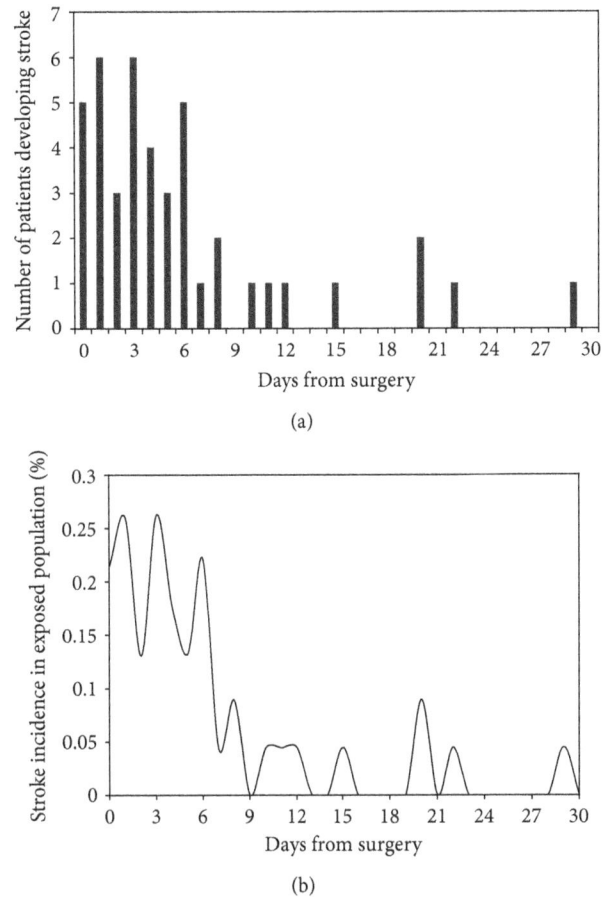

FIGURE 1: (a) Number of patients developing stroke on each day in the 30-day observation period following surgery. (b) Instantaneous stroke incidence per day in the exposed population.

3. Results

A total of 2,313 patients undergoing isolated CABG were included in this analysis. The mean age of the study cohort was 65.9 years (SD: 10.7, range: 25–90) with 1,703 (73.6%) patients being men. The mean preoperative hematocrit concentration was 38.8% (SD: 5.1, range: 12.4–54.9). Forty-three patients developed stroke within 30 days following CABG, corresponding to a 30-day cumulative incidence of 1.9% (95% CI: 1.4–2.5). The median time to development of stroke was 4 days (IQR: 1–7 days, min: same day, max: 29 days), with most patients (74.4%, 95% CI: 59.7–85.0) developing stroke within the first 6 days after surgery (Figure 1). Characteristics of patients who developed and those who did not develop stroke are summarized in Table 1. Patients who developed stroke had a lower mean preoperative hematocrit concentration than those who did not (36.3% versus 38.8%, mean difference: 2.6%, 95% CI: 1.1–4.1).

In an unadjusted analysis, each drop of 1% in preoperative hematocrit concentration (continuous variable) was associated with a 1.09 increased odds of 30-day postoperative stroke (95% CI: 1.04–1.15). The effect was steeper and more certain in men (OR: 1.11, 95% CI: 1.04–1.18) than women (OR: 1.05, 95%

TABLE 1: Patients' characteristics.

Parameter	No stroke $n = 2270$	Stroke $n = 43$
Preoperative hematocrit concentration, mean (SD)	**38.8 (5.1)**	**36.3 (4.9)**
Age in years, mean (SD)	65.9 (10.7)	69.3 (9.2)
Male, n (%)	1,673 (73.7)	30 (69.8)
White race, n (%)	1,866 (82.2)	37 (86.0)
Body mass index $\geq 30\,kg/m^2$, n (%)	974 (42.9)	15 (34.9)
Diabetes, n (%)	831 (36.6)	19 (44.2)
Hypertension, n (%)	1,914 (84.3)	39 (90.7)
Congestive heart failure, n (%)	255 (11.2)	8 (18.6)
Peripheral vascular disease, n (%)	119 (5.2)	2 (4.7)
Currently on dialysis, n (%)	56 (2.5)	4 (9.3)
Current Smoker, n (%)	554 (24.2)	15 (34.9)
Chronic obstructive pulmonary disease, n (%)	237 (10.4)	9 (20.9)
History of transient ischemic attack, n (%)	138 (6.1)	4 (9.3)
History of stroke with neurologic deficit, n (%)	100 (4.4)	4 (9.3)
History of stroke without neurologic deficit, n (%)	91 (4.0)	1 (2.3)
Bleeding disorder, n (%)	366 (16.1)	8 (18.6)
Disseminated cancer, n (%)	3 (0.1)	0 (0.0)
Tumor involving central nervous system, n (%)	1 (0.0)	0 (0.0)

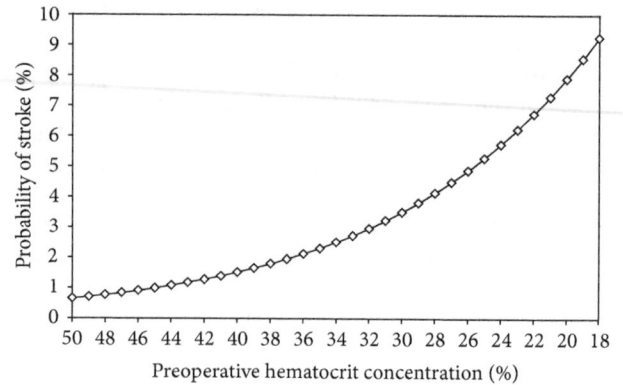

(a)

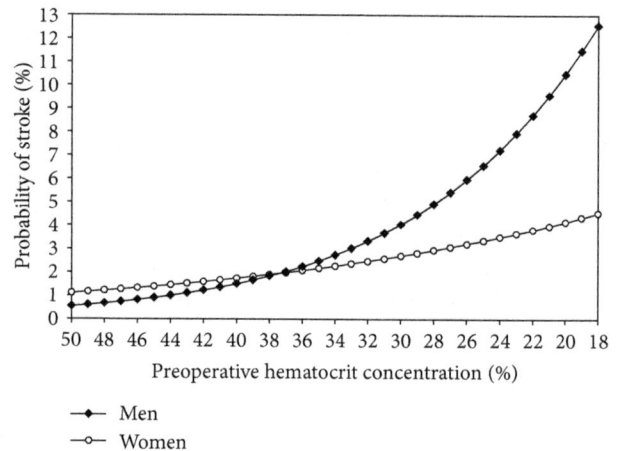

- Men
- Women

(b)

FIGURE 2: Predicted probability of 30-day postoperative stroke as a function of preoperative hematocrit concentration in (a) all patients and (b) men and women.

CI: 0.93–1.17). After adjustment for potential confounders, the effect estimates dropped minimally (OR$_{adj-2}$ 1.07, 95% CI: 1.01–1.13; men, OR$_{adj-2}$: 1.08, 95% CI: 1.01–1.16; women, OR$_{adj-2}$: 1.02, 95% CI: 0.91–1.16) (Table 2).

The predicted probability of stroke for descending preoperative hematocrit concentration values in a clinically relevant range is illustrated in Figure 2(a). The predicted probability of stroke exceeded 2% (cumulative incidence in this study and incidence commonly reported in previous studies) for preoperative hematocrit concentration values <37% (Figure 2(a)). Upon stratification for men and women, the threshold was <37% for men and <38% for women, with a steeper probability increase noted in men beyond the threshold (Figure 2(b)). The adjusted increase in odds of stroke (OR$_{adj-2}$) for men with a preoperative hematocrit concentration <37% compared with ≥37% was 2.39 (95% CI: 1.08–5.26), while the adjusted increase in odds of stroke (OR$_{adj-2}$) for women with a preoperative hematocrit concentration <38% compared with ≥38% was 2.52 (95% CI: 0.53–11.98) (Table 2).

A total of 1,779 (76.9%, 95% CI: 75.2–78.6) patients received intraoperative transfusions (55.1% received 1 or 2 packed red blood cell (pRBC) units and 21.8% received 3 or more pRBC units). The odds of 30-day stroke were more notably increased in patients receiving 3 or more pRBC units (OR: 2.69, 95% CI: 1.04–7.00) than patients receiving 1 or 2 pRBC units (OR: 1.55, 95% CI: 0.62–3.84) when compared to

patients who did not receive intraoperative transfusions. The mean preoperative hematocrit concentration was lower in patients who received 3 or more pRBC units intraoperatively than those who did not (36.1% versus 39.5%, mean difference: 3.4%, 95% CI: 2.9–3.9) (Figure 3(a)). The odds of receiving 3 or more pRBC intraoperatively were 1.14 (95% CI: 1.12–1.17) for each 1% drop in preoperative hematocrit concentration (Figure 3(b)).

The association between preoperative hematocrit concentration (continuous variable) and 30-day postoperative stroke was observed in both patients who received (OR$_{adj-2}$: 1.10, 95% CI: 1.02–1.18) and those who did not receive (OR$_{adj-2}$: 1.04, 95% CI: 1.01–1.08) 3 or more pRBC units intraoperatively, although with higher effect noted in patients who received intraoperative transfusions. This indicated that the effects of preoperative hematocrit concentration on 30-day postoperative stroke are not solely mediated by the use of 3 or more intraoperative pRBC transfusions.

4. Discussion

The incidence of stroke in our study, relying on data from isolated CABG procedures performed in 2008 and 2009,

TABLE 2: Effects of preoperative hematocrit concentration on 30-day postoperative stroke.

Variable	Odds of stroke		
	OR$_{unadj}$ (95% CI)	OR$_{adj-1}$ (95% CI)	OR$_{adj-2}$ (95% CI)
Preoperative hematocrit concentration (continuous variable, per 1% decrease)			
All patients ($n = 2,313$)	1.09 (1.04–1.15)	1.09 (1.03–1.15)	1.07 (1.01–1.13)
Men ($n = 1,703$)	1.11 (1.04–1.18)	1.10 (1.04–1.17)	1.08 (1.01–1.16)
Women ($n = 610$)	1.05 (0.93–1.17)	1.04 (0.92–1.17)	1.02 (0.91–1.16)
Preoperative hematocrit concentration (categorized)			
All patients <37% versus ≥37%	1.92 (1.05–3.51)	1.76 (0.93–3.35)	1.49 (0.76–2.91)
Men <37% versus ≥37%	3.07 (1.49–6.34)	2.80 (1.34–5.88)	2.39 (1.08–5.26)
Women <38% versus ≥38%	2.88 (0.63–13.10)	2.71 (0.59–12.42)	2.52 (0.53–11.98)

OR$_{unadj}$: Unadjusted odds ratio.
OR$_{adj-1}$: Adjusted odds ratio according to Model 1. Adjusted for age, sex, and race.
OR$_{adj-2}$: Adjusted odds ratio according to Model 2. Adjusted for all variables in Table 1.

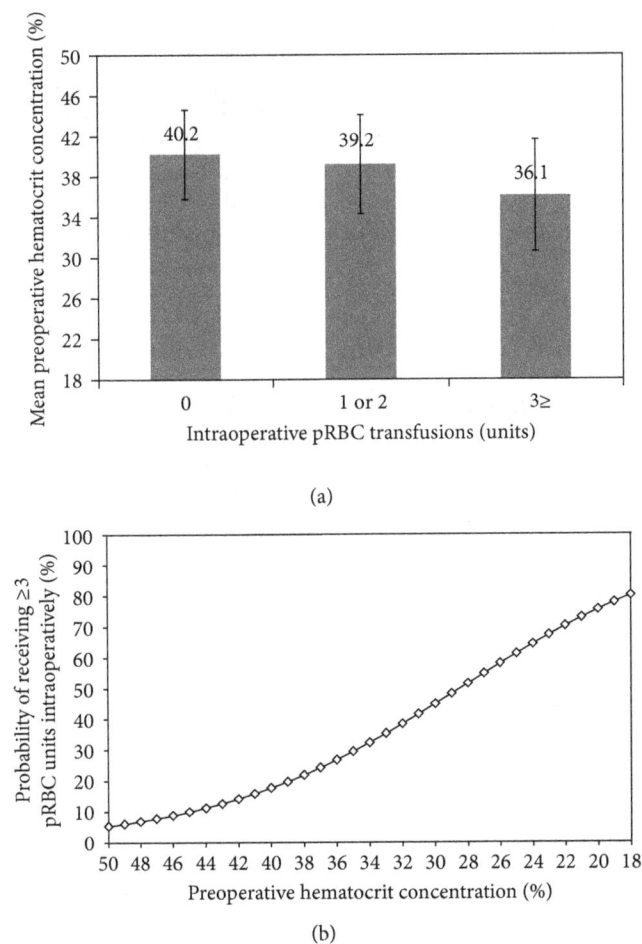

(a)

(b)

FIGURE 3: (a) Bar chart showing mean preoperative hematocrit concentration according to the number of pRBC units transfused intraoperatively, whiskers present standard deviation. (b) Predicted probability of receiving 3 or more pRBC units intraoperatively as a function of preoperative hematocrit concentration. pRBC = packed red blood cell.

was 1.9%, which is in close agreement to recent reports [17]. It should be noted, however, that estimated rates are much higher when asymptomatic infarcts are included in the definition of stroke. In addition, strokes may be missed in the perioperative period, since patients are often receiving pain medications or sedatives, which can mask subtle neurologic signs [1]. The study by Tarakji and colleagues reported an intraoperative occurrence in 40% of overall stroke cases (a total of 705 patients developed stroke among 45432 participants in the study) [17]. None of the 43 cases in this report had stroke documentation intraoperatively, although 5 (11.6%) developed stroke on the same day of surgery. However, the distribution of stroke risk per day in the postoperative period in our study matches that reported by Tarakji and colleagues [17], with a peak incidence during the first 6 days following surgery followed by a decline in risk.

We identified an association between descending preoperative hematocrit concentration values and an increased risk of stroke in the 30-day period following isolated CABG. The increased risk of stroke exceeded 2% in patients with a preoperative hematocrit concentration <37%. Moreover, the increased postoperative stroke risk attributed to declining preoperative hematocrit concentration values was more notable in men than women and was independent of yet augmented by the excessive use of intraoperative pRBC transfusions.

Although numerous studies identified the effects of perioperative hematocrit alterations and pRBC transfusions on morbidity and mortality in cardiac surgery, very few reports evaluated the outcome of stroke in specific. An association between hemodilutional anemia during cardiopulmonary bypass (nadir intraoperative hematocrit levels) and the incidence of stroke was previously demonstrated [18, 19]. One study by Kulier and colleagues showed that both low preoperative hemoglobin (<11.0 g/dl) and intraoperative transfusion requirement are predictors of postoperative adverse noncardiac outcomes (a composite end point of neurological and renal events) in patients undergoing CABG [20]. A more recent study showed that preoperative hemoglobin <12.5 g/dl in both men and women is associated with increased odds of the composite outcome of death, stroke, or acute kidney injury in cardiac surgery patients, irrespective of intraoperative pRBC transfusion use; however, there was no association with the outcome of stroke alone [21]. In this study, we echo these findings and confirm the independent contribution of low preoperative hematocrit concentration on stroke incidence, although a more prominent effect is observed in patients who require intraoperative transfusions of 3 or more pRBC units.

Previous studies suggest that intraoperative hypotension and subsequent hypoperfusion may be a source of neurologic injury in patients undergoing CABG [1, 22, 23]. Preoperative low hematocrit concentration and significant intraoperative blood loss necessitating excessive transfusion [24, 25] may both lead to a state of cerebral hypoperfusion; which in the coexistence of other risk factors (vessel atherosclerosis) may lead to adverse cerebral events. Of note, patients with chronic hypertension may be exposed to relative intraoperative hypotension to the brain if their blood pressure is maintained at a normal or slightly low level during surgery, thus placing them at risk for a watershed stroke [26, 27]. The use of intraoperative transfusions also leads to immunomodulation. Transfusions may lead to immune activation and induce multiple organ failure, despite leukoreduction [28]. In fact, systemic inflammation has been associated with neurologic injury in patients undergoing CABG [1, 22]. Moreover, storage-related posttransfusion hemolysis producing hemoglobin-driven pathophysiology and thrombogenic RBC microparticles in stored blood can lead to target organ damage [29–32]. Thus, our findings support recommendations of a conservative approach to intraoperative blood use in patients undergoing isolated CABG [33] and should lead to a careful consideration of appropriate interventions aimed at correcting preoperatively low hematocrit levels.

Our study carries several limitations. The ACS NSQIP database does not record intraoperative nadir hematocrit or immediate postoperative hematocrit. Thus, we could not evaluate the association between these variables and a stroke outcome. Moreover, the database does not record data on cardiovascular drug use. The ACS NSQIP database also does not document the means by which stroke was diagnosed. The use of magnetic resonance imaging rather than computed tomography may result in higher rates of radiographic infarct. Although the types of imaging techniques used may have affected the observed incidence of stroke in our study, an association between the use of a certain imaging technique and the evaluated risk factors is less likely. Another potential limitation of this study was that we were unable to control for hospital effects owing to the absence of hospital identifiers in our data. There may have been variability in hospital quality or variability in surgical strategy which may have potentially confounded the association between risk factors and outcome. Finally, the possibility of residual confounding is always present in observational studies.

5. Conclusions

Current efforts continue to focus on reducing the embolic burden during CABG, being considered as the primary mechanism through which neurologic injury occurs. Our study shows that other mechanisms of injury could be involved. An increasing number of surgical centers now use preoperative screening to identify patients who have an increased risk for stroke, and to modify surgical conditions according to the results of such screening. This approach should ideally become standard of care.

Conflict of Interests

K. M. Musallam received consultancy fees and travel support from Vifor Pharma Ltd. F. R. Jamali received research funding from Vifor Pharma Ltd. TR department received consultancy fees and research funding from Vifor Pharma Ltd. DRS department received grant support from Vifor SA, Villars-sur-Glâne. D. R. Spahn received honoraria or travel support for consulting or lecturing from the following companies: Galenica AG (including Vifor SA, Villars-sur-Glâne), Janssen-Cilag AG, Janssen-Cilag EMEA, ratiopharm Arzneimittel Vertriebs-GmbH, Roche Pharma (Schweiz) AG, Vifor Pharma Deutschland GmbH, Vifor Pharma Österreich GmbH, Vifor (International) AG. F. R. Rosendaal, K. Khavandi, I. Barakat, B. Demoss, L. A. Lotta, F. Peyvandi, P. M. Sfeir have no relevant conflicts of interest to disclose.

Authors' Contribution

Study conception and design: K. M. Musallam, F. R. Jamali, F. R. Rosendaal and P. M. Sfeir. Statistical analysis: K. M. Musallam. Review and interpretation of data: K. M. Musallam, F. R. Jamali, F. R. Rosendaal, T. Richards, D. R. Spahn, K. Khavandi, I. Barakat, B. Demoss, L. A. Lotta, F. Peyvandi, P. M. Sfeir. Drafting of the manuscript: K. M. Musallam, F. R. Jamali and P. M. Sfeir. Critical revision of the manuscript for important intellectual content: F. R. Rosendaal, T. Richards, D. R. Spahn, K. Khavandi, I. Barakat, B. Demoss, L. A. Lotta, F. Peyvandi. All authors gave final approval of the paper for submission.

References

[1] O. A. Selnes, R. F. Gottesman, M. A. Grega, W. A. Baumgartner, S. L. Zeger, and G. M. McKhann, "Cognitive and neurologic outcomes after coronary-artery bypass surgery," The New England Journal of Medicine, vol. 366, no. 2, pp. 250–257, 2012.

[2] A. L. Shroyer, F. L. Grover, B. Hattler et al., "On-pump versus off-pump coronary-artery bypass surgery," The New England Journal of Medicine, vol. 361, no. 19, pp. 1827–1837, 2009.

[3] C. H. Møller, M. J. Perko, J. T. Lund et al., "No major differences in 30-day outcomes in high-risk patients randomized to off-

pump versus on-pump coronary bypass surgery: the best bypass surgery trial," *Circulation*, vol. 121, no. 4, pp. 498–504, 2010.

[4] W. Hueb, N. H. Lopes, A. C. Pereira et al., "Five-year follow-up of a randomized comparison between off-pump and on-pump stable multivessel coronary artery bypass grafting. The MASS III Trial," *Circulation*, vol. 122, no. 11, pp. S48–S52, 2010.

[5] G. D. Angelini, F. C. Taylor, B. C. Reeves, and R. Ascione, "Early and midterm outcome after off-pump and on-pump surgery in Beating Heart Against Cardioplegic Arrest Studies (BHACAS 1 and 2): a pooled analysis of two randomised controlled trials," *The Lancet*, vol. 359, no. 9313, pp. 1194–1199, 2002.

[6] H. M. Nathoe, D. van Dijk, E. W. Jansen et al., "A comparison of on-pump and off-pump coronary bypass surgery in low-risk patients," *The New England Journal of Medicine*, vol. 348, pp. 394–402, 2003.

[7] C. Muneretto, G. Bisleri, A. Negri et al., "Off-pump coronary artery bypass surgery technique for total arterial myocardial revascularization: a prospective randomized study," *Annals of Thoracic Surgery*, vol. 76, no. 3, pp. 778–783, 2003.

[8] J. F. Légaré, K. J. Buth, S. King et al., "Coronary bypass surgery performed off pump does not result in lower in-hospital morbidity than coronary artery bypass grafting performed on pump," *Circulation*, vol. 109, no. 7, pp. 887–892, 2004.

[9] J. D. Puskas, W. H. Williams, E. M. Mahoney et al., "Off-pump vs conventional coronary artery bypass grafting: early and 1-year graft patency, cost, and quality-of-life outcomes: a randomized trial," *Journal of the American Medical Association*, vol. 291, no. 15, pp. 1841–1849, 2004.

[10] A. Lamy, P. J. Devereaux, D. Prabhakaran et al., "Off-pump or on-pump coronary-artery bypass grafting at 30 days," *The New England Journal of Medicine*, vol. 366, pp. 1489–1497, 2012.

[11] K. M. Musallam, H. M. Tamim, T. Richards et al., "Preoperative anaemia and postoperative outcomes in non-cardiac surgery: a retrospective cohort study," *The Lancet*, vol. 378, no. 9800, pp. 1396–1407, 2011.

[12] S. F. Khuri, W. G. Henderson, J. Daley et al., "The patient safety in surgery study: background, study design, and patient populations," *Journal of the American College of Surgeons*, vol. 204, no. 6, pp. 1089–1102, 2007.

[13] A. S. Fink, D. A. Campbell Jr., R. M. Mentzer et al., "The National Surgical Quality Improvement Program in non-veterans administration hospitals: initial demonstration of feasibility," *Annals of Surgery*, vol. 236, no. 3, pp. 344–354, 2002.

[14] ACS NSQIP, *User Guide for the 2008 Participant Use Data File*, American College of Surgeons, 2009.

[15] M. Limburg, E. F. M. Wijdicks, and H. Li, "Ischemic stroke after surgical procedures: clinical features, neuroimaging, and risk factors," *Neurology*, vol. 50, no. 4, pp. 895–901, 1998.

[16] D. S. Likosky, C. A. S. Marrin, L. R. Caplan et al., "Determination of etiologic mechanisms of strokes secondary to coronary artery bypass graft surgery," *Stroke*, vol. 34, no. 12, pp. 2830–2834, 2003.

[17] K. G. Tarakji, J. F. Sabik III, S. K. Bhudia, L. H. Batizy, and E. H. Blackstone, "Temporal onset, risk factors, and outcomes associated with stroke after coronary artery bypass grafting," *Journal of the American Medical Association*, vol. 305, no. 4, pp. 381–390, 2011.

[18] R. H. Habib, A. Zacharias, T. A. Schwann, C. J. Riordan, S. J. Durham, and A. Shah, "Adverse effects of low hematocrit during, cardiopulmonary bypass in the adult: should current practice be changed?" *Journal of Thoracic and Cardiovascular Surgery*, vol. 125, no. 6, pp. 1438–1450, 2003.

[19] K. Karkouti, G. Djaiani, M. A. Borger et al., "Low hematocrit during cardiopulmonary bypass is associated with increased risk of perioperative stroke in cardiac surgery," *Annals of Thoracic Surgery*, vol. 80, no. 4, pp. 1381–1387, 2005.

[20] A. Kulier, J. Levin, R. Moser et al., "Impact of preoperative anemia on outcome in patients undergoing coronary artery bypass graft surgery," *Circulation*, vol. 116, no. 5, pp. 471–479, 2007.

[21] K. Karkouti, D. N. Wijeysundera, and W. S. Beattie, "Risk associated with preoperative anemia in cardiac surgery: a multicenter cohort study," *Circulation*, vol. 117, no. 4, pp. 478–484, 2008.

[22] S. G. Raja and G. A. Berg, "Impact of off-pump coronary artery bypass surgery on systemic inflammation: current best available evidence," *Journal of Cardiac Surgery*, vol. 22, no. 5, pp. 445–455, 2007.

[23] T. J. Gardner, P. J. Horneffer, T. A. Manolio et al., "Stroke following coronary artery bypass grafting: a ten-year study," *Annals of Thoracic Surgery*, vol. 40, no. 6, pp. 574–581, 1985.

[24] L. T. Goodnough, A. Shander, J. L. Spivak et al., "Detection, evaluation, and management of anemia in the elective surgical patient," *Anesthesia and Analgesia*, vol. 101, no. 6, pp. 1858–1861, 2005.

[25] W. A. van Klei, K. G. M. Moons, A. T. Leyssius, J. T. A. Knape, C. L. G. Rutten, and D. E. Grobbee, "A reduction in type and screen: preoperative prediction of RBC transfusions in surgery procedures with intermediate transfusion risks," *British Journal of Anaesthesia*, vol. 87, no. 2, pp. 250–257, 2001.

[26] J. P. Gold, M. E. Charlson, P. Williams-Russo et al., "Improvement of outcomes after coronary artery bypass: a randomized trial comparing intraoperative high versus low mean arterial pressure," *Journal of Thoracic and Cardiovascular Surgery*, vol. 110, no. 5, pp. 1302–1314, 1995.

[27] R. F. Gottesman, P. M. Sherman, M. A. Grega et al., "Watershed strokes after cardiac surgery: diagnosis, etiology, and outcome," *Stroke*, vol. 37, no. 9, pp. 2306–2311, 2006.

[28] M. Raghavan and P. E. Marik, "Anemia, allogenic blood transfusion, and immunomodulation in the critically ill," *Chest*, vol. 127, no. 1, pp. 295–307, 2005.

[29] D. B. Kim-Shapiro, J. Lee, and M. T. Gladwin, "Storage lesion: role of red blood cell breakdown," *Transfusion*, vol. 51, no. 4, pp. 844–851, 2011.

[30] M. K. Horne III, A. M. Cullinane, P. K. Merryman, and E. K. Hoddeson, "The effect of red blood cells on thrombin generation," *British Journal of Haematology*, vol. 133, no. 4, pp. 403–408, 2006.

[31] T. J. Greenwalt, "The how and why of exocytic vesicles," *Transfusion*, vol. 46, no. 1, pp. 143–152, 2006.

[32] J. H. Baek, F. D'Agnillo, F. Vallelian et al., "Hemoglobin-driven pathophysiology is an in vivo consequence of the red blood cell storage lesion that can be attenuated in guinea pigs by haptoglobin therapy," *The Journal of Clinical Investigation*, vol. 122, no. 4, pp. 1444–1458, 2012.

[33] D. M. Moskowitz, J. N. McCullough, A. Shander et al., "The impact of blood conservation on outcomes in cardiac surgery: is it safe and effective?" *Annals of Thoracic Surgery*, vol. 90, no. 2, pp. 451–458, 2010.

17

Intracranial Blood Flow Velocity in Patients with β-Thalassemia Intermedia Using Transcranial Doppler Sonography

Nahid Ashjazadeh,[1] Sajad Emami,[1] Peyman Petramfar,[1] Ehsan Yaghoubi,[1] and Mehran Karimi[2]

[1] Shiraz Neuroscience Research Center, Department of Neurology, Shiraz University of Medical Sciences, Shiraz, Iran
[2] Hematology Research Center, Shiraz University of Medical Sciences, Shiraz, Iran

Correspondence should be addressed to Mehran Karimi, karimim@sums.ac.ir

Academic Editor: Sezaneh Haghpanah

Introduction. Patients with β-thalassemia intermedia have a higher incidence of thromboembolic events compared to the general population. Previous studies have shown that patients with sickle cell disease, who are also prone to ischemic events, have higher intracranial arterial blood flow velocities measured by transcranial Doppler sonography (TCD). The aim of this study is to evaluate intracranial arterial flow velocities in patients with β-thalassemia intermedia and compare the results with those found in healthy subjects. *Methods.* Sixty-four patients with β-thalassemia intermedia and 30 healthy subjects underwent transcranial Doppler sonography. *Results.* Significantly higher flow velocities were found in intracranial arteries of patients compared to controls ($P = 0.001$). Previously splenectomized patients with thrombocytosis showed higher flow velocities than nonsplenectomized patients without thrombosis. *Conclusion.* The increased flow velocities in patients with β-thalassemia intermedia may point to a higher risk of ischemic events. Preventive measures such as blood transfusion or antiplatelet treatment may be beneficial in these patients.

1. Introduction

Patients with β-thalassemia intermedia (B-TI) seem to show higher rates of thromboembolic events than individuals without thalassemia or patients with β-thalassemia major, in particular if they have been splenectomized [1]. It is estimated that 4% of patients with β-thalassemia intermedia will experience a thromboembolic event [2]. Previous splenectomy and thrombocytosis and/or platelet abnormalities are major factors associated with thromboembolic events in patients with β-thalassemia intermedia [1, 3, 4], and ischemic stroke is increasingly recognized as one of the most devastating complications of this disease [5].

Ischemic stroke is also a known complication of sickle cell disease [6]. In a prospective study in patients with this condition, higher blood flow velocity in the intracranial arteries was associated with a higher risk of ischemic stroke [7]. The stroke prevention trial in sickle cell anemia (STOP) has indicated a role for transcranial Doppler sonography (TCD) in measuring intracranial arterial flow velocities to identify sickle cell patients at a high risk of ischemic stroke [8]. TCD measurement of intracranial flow velocities is of aid in deciding when to start blood transfusion in these patients to reduce the risk of ischemic stroke [8, 9].

An association between TCD findings and stroke risk has been confirmed in sickle cell disease; however, as far as we know, no studies have been conducted to evaluate TCD findings in patients with β-thalassemia intermedia, another high-risk group for ischemic stroke. In the present study, we compared the intracranial arterial flow velocities of β-thalassemia intermedia patients with those of healthy subjects.

2. Patients and Methods

This is a case-control study conducted in a tertiary outpatient clinic affiliated with Shiraz University of Medical Sciences, Southern Iran, for a period of one year during 2009.

Intracranial Blood Flow Velocity in Patients with β-Thalassemia Intermedia Using Transcranial Doppler Sonography

Consecutive patients older than 15 years of age with confirmed β-thalassemia intermedia by complete blood count and hemoglobin electrophoresis who were referred to an outpatient thalassemia clinic enrolled in the study. Diagnosis of B-TI was based on complete blood count, hemoglobin electrophoresis, and initial hemoglobin (Hb) level of 7 gr/dL, and age of diagnosed anemia was after 2. All of them were transfusion independent. Patients were recruited at a routine follow-up visit with a hematologist in the clinic. Exclusion criteria were a history of diabetes mellitus, hypertension, ischemic heart disease, thrombosis, previous cerebrovascular disease, sickle cell anemia, or inadequate temporal window for TCD. The study was approved by the Ethics Committee of Shiraz University of Medical Sciences (no. 2885), and written informed consent to participate was obtained from all patients or their first-degree families. All patients were receiving folic acid (5 mg/day) and hydroxyurea (8–15 mg/kg/day).

For each patient, we completed a data collection form that included age, sex, place of residence, prior splenectomy, prior transfusion, history of thrombosis, previous stroke or transient ischemic attack, and laboratory information (complete blood cell count, ferritin, blood urea nitrogen, creatinine, alanine aminotransferase, aspartate aminotransferase, alkaline phosphatase, and albumin). Thrombocytosis was defined as a platelet count >500,000/dL.

Transcranial Doppler ultrasound was carried out in all patients. All TCD studies were performed by one investigator using a Legend TC22 transcranial Doppler ultrasound unit (Bristol, UK) with a 2-MHz transducer. The two middle cerebral arteries (MCAs), anterior cerebral arteries (ACAs), posterior cerebral arteries (PCAs), and the terminal internal carotid arteries were insonated using a temporal window approach (Eleven patients had poor temporal window who were excluded from the study). The basilar artery (BA) and vertebral arteries were examined through a suboccipital approach in sitting position. The highest mean flow velocity of each artery was recorded separately.

The control group consisted of 30 sex/age-matched subjects with no known hematologic disease. The same exclusion criteria as for the patients were used for the controls. All the control subjects underwent TCD examination with the same protocol.

The Mann-Whitney U test, Pearson correlation coefficient (r), and t-test were used for comparison of the variables between groups. Results are expressed as percentages and absolute frequencies, where appropriate. Descriptive results are presented as the mean ± standard deviation (SD). P values <0.05 were considered significant. Statistical analyses were performed in SPSS version 15.0 (SPSS, Chicago, Ill, USA).

3. Results

After applying the inclusion and exclusion criteria, 64 patients with β-thalassemia intermedia and 30 healthy subjects were recruited. There were no significant differences between patients and controls according to sex (male: 40.6%

TABLE 1: Mean intracranial arterial flow velocities in β-thalassemia intermedia patients with or without splenectomy.

	Without splenectomy	With splenectomy	P value
Left ICA	84.6 ± 24.4	94.1 ± 20.7	0.097
Right ICA	83.1 ± 25.6	86.5 ± 25.1	0.538
Left MCA	66.6 ± 26.9	87.9 ± 23.9	0.001
Right MCA	71.3 ± 28.2	85.8 ± 22.7	0.026
Left ACA	58.2 ± 19.7	73.4 ± 18.3	0.002
Right ACA	57.3 ± 19.0	69.2 ± 18.2	0.013
Left PCA	35.1 ± 11.7	42.1 ± 11.6	0.021
Right PCA	34.8 ± 10.8	41.7 ± 14.3	0.037
Left vertebral artery	52.2 ± 15.0	58.3 ± 14.5	0.102
Right vertebral artery	55.6 ± 15.3	62.4 ± 17.5	0.106
Basilar artery	66.1 ± 17.2	76.7 ± 16.6	0.016

ICA, internal carotid artery; MCA, middle cerebral artery; ACA, anterior cerebral artery; PCA, posterior cerebral artery.

versus 53.3%; $P = 0.251$) or age (23.6 ± 5.2 versus 25.4 ± 5.4; $P = 0.001$). Mean velocities of all mentioned vessels were measured in all patients and control subjects, and no missing vessel was detected. Among the patients, 54.7% (35/64) had undergone splenectomy, and 9.4% (6/64) had received a blood transfusion once or twice a year before the study. None of the control subjects had received transfusion. In patients, mean Hb level was 9.3 ± 1.2 g/dL (range 6.9–12.3), mean white blood cell count was 8873 ± 2004/dL (range 4900–13800), and mean platelet count was $523 \times 10^3 \pm 219 \times 10^3$/dL (range 188×10^3–1035×10^3). There were no significant differences in age, white blood cell count, or Hb level between splenectomized and nonsplenectomized patients ($P > 0.05$). Mean platelet count was significantly higher in patients who had undergone splenectomy ($696 \times 10^3 \pm 129 \times 10^3$/dL versus $315 \times 10^3 \pm 78 \times 10^3$/dL; $P = 0.001$). All the splenectomized patients had thrombocytosis, and none of the nonsplenectomized patients had thrombocytosis. Platelet count correlated with blood flow velocity in the right MCA ($r = 0.291$, $P = 0.020$), left MCA ($r = 0.366$, $P = 0.003$), left ACA ($r = 0.258$, $P = 0.040$), right PCA ($r = 0.270$, $P = 0.031$), left PCA ($r = 0.267$, $P = 0.033$), and BA ($r = 0.300$, $P = 0.016$). There were no correlations between platelet count and blood flow velocities of the other arteries ($P > 0.05$). Mean intracranial arterial flow velocities in β-thalassemia intermedia patients with or without splenectomy are shown in Table 1. There were no significant differences in white blood cell count, Hb levels, or platelet count between patients who had undergone transfusion and those who had not ($P > 0.05$).

Comparison of the mean intracranial artery flow velocities between patients and controls showed significantly higher velocities in all intracranial arteries of patients ($P = 0.001$). Mean flow velocities recorded in patients and controls are shown in Table 2.

TABLE 2: Mean intracranial arterial flow velocities in β-thalassemia intermedia patients and healthy controls.

	Patients	Healthy subjects	P value
Left ICA	89.8 ± 22.8	52.1 ± 8.6	0.001
Right ICA	84.9 ± 21.7	50.0 ± 8.4	0.001
Left MCA	78.3 ± 27.3	49.4 ± 9.1	0.001
Right MCA	79.3 ± 26.2	48.7 ± 7.6	0.001
Left ACA	66.5 ± 20.3	44.4 ± 9.5	0.001
Right ACA	63.8 ± 19.4	42.5 ± 7.8	0.001
Left PCA	38.9 ± 12.1	29.7 ± 6.6	0.001
Right PCA	38.6 ± 13.2	27.3 ± 6.3	0.001
Left vertebral artery	55.5 ± 14.9	29.5 ± 4.6	0.001
Right vertebral artery	59.3 ± 16.8	29.3 ± 4.6	0.001
Basilar artery	71.9 ± 17.6	47.1 ± 8.2	0.001

ICA, internal carotid artery; MCA, middle cerebral artery; ACA, anterior cerebral artery; PCA, posterior cerebral artery.

4. Discussion

In this study, higher blood flow velocities were found in all intracranial arteries of our patients. Flow velocity was higher in most arteries of splenectomized patients compared to nonsplenectomized patients, especially in the anterior circulation. In addition, there was a correlation between platelet count and flow velocities.

Numerous studies in sickle cell anemia have evaluated the role of TCD as a screening tool to identify and followup patients at high risk of ischemic stroke [7–10]. TCD can also detect asymptomatic cerebrovascular disease in patients with sickle β-thalassemia [11], and the findings on TCD study show a good correlation with cerebral angiography [12]. However, no such studies have been performed in β-thalassemia intermedia, another hematologic disease in which there is a substantial associated risk of ischemic stroke. Screening of asymptomatic β-thalassemia intermedia patients by TCD has not been reported previously, and the impact of this measure on further stroke remains to be defined. TI patients are prone to thromboembolic event, especially those patients associated with splenectonomy and thrombocytosis [2, 3].

There is growing evidence that increased intracranial arterial flow velocities associate with a higher risk of ischemic stroke [7, 13]. The recommendation for chronic red blood cell transfusion in patients with high stroke risk is based on findings from the STOP trial, in which patients with high intracranial arterial flow velocities showed a 90% reduction in stroke rate following this treatment [8]. Patients with β-thalassemia intermedia do not regularly receive blood transfusion, and they have a higher risk of ischemic stroke than β-thalassemia major patients, who are often treated with transfusion [3]. In addition, a higher rate of thromboembolic events occurs in splenectomized β-thalassemia intermedia patients [3, 14], who usually have a higher platelet count.

The presence of a high flow velocity in patients with β-thalassemia intermedia may herald a cerebrovascular event and indicate a need for special attention. The association of flow velocity with splenectomy and platelet count suggests that these two factors should also be taken into account when interpreting stroke risk in a patient with β-thalassemia intermedia.

This study has some limitations. Patients were not prospectively followedup to clarify the impact of higher blood flow velocities on the risk of ischemic stroke. The interpretation presented here is based on previous studies, mainly in sickle cell disease, which showed a higher risk of stroke in association with higher flow velocities measured by TCD. Furthermore, we did not measure flow velocities before and after blood transfusion to estimate the impact of this measure on reducing velocities.

In conclusion, in this first study evaluating TCD findings in β-thalassemia intermedia patients, higher intracranial arterial blood flow velocities were found in comparison to normal subjects. These findings may indicate that these patients are at a higher risk of ischemic events and that preventive measures, such as blood transfusion or antiplatelet drug administration, could be beneficial. Nonetheless, prospective randomized clinical trials would be needed to establish recommendations in this regard.

Conflict of Interests

All the authors declare that they have no conflict of interests.

Acknowledgments

This study was financially supported by Shiraz University of Medical Sciences. They thank Shirin Parand at the Hematology Research Center for help with paper preparation, and C. Cavallo (author aid in the Eastern Mediterranean) for editing and improving the use of English in the paper. This paper is relevant to the thesis of S. Emami with Project no. 2885.

References

[1] A. T. Taher, Z. K. Otrock, I. Uthman, and M. D. Cappellini, "Thalassemia and hypercoagulability," *Blood Reviews*, vol. 22, no. 5, pp. 283–292, 2008.

[2] A. Taher, H. Isma'eel, G. Mehio et al., "Prevalence of thromboembolic events among 8,860 patients with thalassaemia major and intermedia in the Mediterranean area and Iran," *Thrombosis and Haemostasis*, vol. 96, no. 4, pp. 488–491, 2006.

[3] M. D. Cappellini, L. Robbiolo, B. M. Bottasso, R. Coppola, G. Fiorelli, and P. M. Mannucci, "Venous thromboembolism and hypercoagulability in splenectomized patients with thalassaemia intermedia," *British Journal of Haematology*, vol. 111, no. 2, pp. 467–473, 2000.

[4] A. Tripodi, M. D. Cappellini, V. Chantarangkul et al., "Hypercoagulability in splenectomized thalassemic patients detected by whole-blood thromboelastometry, but not by thrombin generation in platelet-poor plasma," *Haematologica*, vol. 94, no. 11, pp. 1520–1527, 2009.

[5] M. Karimi, M. Khanlari, and E. A. Rachmilewitz, "Cerebrovascular accident in β-thalassemia major (β-TM) and β-thalassemia intermedia (β-TI)," *American Journal of Hematology*, vol. 83, no. 1, pp. 77–79, 2008.

[6] K. Ohene-Frempong, S. J. Weiner, L. A. Sleeper et al., "Cerebrovascular accidents in sickle cell disease: rates and risk factors," *Blood*, vol. 91, no. 1, pp. 288–294, 1998.

[7] R. J. Adams, V. C. McKie, E. M. Carl et al., "Long-term stroke risk in children with sickle cell disease screened with transcranial Doppler," *Annals of Neurology*, vol. 42, no. 5, pp. 699–704, 1997.

[8] M. T. Lee, S. Piomelli, S. Granger et al., "Stroke prevention trial in sickle cell anemia (STOP): extended follow-up and final results," *Blood*, vol. 108, no. 3, pp. 847–852, 2006.

[9] N. Venketasubramanian, I. Prohovnik, A. Hurlet, J. P. Mohr, and S. Piomelli, "Middle cerebral artery velocity changes during transfusion in sickle cell anemia," *Stroke*, vol. 25, no. 11, pp. 2153–2158, 1994.

[10] J. J. Seibert, C. M. Glasier, R. S. Kirby et al., "Transcranial Doppler, MRA, and MRI as a screening examination for cerebrovascular disease in patients with sickle cell anemia: an 8-year study," *Pediatric Radiology*, vol. 28, no. 3, pp. 138–142, 1998.

[11] D. I. Zafeiriou, M. Prengler, N. Gombakis et al., "Central nervous system abnormalities in asymptomatic young patients with Sβ-thalassemia," *Annals of Neurology*, vol. 55, no. 6, pp. 835–839, 2004.

[12] R. J. Adams, F. T. Nichols, R. Figueroa, V. McKie, and T. Lott, "Transcranial Doppler correlation with cerebral angiography in sickle cell disease," *Stroke*, vol. 23, no. 8, pp. 1073–1077, 1992.

[13] R. Adams, V. McKie, F. Nichols et al., "The use of transcranial ultrasonography to predict stroke in sickle cell disease," *New England Journal of Medicine*, vol. 326, no. 9, pp. 605–610, 1992.

[14] M. Karimi, H. Bagheri, F. Rastgu, and E. A. Rachmilewitz, "Magnetic resonance imaging to determine the incidence of brain ischaemia in patients with β-thalassaemia intermedia," *Thrombosis and Haemostasis*, vol. 103, no. 5, pp. 989–993, 2010.

18

Evaluation of Serum Leptin Levels and Growth in Patients with β-Thalassaemia Major

Lamia Mustafa Al-Naama,[1] **Meaad Kadum Hassan,**[2] **and Muhannad Maki Abdul Karim**[3]

[1]*Department of Biochemistry and Haemoglobinopathy Units, College of Medicine, University of Basrah, Basrah, Iraq*
[2]*Department of Paediatrics and Haemoglobinopathy Units, College of Medicine, University of Basrah, Basrah, Iraq*
[3]*Department of Biochemistry, College of Medicine, University of Basrah, Basrah, Iraq*

Correspondence should be addressed to Lamia Mustafa Al-Naama; lamia_alnaama@yahoo.com

Academic Editor: Aurelio Maggio

Background. Iron deposition in the body can damage the endocrine glands of patients with β-thalassaemia major (β-TM). Leptin plays a key role in the regulation of appetite, body fat mass, and endocrine function. *Objectives.* This study aimed to evaluate the relationship between serum leptin and growth and pubertal development in patients with β-TM, as well as whether serum leptin can predict growth retardation and delayed puberty in these patients. *Methods.* Fifty β-TM patients (aged 8–20 years) and 75 age-matched healthy controls were recruited. Anthropometric data and sexual maturity ratings were assessed. Serum leptin was measured by ELISA. *Results.* Serum leptin levels were significantly lower in patients with β-TM than in healthy individuals ($P < 0.001$). Leptin levels were also significantly reduced in female patients with short stature ($P < 0.002$) and in patients who displayed delayed puberty ($P = 0.032$) compared to those with normal stature who had reached puberty. The sensitivity of leptin for predicting short stature and delayed puberty among patients was 84.6% and 92.3%, respectively. *Conclusion.* Low serum leptin is sensitive to predict short stature and significant in β-TM females only. This link could thus be used as a guide for further therapeutic or hormonal modulation.

1. Introduction

Short stature among patients with thalassaemia is a problem in developing countries due to several factors, such as inadequate blood transfusion, iron overload, abnormal growth hormone (GH) secretion, hypothyroidism, zinc deficiency, deferoxamine toxicity, inadequate treatment, and noncompliance of patients [1].

Leptin, an adipokine that is synthesized and released from adipocytes in response to changes in body fat [2], binds receptors within the hypothalamus to control appetite [2–4]. Moreover, leptin stimulates the secretion of luteinising hormone (LH) by activating nitric oxide synthase in gonadotropes and in the hypothalamus, which in turn stimulates the release of gonadotropin-releasing hormone (GnRH) [5, 6]. Leptin has been proposed as a physiological link between nutritional status and reproductive maturation and function [2]. Therefore, leptin may serve as a trigger or metabolic gate

for sexual development [7–9]. The importance of leptin in regulating sexual maturation is supported by data showing that alterations in the leptin receptor or deletion of the leptin gene results in infertility [10], whereas the administration of leptin to leptin-deficient patients reportedly led to increased serum gonadotropin hormone levels [11].

Previous studies have demonstrated that leptin can be considered one of the many metabolic signals that can regulate growth hormone (GH) secretion [12]. In rats, the central administration of leptin completely prevents the disappearance of pulsatile GH secretion that occurs after 3 days of fasting [12].

Beta-thalassaemia (β-TM) is a hereditary disorder that is highly prevalent worldwide and in our local community of Basrah, Iraq [13], due to high rates of relative marriages. Therefore, we conducted this study to evaluate whether serum leptin levels in Iraqi patients with β-TM from Basrah correlate with short stature, body mass index (BMI), and delayed puberty relative to normal children as well as study the independent effects of selected risk factors on serum leptin levels. Furthermore, we examined the sensitivity of serum leptin levels in predicting growth retardation and delayed puberty in patients with β-TM.

2. Patients and Methods

2.1. Patients. This case-control study was conducted between December 1, 2008, and March 31, 2010. The Council and the Ethical Committee of the College of Medicine at the University of Basrah approved the protocol for this study. The study was explained to the young adult patients or controls and their parents/relatives or guardian, and appropriate written consent was obtained.

The patient group comprised 50 patients (27 males and 23 females) diagnosed with β-TM using HPLC Variant (Bio-Rad, USA) who were registered at the Center for Hereditary Blood Diseases in Basrah, Iraq. Patients undergoing hormonal or zinc therapy were excluded.

The control group included 75 age-matched healthy individuals (41 males and 34 females) with normal haemoglobin (Hb AA) and no previous history of relevant medical illnesses, such as a history of anaemia.

2.2. Anthropometry. Body weight, height, body mass index (BMI), and BMI Z-score (BMIZ) were assessed and plotted on age- and sex-appropriate growth charts. Short stature was defined according to the Centers for Disease Control and Prevention (CDC) as height or stature below the 5th percentile on the CDC age- and gender-specific height or stature reference [14]. BMI and BMI Z-score were calculated for all patients according to the WHO 2006/2007 reference values [15]. BMI Z-scores were used to determine the severity of wasting. Pubertal staging was assessed using the sex maturity rating (SMR) according to Tanner classification [16], wherein any person with signs of stage 2 or greater, plus breast development in girls or genital development in boys, was allocated to pubertal groups. An individual was considered to have delayed puberty when a girl of 13 or a boy of 14 did not exhibit signs of pubertal development, that is, the absence of breast development in a girl by the age of 13 or a testicular volume of less than 4 mL in a boy by the age of 14. Other definitions of delayed puberty included the absence of menarche by 16 years of age or a prolonged rate of pubertal progression with more than 5 years from pubertal onset to completion [16].

2.3. Laboratory Analysis. Blood samples were collected after overnight fast from 8:30 to 9:30 a.m. to ensure uniform timing for sample collection. The blood was centrifuged, and the sera were stored at −18°C until assayed.

Serum leptin was measured in duplicate by enzyme-linked immunosorbent assay (ELISA) using a kit from DRG (Germany). The inter- and intra-assay coefficients of variation were 5.3% and 4.9%, respectively. Based on the values of the control individuals, the reference values for males and females were 3.92 ± 1.22 ng/mL and 5.95 ± 2.43 ng/mL, respectively. A low serum leptin level is defined as a value

below the 95% confidence intervals of the mean values of the control group according to the sex. Serum ferritin levels were estimated by ELISA using a kit from HUMAN (Germany).

2.4. Statistical Analysis. Data were analysed using Statistical Package for the Social Sciences (SPSS) software version 15 (IBM, Chicago, Illinois, USA), and the results are presented as tables or figures. For continuous variables, means and standard deviations were used to present the data, and analysis was performed using independent Student's *t*-test. The strength and direction of linear relationships between variables were evaluated using Pearson's correlation coefficient. A linear multiple regression analysis was used to identify significant predictors of changes in serum leptin. The validity of serum leptin estimation as a predicator of short stature and delayed puberty among β-TM patients was assessed using receiver operating characteristic (ROC) analyses, and the area under the curve (AUC) was calculated. $P < 0.05$ was considered statistically significant.

3. Results

The mean serum leptin level, BMI, BMI Z-score, height, and weight were significantly lower in patients of both sexes with β-TM than in controls ($P < 0.014$ to $P < 0.001$) (Table 1). The mean serum leptin level was significantly higher in female β-TM patients than in male β-TM patients ($P < 0.001$). However, within the patient group, there were no significant differences in BMI, BMI Z-score, and weight between males and females. As expected, serum ferritin levels were significantly higher ($P = 0.001$) in β-TM patients relative to healthy control individuals, with no significant difference ($P > 0.05$) between male and female patients (Table 1).

Concerning delayed puberty, 7 of 11 (63%) male patients at least 14 years of age and 6 of 11 (54.5%) female patients at least 13 years of age showed signs of delayed puberty. In contrast, all individuals in the control group exhibited normal pubertal development. All male β-TM patients with delayed puberty (100%) and 5 of 6 females with delayed puberty (83.3%) had low serum leptin levels. The mean serum leptin level was significantly lower in all patients with delayed puberty ($P = 0.032$) (Table 2).

Short stature was observed in 26 of 50 (52%) patients with β-TM. Low serum leptin levels were detected in 33 of 50 (66%) β-TM patients, of whom 22 (67%) had short stature, whereas the rest had normal stature. The mean serum leptin level was significantly lower only in female patients with short stature ($P = 0.002$) (Table 3).

In β-TM patients, a significant positive correlation was observed between serum leptin levels and BMI ($r = 0.353$, $P = 0.012$) (Figure 1), as well as with the BMI Z-score ($r = 0.404$, $P = 0.004$) (Figure 2).

To study the independent effects of selected risk factors on serum leptin levels, a stepwise linear multiple regression analysis was performed (Table 4). The factors examined were age, sex, β-TM status, BMI Z-score, and BMI. β-TM, sex, and BMI were significantly correlated with serum leptin levels, with β-TM appearing to be the strongest variable, accounting

Table 1: Serum leptin, ferritin, age, weight, height, BMI Z-score, BMI, and IGF-1 in β-TM patients and controls according to sex.

Variables	Sex	β-TM patients	Controls	P value
	M/F	27/23	41/34	
Age (years)	Male	13.6 ± 3.4	13.7 ± 3.1	>0.05
	Female	12.3 ± 3.3	12.6 ± 3.0	>0.05
Height (cm)	Male	141.93 ± 15.54^{b}	156.99 ± 16.07^{b}	<0.001
	Female	132.11 ± 12.58	147.82 ± 14.45	<0.001
Weight (kg)	Male	34.81 ± 11.78	54.05 ± 19.55^{b}	<0.001
	Female	30.52 ± 8.94	44.62 ± 15.96	<0.001
BMI Z-score	Male	-1.22 ± 1.15	0.42 ± 1.38	<0.001
	Female	-0.68 ± 1.04	0.09 ± 1.11	<0.004
BMI (kg/m^2)	Male	16.79 ± 2.12	21.2 ± 4.65	<0.001
	Female	17.12 ± 2.62	19.85 ± 4.67	<0.014
S. leptin (ng/mL)	Male	1.71 ± 1.27^{a}	3.92 ± 1.22^{a}	<0.001
	Female	3.27 ± 1.97	5.95 ± 2.43	<0.001
S. ferritin (ng/mL)	Male	5285.5 ± 3220.2	114.14 ± 65.31^{a}	<0.001
	Female	5084.0 ± 3260.5	67.74 ± 30.54	<0.001

The significant sex differences (males versus females) for the above parameters within each group of β-TM and controls were assessed as follows: [a]$P \leq 0.001$, [b]$P < 0.03$.

Table 2: Serum leptin levels in patients with β-TM with delayed and normal puberty according to gender.

	Serum leptin levels (ng/mL)				
β-TM patients	Delayed puberty		Normal puberty		P value
	N	Mean $\pm$ SD	N	Mean $\pm$ SD	
Males ($N = 11$)	7	0.89 ± 0.66	4	1.68 ± 1.08	0.16
Females ($N = 11$)	6	2.32 ± 1.59	5	4.1 ± 1.88	0.12
All ($N = 22$)	13	1.55 ± 1.35	9	3.02 ± 1.96	0.032

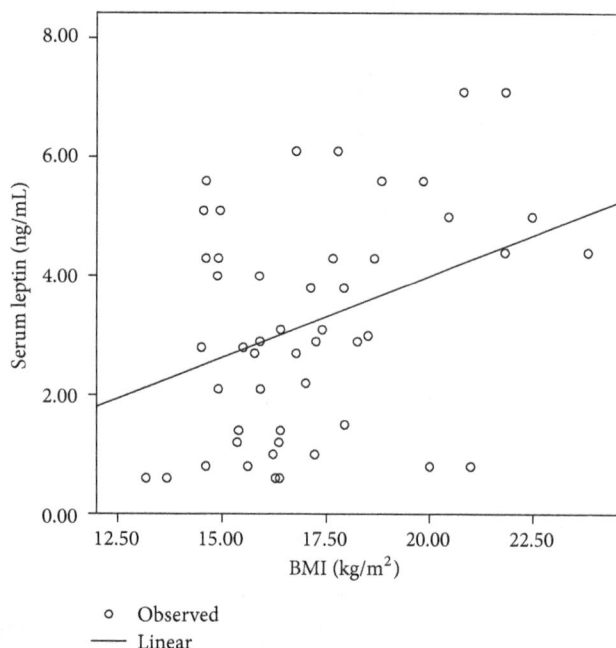

Figure 1: Correlation between serum leptin levels (ng/mL) and BMI (kg/m^2) in β-TM patients. Pearson correlation coefficient ($r = 0.353$, $P = 0.012$).

for 25.1% of the variability in serum leptin levels. Combined variables (β-TM, sex, and BMI) explained 45.6% of the variation in serum leptin levels, whereas 54.4% of the variation remained unaccounted for.

To assess the validity of low serum leptin levels as a predicator of short stature and delayed puberty in β-TM patients, cut-off values of 3.34 ng/mL and 4.52 ng/mL were selected for serum leptin in female patients aged ≤13 years and >13 years, respectively, whereas, for male β-TM patients, the threshold values for ≤13 years and >13 years were set at 2.45 and 3.09 ng/mL, respectively. Accordingly, the use of serum leptin to predict short stature showed sensitivity and specificity of 83.3% and 40% for male and 85.7% and 77.8% for female β-TM patients, whereas, for delayed puberty, sensitivity and specificity of 100% and 25% for male and 60% and 92.3% for female β-TM patients were observed. The receiver operating characteristic (ROC) curves for serum leptin in β-TM patients with short stature and delayed puberty are shown in Figures 3 and 4.

4. Discussion

Leptin plays a key role in controlling reproduction and the hypothalamic-pituitary-gonadal (HPG) axis, and the level

TABLE 3: Serum leptin levels in β-TM patients with normal and short stature according to gender.

| β-TM patients | Serum leptin levels (ng/mL) | | | | | P value |
| | Short stature | | Normal stature | | | |
	N	Mean ± SD	N	Mean ± SD		
Males ($N = 27$)	12	1.33 ± 1.07	15	2.0 ± 1.37		0.18
Females ($N = 23$)	14	2.32 ± 1.41	9	4.75 ± 1.83		0.002
All ($N = 50$)	26	1.87 ± 1.34	24	3.03 ± 2.04		0.021

TABLE 4: Stepwise multiple regression analysis between serum leptin levels and different variables in β-TM patients.

Variable	Beta	R^2	P value
Thalassaemia alone	0.512	0.256	<0.001
Thalassaemia + sex	0.399	0.413	<0.001
Thalassaemia + sex + BMI	0.289	0.478	<0.001

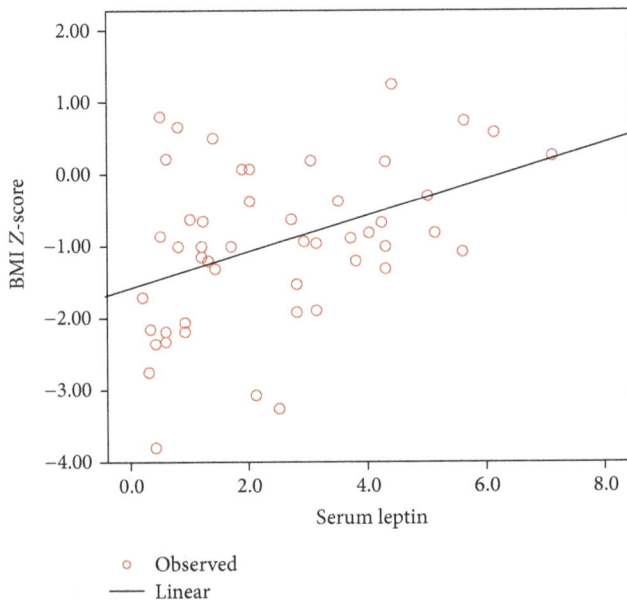

FIGURE 2: Correlation between serum leptin levels (ng/mL) and the BMI Z-score in β-TM patients. Pearson correlation coefficient ($r = 0.404$, $P = 0.004$).

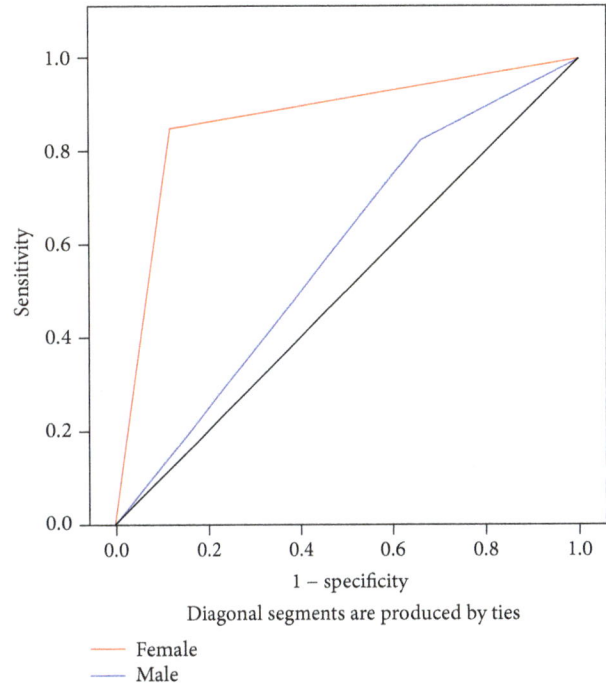

FIGURE 3: Receiver operating characteristic (ROC) curves of serum leptin levels and short stature in β-TM patients using cut-off values mentioned in the text. The red and blue lines indicate female and male β-TM patients, respectively. The AUCs (±SE) and P values for female and male β-TM patients are 0.822 (±0.095), $P = 0.009$ and 0.638 (±0.116), $P = 0.265$, respectively.

of circulating leptin may affect the HPG axis [17]. These effects may highlight an essential role for leptin in regulating reproductive function [8, 9, 17], supporting the hypothesis that leptin is one of the factors mediating reproductive abnormalities in several disease states [18]. In addition, leptin is also part of a complex network of endocrine signals that includes several hormones and vitamin D, which governs the process of longitudinal bone growth [19].

The mean serum leptin level was found to be significantly lower in our β-TM patients than in control patients. Similar findings were reported for β-TM patients of different age groups [20–22]. A significantly lower level of serum leptin was also observed in our stunted β-TM patients. In addition, the low BMI values observed in our β-TM patients probably reflect a reduction in fat mass in these patients, resulting in

low levels of leptin secretion. These associations may explain the importance of adipose tissue-dependent leptin secretion in normal growth.

Blüher and Mantzoros [18] found that, during early childhood, individuals who present a congenital leptin deficiency may demonstrate significant growth delay due to the decreased secretion of GH and decreases in the levels of IGF-1 and IGF-BP3. These results might suggest that leptin has both direct and indirect effects on the GH-IGF-I-insulin-like growth factor binding protein (IGF-BP) axis. Serum leptin has also been found to indirectly stimulate growth as a trigger for sexual development and, thus, the induction of the pubertal growth spurt [7].

The current study showed that β-TM patients with delayed puberty had significantly lower serum leptin levels than both β-TM patients with normal puberty and the control group. These findings are similar to those reported by Perrone et al. [20], who concluded that, in patients with β-TM,

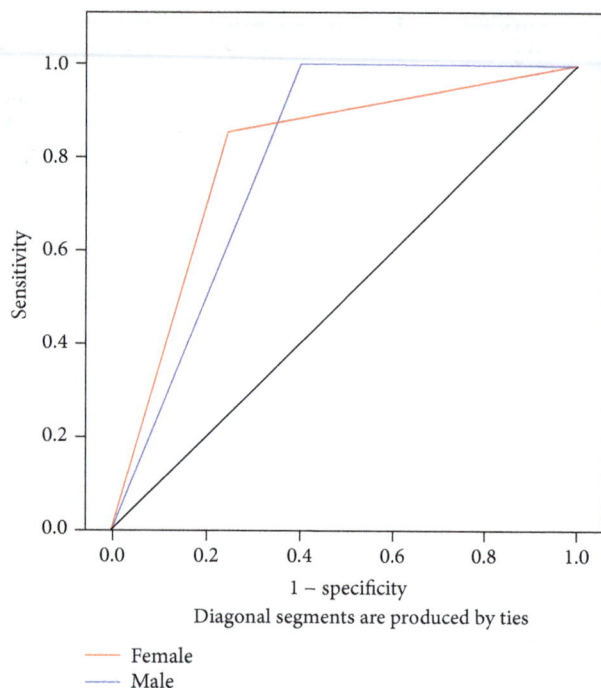

FIGURE 4: Receiver operating characteristic (ROC) curves of serum leptin and delayed puberty in β-TM patients with cut-off vales mentioned in the text. The red and blue lines indicate female and male β-TM patients, respectively. The AUCs ($\pm$SE) and P values for female and male β-TM patients are 0.717 ($\pm$0.166), $P = 0.235$ and 0.553 ($\pm$0.191), $P = 0.777$, respectively.

adipose tissue cannot ensure adequate leptin production when the highest leptin secretion levels are required during development. These authors suggested that the lack of leptin production might be a cofactor for the dysfunction in pubertal timing observed in patients with β-TM.

The present findings of significantly lower serum leptin levels in males with β-TM relative to females are similar to results observed in Greece [23] and Iran [24]. Serum leptin levels were found to be two- to threefold higher in pubertal girls relative to pubertal boys [25], which is also associated with a rise in oestrogen levels [26]. Androgens are thought to provoke a reduction in leptin production, which may explain the low levels of serum leptin observed in male individuals [27]. However, the difference in the serum leptin concentrations in both sexes also occurred during prepubertal age, implying that factors other than sex steroid hormones (e.g., fat mass in the body and energy expenditure) may cause a fluctuation in serum leptin concentrations [28, 29].

Linear multiple regression analysis showed a positive association between serum leptin levels and sex, BMI, and β-TM. Many studies [30, 31] showed that BMI is positively associated with high serum leptin levels. Gender also affects serum leptin levels [32] as leptin is higher in females than in males. The sex differences are probably due to different amounts of subcutaneous adipose tissue [33] and hormonal concentrations [26, 28]. However, β-TM appears to be an even stronger factor than sex as β-TM accounts for one-quarter (25.1%) of the variation in serum leptin levels. However, other reports mentioned that other factors can affect serum leptin levels, including lifestyle variables, serum lipid patterns, and iron overload [30, 34, 35]. Iron overload typically occurs in patients with β-TM due to repeated blood transfusions, which is accompanied by increased serum ferritin, a condition observed in our β-TM patients. Although iron is indispensable for life, it can act as a potent and potentially dangerous oxidant. Thus, iron overload followed by iron deposition in fat cells is harmful and toxic because of the free radical formation that causes the destruction of the adipocyte membrane and inhibits the activity of adipose cells [36]. The leptin receptor is also found on haematopoietic and bone marrow cells; hence, in β-TM patients, who display a high haemolytic rate due to an abnormal Hb structure, a defect in haematopoietic cells may result in decreased serum leptin levels [36]. Kyriakou and Skordis stated that the hypogonadotropic hypogonadism observed in β-TM is associated not only with the toxic effect of iron on gonadotroph cells but also with iron toxicity in adipocytes, thereby altering the physiological role of leptin in sexual maturation and fertility [37]. Dedoussis et al. found a negative correlation between soluble transferrin receptor levels, a clinical marker for total body iron stores, and plasma leptin in β-TM patients [38]. They reported that these findings enhance previous results indicating that leptin may play some role in haematopoiesis and could associate the pathophysiology of β-TM patients with the effect of leptin in triggering reproductive ability.

Recently, a direct relationship between iron and leptin was suggested [35]. This relationship is based on the observation that the absence of adipocyte ferroportin (iron-regulated transporter 1) results in increased levels of iron in the adipose tissue together with reduced serum leptin and the demonstration that the decreased leptin mRNA levels are due to decreased transcription, indicating that iron directly regulates leptin synthesis [35]. Whether such observation and results are applicable in β-TM patients requires further study.

Data from the HELENA study [39] of 967 healthy adolescents suggested that serum leptin levels could be used as a marker for the prediction of early-onset puberty. In our study, the sensitivity and specificity of serum leptin levels as a predicator of short stature and delayed puberty in β-TM patients were assessed using ROC analysis, which is considered a useful tool for evaluating the performance of diagnostic tests [40]. This analysis revealed higher sensitivity and specificity in β-TM females relative to males which was significant only in short-stature β-TM females. We are unable to explain the lower specificity of leptin levels in males with short stature or delayed puberty apart from differences in body fat distribution, particularly in the amount of subcutaneous fat, and sex hormones. The small sample size could also be a factor, particularly regarding delayed puberty. However, other factors cannot be excluded; thus, further investigation is required. Ganji et al. [41] suggested that physiological and/or metabolic differences could be the cause of variations in serum leptin levels between males and females.

Low serum leptin has implications for growth and pubertal development in normal children and adolescents [42].

These effects would likely be more pronounced in patients with β-TM. More data are required for an effective interpretation of our results. Furthermore, the interplay of leptin with the metabolism of energy balance and reproduction is well reviewed and discussed in several recent studies [8, 9, 17, 43] that investigated the mechanisms of leptin signalling through kisspeptin-dependent and kisspeptin-independent pathways and through leptin receptors. Whether these mechanisms are interrupted or amplified in thalassaemia patients remains an open question.

Our study has the following limitations. First, the sample size was small, which could affect our analysis and conclusions. Second, sex hormone profiles and measurements of fat distribution were not performed. Third, levels of the peptide hormone hepcidin, which is secreted by the liver and acts as a key regulator of iron metabolism in the body, as well as leptin receptor levels, were not determined. Despite these limitations, the results of our study are comparable to published findings and, to the best of our knowledge, our study is the first of its kind to be conducted in Arab patients with β-TM.

Importantly, every β-TM patient requires proper management and strict follow-up. Early diagnosis and treatment with chelating agents to prevent hypogonadism are essential for a better quality of life. A deeper knowledge of the pathogenesis and manifestation of β-TM, combined with innovative new treatments to prevent endocrine complications and iron overload toxicity, will result in better life for β-TM patients.

5. Conclusion

In conclusion, the association and interaction between serum leptin levels, growth retardation, and pubertal development in patients with β-TM suggested that serum leptin can be used to predict short stature in β-TM patients and as a guide for further therapeutic or hormonal modulation, particularly in females. Furthermore, additional research is required to elucidate the biochemical and physiological changes in subjects with β-TM that affect the levels of serum leptin.

Competing Interests

The authors declare no competing financial interests.

Authors' Contributions

Lamia Mustafa Al-Naama and Meaad Kadum Hassan designed the study, interpreted the data, and cowrote and gave the final approval for publication of the paper. Muhannad Maki Abdul Karim collected and analysed the data and wrote the paper.

Acknowledgments

The authors thank Professor Dr. Jasim Al Asadi, Department of Community Medicine, College of Medicine, University of Basrah, for his valuable remarks, criticism, and assistance in the linear regression analysis. Thanks are due to the study participants and their families, who made this work possible.

References

[1] P. J. Giardina and B. G. Forget, "Thalassemia syndromes," in Haematology, Basic Principles and Practice, R. Hoffman, E. J. Benz Jr., S. J. Shattil et al., Eds., chapter 41, pp. 535–564, Churchill Livingstone, New York, NY, USA, 5th edition, 2008.

[2] L. Gautron and J. K. Elmquist, "Sixteen years and counting: an update on leptin in energy balance," Journal of Clinical Investigation, vol. 121, no. 6, pp. 2087–2093, 2011.

[3] R. S. Ahima, C. B. Saper, J. S. Flier, and J. K. Elmquist, "Leptin regulation of neuroendocrine systems," Frontiers in Neuroendocrinology, vol. 21, no. 3, pp. 263–307, 2000.

[4] J. W. Hill, J. K. Elmquist, and C. F. Elias, "Hypothalamic pathways linking energy balance and reproduction," The American Journal of Physiology—Endocrinology and Metabolism, vol. 294, no. 5, pp. E827–E832, 2008.

[5] S. N. De Biasi, L. I. Apfelbaum, and M. E. Apfelbaum, "In vitro effect of leptin on LH release by anterior pituitary glands from female rats at the time of spontaneous and steroid-induced LH surge," European Journal of Endocrinology, vol. 145, no. 5, pp. 659–665, 2001.

[6] W. H. Yu, A. Walczewska, S. Karanth, and S. M. McCann, "Nitric oxide mediates leptin-induced luteinizing hormone-releasing hormone (LHRH) and LHRH and leptin-induced LH release from the pituitary gland," Endocrinology, vol. 138, no. 11, pp. 5055–5058, 1997.

[7] D. R. Mann, A. O. K. Johnson, T. Gimpel, and V. D. Castracane, "Changes in circulating leptin, leptin receptor, and gonadal hormones from infancy until advanced age in humans," Journal of Clinical Endocrinology and Metabolism, vol. 88, no. 7, pp. 3339–3345, 2003.

[8] C. F. Elias and D. Purohit, "Leptin signaling and circuits in puberty and fertility," Cellular and Molecular Life Sciences, vol. 70, no. 5, pp. 841–862, 2013.

[9] M. A. Sanchez-Garrido and M. Tena-Sempere, "Metabolic control of puberty: roles of leptin and kisspeptins," Hormones and Behavior, vol. 64, no. 2, pp. 187–194, 2013.

[10] M. E. Wilson, J. Fisher, K. Chikazawa et al., "Leptin administration increases nocturnal concentrations of luteinizing hormone and growth hormone in juvenile female rhesus monkeys," Journal of Clinical Endocrinology and Metabolism, vol. 88, no. 10, pp. 4874–4883, 2003.

[11] C. G. D. Brook and R. S. Brown, "Problems of puberty and adolescence," in Handbook of Clinical Paediatric Endocrinology, C. G. D. Brook and R. S. Brown, Eds., pp. 63–70, Blackwell Publishing, Oxford, UK, 1st edition, 2008.

[12] D. Cocchi, V. De Gennaro Colonna, M. Bagnasco, D. Bonacci, and E. E. Müller, "Leptin regulates GH secretion in the rat by acting on GHRH and somatostatinergic functions," Journal of Endocrinology, vol. 162, no. 1, pp. 95–99, 1999.

[13] M. K. Hassan, J. Y. Taha, L. M. Al-Naama, N. M. Widad, and S. N. Jasim, "Frequency of β-thalassaemia, haemoglobin S and glucose-6-phosphate dehydrogenase deficiency in Basra

governorate, Iraq," *The Eastern Mediterranean Health Journal*, vol. 9, no. 1-2, pp. 45–54, 2003.

[14] Centers for Disease Control (CDC), "Ped NSS Health Indicators," 2009, http://www.cdc.gov/pednss/what_is/pednss_health_indicators.htm.

[15] World Health Organization, "The WHO child growth standard," 2006, http://www.who.int/growthref/en/, http://www.who.int/childgrowth/en/.

[16] D. Styne, "Puberty," in *Greenspan's Basic and Clinical Endocrinology*, D. G. Gardner and D. Shoback, Eds., pp. 620–630, McGraw-Hill Companies, New York, NY, USA, 8th edition, 2007.

[17] M. Tena-Sempere, "Interaction between energy homeostasis and reproduction: central effects of leptin and ghrelin on the reproductive axis," *Hormone and Metabolic Research*, vol. 45, no. 13, pp. 919–927, 2013.

[18] S. Blüher and C. S. Mantzoros, "Leptin in humans: lessons from translational research," *The American Journal of Clinical Nutrition*, vol. 89, no. 3, pp. 991S–997S, 2009.

[19] O. Nilsson, R. Marino, F. De Luca, M. Phillip, and J. Baron, "Endocrine regulation of the growth plate," *Hormone Research*, vol. 64, no. 4, pp. 157–165, 2005.

[20] L. Perrone, S. Perrotta, P. Raimondo et al., "Inappropriate leptin secretion in thalassemia: a potential cofactor of pubertal timing derangement," *Journal of Pediatric Endocrinology and Metabolism*, vol. 16, no. 6, pp. 877–881, 2003.

[21] G.-R. Moshtaghi-Kashanian and F. Razavi, "Ghrelin and leptin levels in relation to puberty and reproductive function in patients with beta-thalassemia," *Hormones*, vol. 8, no. 3, pp. 207–213, 2009.

[22] H. Choobineh, S. J. Dehghani, S. Alizadeh et al., "Evaluation of leptin levels in major beta-thalassemic patients," *International Journal of Hematology-Oncology and Stem Cell Research*, vol. 3, no. 4, pp. 1–4, 2009.

[23] F. Karachaliou, E. Vlachopapadopoulou, M. Theochari, E. Konstandellou, and S. Michalacos, "Leptin levels in patients with thalassemia major," *Minerva Pediatrica*, vol. 58, no. 4, pp. 373–378, 2006.

[24] I. Shahramian, N. M. Noori, A. Teimouri, E. Akhlaghi, and E. Sharafi, "The correlation between serum level of leptin and troponin in children with major beta-Thalassemia," *Iranian Journal of Pediatric Hematology and Oncology*, vol. 5, no. 1, pp. 11–17, 2015.

[25] P. E. Clayton, M. S. Gill, C. M. Hall, V. Tillmann, A. J. Whatmore, and D. A. Price, "Serum leptin through childhood and adolescence," *Clinical Endocrinology*, vol. 46, no. 6, pp. 727–733, 1997.

[26] M. F. Saad, S. Damani, R. L. Gingerich et al., "Sexual dimorphism in plasma leptin concentration," *Journal of Clinical Endocrinology and Metabolism*, vol. 82, no. 2, pp. 579–584, 1997.

[27] M. Wabitsch, W. F. Blum, R. Muche et al., "Contribution of androgens to the gender difference in leptin production in obese children and adolescents," *The Journal of Clinical Investigation*, vol. 100, no. 4, pp. 808–813, 1997.

[28] J. N. Roemmich, P. A. Clark, S. S. Berr et al., "Gender differences in leptin levels during puberty are related to the subcutaneous fat depot and sex steroids," *The American Journal of Physiology—Endocrinology and Metabolism*, vol. 275, no. 3, pp. E543–E551, 1998.

[29] F. B. Slama, N. Jridi, M. C. B. Rayana, A. Trimeche, M. Hsairi, and O. Belhadj, "Plasma levels of leptin and ghrelin and their correlation with BMI, and circulating lipids and glucose in obese Tunisian women," *Asian Biomedicine*, vol. 9, no. 2, pp. 161–168, 2015.

[30] M. Y. Al Maskari and A. A. Alnaqdy, "Correlation between serum leptin levels, body mass index and obesity in Omanis," *Sultan Qaboos University Medical Journal*, vol. 6, no. 2, pp. 27–31, 2006.

[31] R. F. Paul, M. Hassan, H. S. Nazar, S. Gillani, and N. Afzal, "Effect of body mass index on serum leptin levels," *Journal of Ayub Medical College, Abbottabad*, vol. 23, no. 3, pp. 40–43, 2011.

[32] W. T. Ambrosius, J. A. Compton, R. R. Bowsher, and J. H. Pratt, "Relation of race, age, and sex hormone differences to serum leptin concentrations in children and adolescents," *Hormone Research*, vol. 49, no. 5, pp. 240–246, 1998.

[33] R. N. Bawngartner, R. R. Ross, D. L. Waters et al., "Serum leptin in elderly people: associations with sex hormones, insulin, and adipose tissue volumes," *Obesity Research*, vol. 7, no. 2, pp. 141–149, 1999.

[34] R. Olstad, J. Florholmen, J. Svartberg, J. H. Rosenvinge, and G. S. Birketvedt, "Leptin in the general population, differences in sex hormones, blood lipids, gender and life style characteristics," *The Open Behavioral Science Journal*, vol. 5, pp. 8–15, 2011.

[35] Y. Gao, Z. Li, J. S. Gabrielsen et al., "Adipocyte iron regulates leptin and food intake," *The Journal of Clinical Investigation*, vol. 125, no. 9, pp. 3681–3691, 2015.

[36] I. Shahramian, E. Akhlaghi, A. Ramezani, A. Rezaee, N. M. Noori, and E. Sharafi, "A Study of leptin serum concentrations in patients with major beta-Thalassemia," *Iranian Journal of Pediatric Hematology and Oncology*, vol. 3, no. 2, pp. 59–63, 2013.

[37] A. Kyriakou and N. Skordis, "Thalassaemia and aberrations of growth and puberty," *Mediterranean Journal of Hematology and Infectious Diseases*, vol. 1, no. 1, Article ID e2009003, 2009.

[38] G. V. Dedoussis, M. C. Kyrtsonis, N. E. Andrikopoulos, E. Voskaridou, and A. Loutradis, "Inverse correlation of plasma leptin and soluble transferrin receptor levels in β-thalassemia patients," *Annals of Hematology*, vol. 81, no. 9, pp. 543–547, 2002.

[39] T. Koester-Weber, J. Valtuena, C. Breidenassel et al., "Reference values for leptin, cortisol, insulin and glucose, among european adolescents and their association with adiposity: the HELENA study," *Nutricion Hospitalaria*, vol. 30, no. 5, pp. 1181–1190, 2014.

[40] K. H. Zou, A. J. O'Malley, and L. Mauri, "Receiver-operating characteristic analysis for evaluating diagnostic tests and predictive models," *Circulation*, vol. 115, no. 5, pp. 654–657, 2007.

[41] V. Ganji, M. R. Kafai, and E. McCarthy, "Serum leptin concentrations are not related to dietary patterns but are related to sex, age, body mass index, serum triacylglycerol, serum insulin, and plasma glucose in the US population," *Nutrition and Metabolism*, vol. 6, article 3, 2009.

[42] A. T. Soliman, M. Yasin, and A. Kassem, "Leptin in pediatrics: a hormone from adipocyte that wheels several functions in children," *Indian Journal of Endocrinology and Metabolism*, vol. 16, supplement 3, pp. S577–S587, 2012.

[43] D. Garcia-Galiano, S. J. Allen, and C. F. Elias, "Role of the adipocyte-derived hormone leptin in reproductive control," *Hormone Molecular Biology and Clinical Investigation*, vol. 19, no. 3, pp. 141–149, 2014.

19

Towards a Molecular Understanding of the Fanconi Anemia Core Complex

Charlotte Hodson and Helen Walden

Protein Structure and Function Laboratory, Lincoln's Inn Fields Laboratories, London Research Institute, Cancer Research UK, 44 Lincoln's Inn Fields, London WC2A 3LY, UK

Correspondence should be addressed to Helen Walden, helen.walden@cancer.org.uk

Academic Editor: Stefan Meyer

Fanconi Anemia (FA) is a genetic disorder characterized by the inability of patient cells to repair DNA damage caused by interstrand crosslinking agents. There are currently 14 verified FA genes, where mutation of any single gene prevents repair of DNA interstrand crosslinks (ICLs). The accumulation of ICL damage results in genome instability and patients having a high predisposition to cancers. The key event of the FA pathway is dependent on an eight-protein core complex (CC), required for the monoubiquitination of each member of the FANCD2-FANCI complex. Interestingly, the majority of patient mutations reside in the CC. The molecular mechanisms underlying the requirement for such a large complex to carry out a monoubiquitination event remain a mystery. This paper documents the extensive efforts of researchers so far to understand the molecular roles of the CC proteins with regard to its main function in the FA pathway, the monoubiquitination of FANCD2 and FANCI.

1. Introduction

Fanconi Anemia (FA) patients present a variety of symptoms including skeletal and developmental defects, bone marrow failure, and a high predisposition to cancer [1]. The predisposition to cancer is attributed to the FA pathway being involved in DNA damage repair, particularly interstrand crosslinks (ICLs). FA patients are highly susceptible to crosslinking agents such as mitomycin C (MMC) and cisplatin. Such treatment results in chromosome abnormalities, and sensitivity to these agents is used as a diagnostic tool for FA [2]. Currently there are 14 verified FA genes [3–22], with a possible additional gene FANCO/Rad51C [23, 24], that make up the FA pathway. Mutations in any of the 15 genes results in the loss of ICL repair. The key event of the FA pathway is the monoubiquitination of FANCD2 and FANCI [4–7], which triggers the downstream factors, FANCP/SLX4, FANCD1/BRCA2, FANCJ/BRIP1, FANCN/PALB2 [9, 10, 17–22] to repair DNA damage (Figure 1). Only one protein to date has been shown to have E3 ubiquitin ligase activity, FANCL [8]. FANCL is a member of the Fanconi Anemia Core Complex (CC), consisting of 7 other FA proteins: FANCA, FANCB, FANCC, FANCE, FANCF, FANCG, and FANCM (Figure 1) [3, 25–28]. Additionally, there are the Fanconi Anemia Associated Proteins (FAAPs), which are not yet found mutated in patients but form part of the CC: FAAP100, FAAP24, and most recently FAAP20 [29–33]. MHF1 and MHF2 (also known as FAAP16 and FAAP10) have also been implicated in the FA pathway through their association with FANCM [34, 35]. Approximately 90% of patient mutations reside in the CC, most of which are found in FANCA (60%) (Table 1) [36]. Importantly a single mutation in any of the 8 genes that make up the CC prevents the key monoubiquitination event from occurring. Extensive research efforts have been made to understand the role of the individual CC proteins and the requirement of all CC proteins for the monoubiquitination event. This paper outlines our current understanding of the molecular interactions within the core complex and highlights key remaining questions for a full molecular understanding of the CC.

2. E3 Ligase Function of the CC

Patient mutations in any member of a CC protein result in the loss of the critical monoubiquitination of the

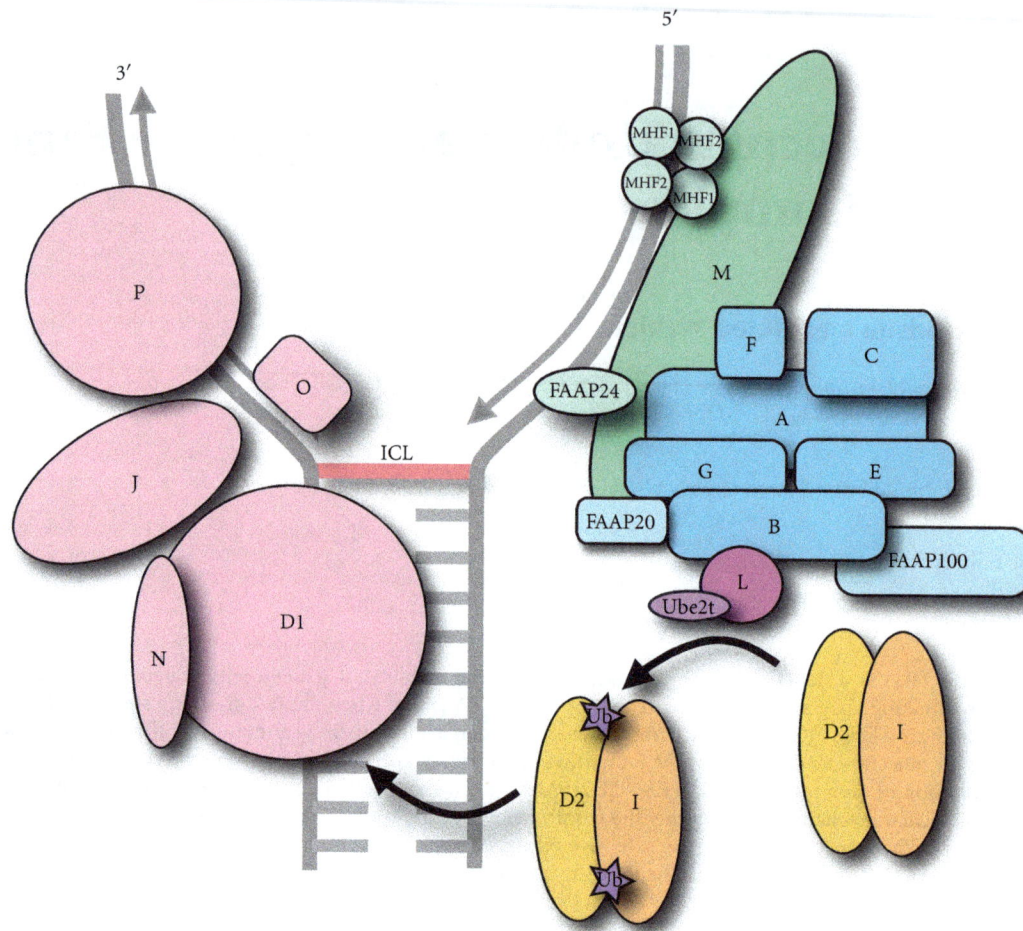

FIGURE 1: The Fanconi Anemia Pathway. A model of the Fanconi Anemia Pathway at a stalled DNA (grey) replication fork, caused by an interstrand crosslink (ICL). FANCM and its associated genes are coloured green, which assemble on DNA at the stalled replication fork. The other CC proteins are represented by blue with FANCL as the E3 ligase of the CC represented by mauve. The substrates for ubiquitination FANCD2 and FANCI are coloured gold and peach, respectively, with their associated ubiquitins represented by purple stars. The DNA repair machinery is coloured pink.

FANCI/FANCD2 complex. All CC proteins appear to be required for this event *in vivo;* therefore, historically the CC has been regarded as a multisubunit E3 ligase. Multisubunit E3 ligases such as the Cullin-RING ligases (CRLs) and the Anaphase Promoting Complex (APC) are well understood at the molecular level, with their modularity essential for function.

The CRLs consist of a Cullin scaffold protein, which associates with either Rbx1 or Rbx2 RING proteins, the subunit responsible for binding the E2 carrying the activated ubiquitin moiety [37]. The Cullin and RING therefore form the catalytic unit of the CRL. In order for a substrate to become ubiquitinated, it must be recognised by the CRL. This is achieved by the substrate receptor proteins, which associate through an adaptor protein onto the Cullin scaffold, forming the complete CRL (Figure 2(a)) [37]. A plethora of different substrate recognition proteins for a

single Cullin achieves flexibility within the CRLs to target a repertoire of substrates.

The APC also targets a variety of substrates to control cell cycle progression from metaphase to anaphase. Similarly to the CRLs the APC comprises of a Cullin repeat protein Apc2, which binds the RING protein Apc11, and also Apc10 involved in substrate association. Together, these 3 subunits form the catalytic unit. However, in contrast to CRLs the APC contains an additional 10 proteins (Figure 2(b)). Apc9 and 13 and Cdc26 are structural stabilizers, whereas Apc1, 4, and 5 form a scaffold platform for the catalytic unit [38]. The scaffold platform along with the tetratricopeptide repeat (TPR) proteins Cdc23, Cdc27, Cdc16, and structural stabilizer Cdc26 forms the TPR subcomplex, orientating the catalytic unit for its association with coactivators, Cdc20 and Cdh1 [38]. The co-activators are required along with Apc10 for substrate recognition [38–40]. In common with

TABLE 1: Fanconi Anemia genes and their products.

Gene	MW (kDa)	No. of amino acids	Patient mutations
A	163	1455	60%
B	98	859	2%
C	63	558	13%
D1	384	3418	2%
D2	164	1451	3%
E	59	536	3%
F	42	374	3%
G	68	622	9%
I	150	1328	1%
J	141	1249	2%
L	42	375	0.2%
M	232	2048	0.2%
N	131	1186	0.6%
O	42	376	0.5%
P	200	1834	0.5%
FAAP24	24	215	—
FAAP100	100	881	—
MHF1	16	138	—
MHF2	10	81	—

Amino acids numbers were taken from the NCBI webserver, and patient mutational information was obtained from the Rockerfeller FA Mutations Database and was calculated as a percentage of all individuals recorded in the database.

the CRLs, this ensemble allows flexibility and diversity in substrate recognition.

By contrast, the CC has one subunit with E3 ligase activity, FANCL [8] (Figure 2(c)), shown to be the only subunit of the CC required for FANCD2 monoubiquitination *in vitro* [41]. FANCL is a RING E3 ligase [42], which binds the E2 of the FA pathway, Ube2t [41, 43] in a canonical fashion through its RING domain [43, 44]. Earlier *in vitro* and *in vivo* work indicated a FANCE-FANCD2 interaction [45] and a series of yeast and mammalian 2-hybrid studies further support this interaction [46–48]. The interaction of FANCD2 with a CC component prompted the idea that FANCE may bring the substrates FANCD2 and FANCI into close proximity of FANCL for their subsequent monoubiquitination. As with other multisubunit E3 ligases, this would leave FANCL as the "catalytic" subunit, indirectly ubiquitinating substrates through its interaction with E2. However, not only is FANCL sufficient *in vitro* for the monoubiquitination event [41], but also has been shown to interact directly with both FANCD2 and FANCI *in vitro* [42, 44], and with FANCD2 in cells [49]. Although mutations in other CC proteins result in a loss of the monoubiquitination event, these more recent findings suggest FANCL possesses all the requirements to be able to carry out the monoubiquitination, unlike the multisubunit E3 ligases.

3. Protein-Protein Interactions Required for CC Stability

Although the monoubiquitination event *in vitro* requires only FANCL, it is clear from patient mutations that all members of the CC are required *in vivo*. The reasons for this are not clear, although numerous groups have shown the CC proteins interact with one another and are required to form a stable CC. Part of the challenge of gaining a molecular understanding of the core complex lies in the lack of obvious domain structures from primary sequences in any of the proteins except FANCL and FANCM. This section will describe the efforts to understand the molecular biology of the core complex to date.

3.1. FANCG-FANCA CC Interactions. FANCG and FANCA have been shown to interact directly and indirectly through yeast 2-hybrid, co-immunoprecipitations (co-IPs), cell-based studies, and *in vitro* translational (IVT) work [25, 26, 46, 50–55] (Figure 3). Co-IPS and IVT studies suggested the N-terminal 300 residues of FANCA bind FANCG [50, 51]. This region has been further narrowed down to the first 40 amino acids by a yeast 2-hybrid assay and the first 37 amino acids by a co-IP study [25, 46], with a requirement for basic amino acids within this region for the interaction [25]. IVT studies indicate residues 18–29 of FANCA are sufficient for a FANCG interaction, specifically Arginine 18, Arginine 19, and Leucine 25 [50]. Studies aimed at identifying the regions of FANCG involved in a FANCA interaction are more conflicting. Hussain et al. [55] reported via yeast 2-hybrid analysis that the predicted TPR motifs 5 and 6 of FANCG, which reside in the C-terminal 170 residues, were required for the interaction. Consistent with this finding, IVT assays also revealed two FANCA binding regions in the C-terminal 222 residues of FANCG: one encompassing the same predicted TPR motifs 5 and 6, and the second

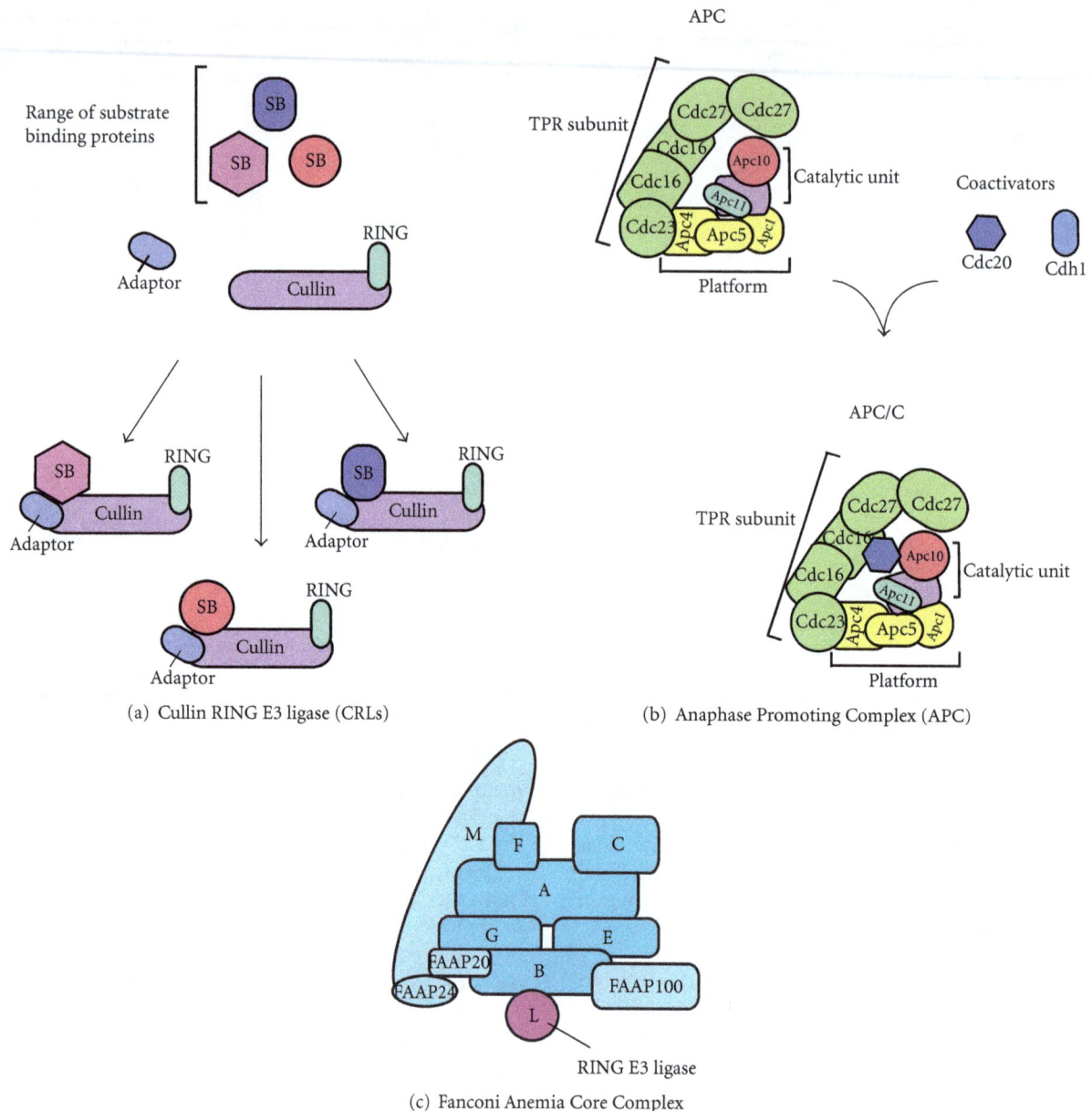

FIGURE 2: Models of multisubunit E3 ligases. (a) A model of the proteins that make a Cullin-RING E3 ligase (CRL). The Cullin protein (lilac) acts as scaffold and binds the RING domain (cyan) required for E2 binding and the substrate binding proteins (pink, red, blue) via an adaptor. The variety of substrate binding proteins allows the CRLs flexibility in binding a range of substrates. (b) A model of the Anaphase Promoting Complex (APC). The catalytic core consists of a Cullin repeat protein Apc2 (lilac), which acts a scaffold for the RING protein, Apc11 (cyan), and the substrate binding protein Apc10 (red). For substrate recognition the APC also binds coactivators (dark blue). The APC also consists of a TPR subcomplex (green) and a platform (yellow) which orient the catalytic unit and aid binding to the co-activators. The range of subunits allows a variety of substrates to be recognised. (c) A model of the Fanconi Anemia Core Complex. The catalytic activity resides in one protein FANCL (mauve). The rest of the CC proteins are coloured blue, with light blue representing proteins associated with the CC.

residing in the last 37 residues of FANCG [50]. However, in contrast, a yeast 2-hybrid study found the C-terminal 142 amino acids of FANCG to be dispensable for interaction with FANCA [46]. To add to the complexity, other studies report a requirement for additional regions throughout FANCG for a FANCA interaction [52, 54, 56] with Wilson et al.'s [56] *in vivo* study indicating several regions, TPR motifs 1, 2, 5, and 6 throughout FANCG are required.

FANCG null lymphoblasts have a defect in FANCA nuclear accumulation, which can be rescued by the addition of FANCG, suggesting that FANCG plays a role in the subcellular localization of FANCA [26]. Indeed, the FANCG interaction with FANCA appears to promote FANCA nuclear accumulation [26]. However, a thorough analysis of multiple FANCA patient mutations suggests that FANCG binds FANCA even when the nuclear localisation of FANCA

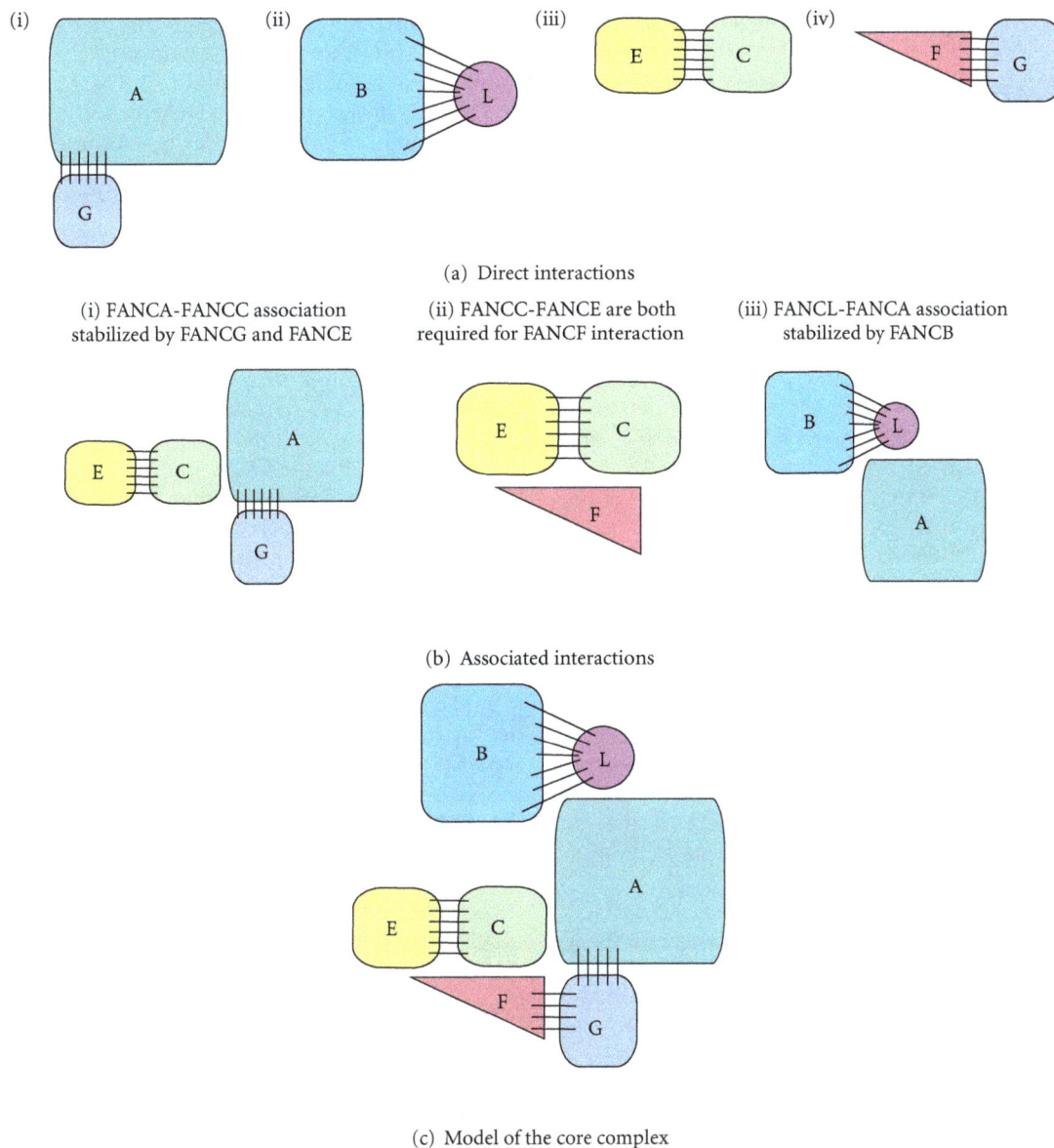

(a) Direct interactions

(i) FANCA-FANCC association stabilized by FANCG and FANCE

(ii) FANCC-FANCE are both required for FANCF interaction

(iii) FANCL-FANCA association stabilized by FANCB

(b) Associated interactions

(c) Model of the core complex

FIGURE 3: A model of CC interactions. (a) Models of the CC proteins that directly interact with one another, represented by black lines. Yeast and mammalian 2-hybrid and *in vitro* and translational studies have shown these interactions. (b) Associated CC interactions as shown by mammalian and yeast 3-hybrid experiments. (c) A model of how all the CC proteins interact to from the full CC, the requirement for the monoubiquitination event.

is lost [57]. The FANCA extreme N-terminus contains a nuclear localisation signal (NLS) [25, 58]. FANCA patient mutations are varied and account for 60% of all FA cases (Table 1) and predominantly result in loss of FANCA nuclear accumulation [57]. It appears likely that a combination of the NLS on FANCA and FANCG-binding stabilise, and supports the nuclear subcellular localisation of the core complex.

These studies all indicate a likely physical interaction between FANCG, and FANCA, but the molecular details have yet to be fully resolved.

3.2. FANCF CC Interactions. FANCF has been implicated in the physical stability of the majority of other CC proteins,

FANCC, FANCE, FANCG and FANCA by several groups [27, 28, 59, 60]. X-ray crystallographic analysis of a C-terminal portion of FANCF (residues 156–357) revealed an architecture of helical repeats [60], similar to those found in scaffolding proteins. Structure-based mutations were then generated for use in mammalian co-IP assays. Using both point mutations L209R and F251R and a hydrophobic patch mutation Y287A/L289A/F339A/V341A/L344A, Kowal and coworkers [60] verified and provided the molecular details of the FANCF associations with FANCA and FANCC reported from earlier co-IP studies [27]. In addition, a further association with FANCE was identified [60]. In contrast to the structure-based analysis, Léveillé et al. [59]

use coimmunoprecipitation from cultured lymphoblasts and report the requirement of the last 31 amino acids (343–374) of FANCF for a FANCG and FANCA interaction and additionally report that the first 15 N-terminal amino acids are required for a FANCE and FANCC interaction.

Yeast and mammalian 3-hybrids revealed that a FANCC-FANCE interaction was required for a direct interaction with FANCF [59, 61]. In accordance with their co-IP studies, Léveillé et al. [59] show residues Leu5/Leu8/Leu15 are required for a FANCC-FANCE interaction in their mammalian 3-hybrid assay and report two additional regions, Arg10/Phe11/Arg47/Phe48 and Ser18/Ser19/Thr20/Thr21, also required for this interaction [59]. Whilst these findings are not necessarily incompatible, the molecular details of the interactions between FANCF and FANCG, FANCA and FANCE are still unresolved.

The FANCA-FANCF interaction is mediated by FANCG, from yeast 3-hybrid analyses [46]; conversely co-IP studies indicate a FANCA-FANCG interaction is stabilized by FANCF [27]. Both these observations are supported by yeast 2-hybrid experiments that show a direct interaction of FANCG with FANCF [28, 46, 55, 59]. Gordon and Buchwald [46] show that this interaction resides in the last 131 C-terminal residues of FANCF, and Léveillé et al. [59] narrow this down to the last 40 amino acids in their yeast 2-hybrid assay. Several groups have attempted to map the region of FANCG responsible for a FANCF interaction by yeast 2-hybrid analysis, all of which conclude that several sites are required throughout the full amino acid sequence of FANCG [46, 52, 55].

Importantly, structure-guided mutagenesis of FANCF increased MMC sensitivity, thereby directly showing FANCF interactions are critical [60]. Although there are conflicting results regarding FANCF associations with other CC members, numerous studies all support the role for FANCF in coordinating and stabilizing other CC proteins, as seen for FANCG.

3.3. FANCE-FANCC CC Interactions. A FANCC-FANCE interaction and their association with other members of the CC have been documented by yeast and mammalian 2- and 3-hybrid assays, IVT studies and co-IPs [28, 45–47, 59, 62]. The central part of FANCE, residues 149–371, is required for the FANCC interaction as seen by yeast and mammalian 2-hybrid experiments [46, 47]. However, the corresponding regions of FANCC required for the interaction were not determined. More recent studies employing mammalian and yeast 3-hybrid assays indicate the importance of a FANCC-FANCE interaction to facilitate a direct interaction with FANCF [59, 61]. This interaction of FANCE with FANCF explains early co-IP findings of FANCEs associations with FANCA, FANCG, and FANCF [45, 62], as FANCF has been shown to directly interact with FANCG, and FANCG directly interacts with FANCA, indicating a possible indirect association of these proteins.

3.4. FANCL-FANCB CC Interactions. Research has indicated FANCL is required to form a stable CC using co-IP

experiments and size exclusion chromatography [63, 64]. Alpi et al. [64] show that in a wild-type chicken DT40 lymphoblastoid cell line, a complex of 1.5 MDa pulled out using a Tandem-affinity tagged FANCC exists. In corresponding FANCL-null cells, this complex is both less abundant and a lower molecular weight. However, the 1.5 MDa complex is established again upon expressing FANCL [64]. Consistent with these data, co-IPs in FANCL-null cells show a disruption of the interactions of FA CC proteins [63]. In the same study, a mammalian 2-hybrid assay indicates that FANCL forms a direct interaction with the CC via FANCB [63] (Figure 3). Medhurst et al. [63] also suggest that FANCL-FANCA interactions are mediated through FANCB and that FANCG is required to stabilize FANCA in this interaction. Additionally Alpi et al. [64] demonstrate that the stabilizing role of FANCL for the CC is independent from its E3 ligase activity, as point mutations that disrupt the RING domain and inhibit the monoubiquitination activity can still form a stable CC when introduced into the FANCL-null cell line. It is clear that FANCL is an important member of the CC for stability; however, molecular details, including the stoichiometry and domain requirements of how FANCL interacts with the CC are still lacking.

The intricacy of, these CC protein-protein interactions is further complicated by the findings that a FANCA-FANCG interaction is required in stabilizing a FANCC-FANCA interaction and the need for FANCE to support the FANCA-FANCC interaction [25, 62].

The extensive research described here reflects a complex network of interactions between the CC proteins (summarized in Figure 3), all of which seem to be a requirement for a fully stable CC.

4. Subcomplexes, Stoichiometry, and Assembly of the CC

As discussed above FANCA has an NLS and monoubiquitinated FANCD2 locates at nuclear foci on chromatin as seen by fluorescent microscopy and co-IP studies [7, 65, 66]. However, FANCD2 has also been located in the cytoplasm [67–70] as have several of the CC components [8, 27, 51, 71]. Such findings give rise to the possibility that subcomplexes of the CC exist and localize in different cellular regions.

Meetei et al. [72] reported different ratios of CC proteins observed in their co-IPs studies suggesting the idea of subcomplexes, although this could also reflect different stoichiometry of the CC proteins. An analysis of CC proteins isolated from the cytoplasm at different stages of the cell cycle revealed different molecular weight protein complexes by size exclusion chromatography [73]. A complex that consists of a single copy of each FA protein of the CC would give an approximate 737 kDa complex, which would increase to 861 kDa if FAAP24 and FAAP100 were included. Thomashevski et al. [73] report a 600 kDa cytoplasmic complex that increases to a 750 kDa complex during mitosis, supporting the idea of subcomplexes. One study documents such a subcomplex: FANCL-FANCB-FAAP100, which was tandem affinity purified from HeLa cell extracts [29].

Ling et al. [29] also suggest this subcomplex has a stoichiometric ratio of 1 : 1 : 1 in both cytoplasmic and nuclear extracts, with a more prominent association with FANCA in the nucleus. They speculate FANCA along with FANCM may localize the FANCL-FANCB-FAAP100 subcomplex to the nucleus [29]. Medhurst et al. [63] also support the idea of subcomplexes as they reveal from immunoprecipitation experiments of FANCG that FANCA and FANCL are coprecipitated independently of FANCE, FANCC, and FANCF. Studies identifying the localization of individual CC proteins by fluorescence microscopy in cells indicate FANCF and FANCE, which give a joint molecular weight of 101 kDa, are predominantly located in the nucleus, independently of any other CC proteins [27, 45, 47, 62]. FANCEs absence from any cytoplasmic complex described by Thomashevski et al. [73] further supports FANCEs localization in the nucleus. As a full complement of CC proteins is required for the monoubiquitination event, the observations of cytoplasmic subcomplexes and nuclear localization of certain CC proteins prompt the idea of the assembly of the full CC in the nucleus.

The study by Thomashevski et al. [73] supports the idea of the full CC residing in the nucleus, as they report a large nuclear complex of 2 MDa and a 1 MDa chromatin associated complex, both containing CC proteins. As stated above, a CC consisting of one copy of each protein would give an approximate molecular weight of 861 kDa (including FAAP24 and FAAP100). Their reports suggest the nuclear and chromatin complexes may contain multiple copies of CC proteins and indicate the associations of the CC proteins and their stoichiometry differ between the two nuclear and chromatin complexes. Additionally components of these large nuclear complexes are likely to include other nuclear proteins, such as the BLM proteins and MHF1 and MHF2. Meetei et al. [72] report a 1.5–2 MDa complex when immunoprecipitating the BLM complex and found this complex to contain CC proteins. FANCM has since been appointed the CC protein interacting with the BLM proteins, as shown by co-IPs, *in vitro* translational work and fluorescence microscopy [74]. Likewise, Yan et al. [35] report a 1 MDa complex containing CC proteins and the FANCM-associated histone-fold proteins 1 and 2 (MHF1 and MHF2). Elucidating the existence of subcomplexes and a large nuclear CC certainly complicates the understanding of the CC. However, these studies highlight the importance of understanding both the assembly and stoichiometry of the CC and its subcomplexes. Whether there are additional roles for the subcomplexes is not yet understood.

5. FANCM: A Member of the CC?

FANCM is considered a member of the CC, as it coimmunoprecipitates with other CC proteins and the loss of FANCM results in a loss of DNA damaged induced monoubiquitination and nuclear localization of other CC proteins [3, 30, 75, 76]. Indeed FANCM is thought to promote DNA damage-induced monoubiquitination of FANCD2 by recruitment of the CC via FANCF through its MM1 region [74]. Deans and West [74] also show deletions

of regions throughout FANCF reduce an interaction with FANCM and deletion of FANCF residues 1–158 completely disrupt this interaction. The C-terminal end of FANCM associates with FAAP24 and both are thought to stabilize one another, [30, 76]. Ciccia et al. [30] also suggest the stability of FANCM-FAAP24 complex may be dependent on FANCB. However, Kim et al. [77] suggest FANCM recruits the CC proteins to chromatin and is not required for a stable CC. The histone-fold proteins MHF1 and MHF2 form another complex with FANCM [78] and are suggested to aid with the remodelling of DNA, as seen by co-IPs, size exclusion chromatography and DNA binding assays [34, 35]. Although the loss of MHF1 and MHF2 results in a loss of FANCD2 DNA damage inducible monoubiquitination, in agreement with Kim et al. [77], Yan et al. [35] report more than 70% of this complex is independent from the CC. A recent structural analysis reveals that MHF1 and MHF2 form a heterotetrameric complex and that disrupting the heterotetrameric interfaces results in an increased sensitivity to DNA damaging agents as seen by methyl methanesulfonate (MMS) treatment sensitivity assays in yeast [78]. A loss of FANCM has shown a loss of DNA damage inducible monoubiquitination of FANCD2 and many groups have suggested its role as a member of the CC; however, evidence is directing its role upstream of the CC suggesting it acts as a platform to recruit proteins to DNA. Additional evidence shows the FANCM-FAAP24 subcomplex has also been associated with interactions of the BLM complex [30, 74]. The role of FANCM in both Bloom syndrome and FA explains the similarities of the BLM and FA patients' high predisposition to cancer. Additionally the FANCM-FAAP24 subcomplex has also been implicated in ataxia telangiectasia and Rad3-related protein (ATR), a protein kinase associated with cell cycle arrest and checkpoint signalling independently from the rest of the CC proteins, through binding HCLK2 [79].

6. Discussion

The FA pathway has rapidly expanded over the last 15 years to a current count of 15 proteins. The number of FA proteins reflects the complicated nature of understanding the FA pathway, particularly the CC, which consists of over half of the FA proteins. Ascertaining functions for the FA proteins have been exceptionally challenging due to the lack of information divulged from the primary amino acid sequences. Extensive efforts have been made by researchers to define the roles of the individual CC proteins within the CC and to understand the need for such a large CC. However, there are still many remaining questions.

(1) How does the CC support FANCLs E3 ligase activity? Is there a requirement for other CC proteins to localize FANCL to the nucleus? Or do the other CC proteins act as a structural scaffold for the monoubiquitination event?

(2) Do the subcomplexes come together to form a full CC? If so how and where does the assembly take place? And are there independent roles for the subcomplexes?

(3) What are the molecular and stoichiometric details of the CC? The requirement for all CC proteins for the monoubiquitination event is clear from patients with defects in the CC. Therefore, understanding the molecular details of the protein interactions that occur in the CC is key, because therapeutics could be designed to restore or diminish these interactions and furthermore tailored to the different FA complementation groups. The combination of biochemical, biophysical, clinical, and cell work will in time answer these questions.

References

[1] B. P. Alter, "Fanconi's anemia and malignancies," *American Journal of Hematology*, vol. 53, no. 2, pp. 99–110, 1996.

[2] J. German, S. Schonberg, and S. Caskie, "A test for Fanconi's anemia," *Blood*, vol. 69, no. 6, pp. 1637–1641, 1987.

[3] A. R. Meetei, A. L. Medhurst, C. Ling et al., "A human ortholog of archaeal DNA repair protein Hef is defective in Fanconi anemia complementation group M," *Nature Genetics*, vol. 37, no. 9, pp. 958–963, 2005.

[4] A. Smogorzewska, S. Matsuoka, P. Vinciguerra et al., "Identification of the FANCI protein, a monoubiquitinated FANCD2 paralog required for DNA repair," *Cell*, vol. 129, no. 2, pp. 289–301, 2007.

[5] A. E. Sims, E. Spiteri, R. J. Sims et al., "FANCI is a second monoubiquitinated member of the Fanconi anemia pathway," *Nature Structural and Molecular Biology*, vol. 14, no. 6, pp. 564–567, 2007.

[6] C. Timmers, T. Taniguchi, J. Hejna et al., "Positional cloning of a novel Fanconi anemia gene, FANCD2," *Molecular Cell*, vol. 7, no. 2, pp. 241–248, 2001.

[7] I. Garcia-Higuera, T. Taniguchi, S. Ganesan et al., "Interaction of the Fanconi anemia proteins and BRCA1 in a common pathway," *Molecular Cell*, vol. 7, no. 2, pp. 249–262, 2001.

[8] A. R. Meetei, J. P. de Winter, A. L. Medhurst et al., "A novel ubiquitin ligase is deficient in Fanconi anemia," *Nature Genetics*, vol. 35, no. 2, pp. 165–170, 2003.

[9] M. Levitus, Q. Waisfisz, B. C. Godthelp et al., "The DNA helicase BRIP1 is defective in Fanconi anemia complementation group J," *Nature Genetics*, vol. 37, no. 9, pp. 934–935, 2005.

[10] N. G. Howlett, T. Taniguchi, S. Olson et al., "Biallelic inactivation of BRCA2 in Fanconi anemia," *Science*, vol. 297, no. 5581, pp. 606–609, 2002.

[11] J. P. de Winter, Q. Waisfisz, M. A. Rooimans et al., "The Fanconi anaemia group G gene FANCG is identical with XRCC9," *Nature Genetics*, vol. 20, no. 3, pp. 281–283, 1998.

[12] J. P. de Winter, M. A. Rooimans, L. van der Weel et al., "The Fanconi anaemia gene FANCF encodes a novel protein with homology to ROM," *Nature Genetics*, vol. 24, no. 1, pp. 15–16, 2000.

[13] A. R. Meetei, M. Levitus, Y. Xue et al., "X-linked inheritance of Fanconi anemia complementation group B," *Nature Genetics*, vol. 36, no. 11, pp. 1219–1224, 2004.

[14] J. R. L. T. Foe, M. A. Rooimans, L. Bosnoyan-Collins et al., "Expression cloning of a cDNA for the major Fanconi anaemia gene, FAA," *Nature Genetics*, vol. 14, no. 3, pp. 320–323, 1996.

[15] C. A. Strathdee, A. M. V. Duncan, and M. Buchwald, "Evidence for at least four Fanconi anaemia genes including FACC on chromosome 9," *Nature Genetics*, vol. 1, no. 3, pp. 196–198, 1992.

[16] M. Levitus, M. A. Rooimans, J. Steltenpool et al., "Heterogeneity in Fanconi anemia: evidence for 2 new genetic subtypes," *Blood*, vol. 103, no. 7, pp. 2498–2503, 2004.

[17] O. Levran, C. Attwooll, R. T. Henry et al., "The BRCA1-interacting helicase BRIP1 is deficient in Fanconi anemia," *Nature Genetics*, vol. 37, no. 9, pp. 931–933, 2005.

[18] R. Litman, M. Peng, Z. Jin et al., "BACH1 is critical for homologous recombination and appears to be the Fanconi anemia gene product FANCJ," *Cancer Cell*, vol. 8, no. 3, pp. 255–265, 2005.

[19] S. Reid, D. Schindler, H. Hanenberg et al., "Biallelic mutations in PALB2 cause Fanconi anemia subtype FA-N and predispose to childhood cancer," *Nature Genetics*, vol. 39, no. 2, pp. 162–164, 2007.

[20] B. Xia, J. C. Dorsman, N. Ameziane et al., "Fanconi anemia is associated with a defect in the BRCA2 partner PALB2," *Nature Genetics*, vol. 39, no. 2, pp. 159–161, 2007.

[21] Y. Kim, F. P. Lach, R. Desetty, H. Hanenberg, A. D. Auerbach, and A. Smogorzewska, "Mutations of the SLX4 gene in Fanconi anemia," *Nature Genetics*, vol. 43, no. 2, pp. 142–146, 2011.

[22] C. Stoepker, K. Hain, B. Schuster et al., "SLX4, a coordinator of structure-specific endonucleases, is mutated in a new Fanconi anemia subtype," *Nature Genetics*, vol. 43, no. 2, pp. 138–141, 2011.

[23] A. Meindl, H. Hellebrand, C. Wiek et al., "Germline mutations in breast and ovarian cancer pedigrees establish RAD51C as a human cancer susceptibility gene," *Nature Genetics*, vol. 42, no. 5, pp. 410–414, 2010.

[24] F. Vaz, H. Hanenberg, B. Schuster et al., "Mutation of the RAD51C gene in a Fanconi anemia-like disorder," *Nature Genetics*, vol. 42, no. 5, pp. 406–409, 2010.

[25] I. Garcia-Higuera, Y. Kuang, D. Näf, J. Wasik, and A. D. D'Andrea, "Fanconi anemia proteins FANCA, FANCC, and FANCG/XRCC9 interact in a functional nuclear complex," *Molecular and Cellular Biology*, vol. 19, no. 7, pp. 4866–4873, 1999.

[26] I. Garcia-Higuera, Y. Kuang, J. Denham, and A. D. D'Andrea, "The Fanconi anemia proteins FANCA and FANCG stabilize each other and promote the nuclear accumulation of the Fanconi anemia complex," *Blood*, vol. 96, no. 9, pp. 3224–3230, 2000.

[27] J. P. de Winter, L. van der Weel, J. De Groot et al., "The Fanconi anemia protein FANCF forms a nuclear complex with FANCA, FANCC and FANCG," *Human Molecular Genetics*, vol. 9, no. 18, pp. 2665–2674, 2000.

[28] A. L. Medhurst, P. A. J. Huber, Q. Waisfisz, J. P. de Winter, and C. G. Mathew, "Direct interactions of the five known Fanconi anaemia proteins suggest a common functional pathway," *Human Molecular Genetics*, vol. 10, no. 4, pp. 423–429, 2001.

[29] C. Ling, M. Ishiai, A. M. Ali et al., "FAAP100 is essential for activation of the Fanconi anemia-associated DNA damage response pathway," *The EMBO Journal*, vol. 26, no. 8, pp. 2104–2114, 2007.

[30] A. Ciccia, C. Ling, R. Coulthard et al., "Identification of FAAP24, a Fanconi anemia core complex protein that interacts with FANCM," *Molecular Cell*, vol. 25, no. 3, pp. 331–343, 2007.

[31] H. Kim et al., "Regulation of Rev1 by the Fanconi anemia core complex," *Nature Structural and Molecular Biology*, vol. 19, no. 2, pp. 164–170, 2012.

[32] A. M. Ali et al., "FAAP20: a novel ubiquitin-binding FA nuclear core complex protein required for functional integrity

of the FA-BRCA DNA repair pathway," *Blood*, vol. 119, no. 14, pp. 3285–3294, 2012.

[33] J. W. C. Leung, Y. Wang, K. W. Fong, M. S. Y. Huen, L. Li, and J. Chen, "Fanconi anemia (FA) binding protein FAAP20 stabilizes FA complementation group A (FANCA) and participates in interstrand cross-link repair," *Proceedings of the National Academy of Sciences*, vol. 109, no. 12, pp. 4491–4496, 2012.

[34] T. R. Singh, D. Saro, A. M. Ali et al., "MHF1-MHF2, a histone-fold-containing protein complex, participates in the Fanconi anemia pathway via FANCM," *Molecular Cell*, vol. 37, no. 6, pp. 879–886, 2010.

[35] Z. Yan, M. Delannoy, C. Ling et al., "A histone-fold complex and FANCM form a conserved DNA-remodeling complex to maintain genome stability," *Molecular Cell*, vol. 37, no. 6, pp. 865–878, 2010.

[36] G. L. Moldovan and A. D. D'Andrea, "How the Fanconi anemia pathway guards the genome," *Annual Review of Genetics*, vol. 43, no. 1, pp. 223–249, 2009.

[37] E. S. Zimmerman, B. A. Schulman, and N. Zheng, "Structural assembly of cullin-RING ubiquitin ligase complexes," *Current Opinion in Structural Biology*, vol. 20, no. 6, pp. 714–721, 2010.

[38] A. Schreiber, F. Stengel, Z. Zhang et al., "Structural basis for the subunit assembly of the anaphase-promoting complex," *Nature*, vol. 470, no. 7333, pp. 227–232, 2011.

[39] B. A. Buschhorn, G. Petzold, M. Galova et al., "Substrate binding on the APC/C occurs between the coactivator Cdh1 and the processivity factor Doc1," *Nature Structural and Molecular Biology*, vol. 18, no. 1, pp. 6–13, 2011.

[40] P. C. A. da Fonseca, E. H. Kong, Z. Zhang et al., "Structures of APC/C^{Cdh1} with substrates identify Cdh1 and Apc10 as the D-box co-receptor," *Nature*, vol. 470, no. 7333, pp. 274–278, 2011.

[41] A. F. Alpi, P. E. Pace, M. M. Babu, and K. J. Patel, "Mechanistic insight into site-restricted monoubiquitination of FANCD2 by Ube2t, FANCL, and FANCI," *Molecular Cell*, vol. 32, no. 6, pp. 767–777, 2008.

[42] A. R. Cole, L. P. C. Lewis, and H. Walden, "The structure of the catalytic subunit FANCL of the Fanconi anemia core complex," *Nature Structural and Molecular Biology*, vol. 17, no. 3, pp. 294–298, 2010.

[43] Y. J. Machida, Y. Machida, Y. Chen et al., "UBE2T is the E2 in the Fanconi anemia pathway and undergoes negative autoregulation," *Molecular Cell*, vol. 23, no. 4, pp. 589–596, 2006.

[44] C. Hodson, A. R. Cole, L. P. C. Lewis, J. A. Miles, A. P. Trew, and H. Walden, "Structural analysis of human FANCL, the E3 ligase in the Fanconi anemia pathway," *The Journal of Biological Chemistry*, vol. 286, no. 37, pp. 32628–32637, 2011.

[45] P. Pace, M. Johnson, W. M. Tan et al., "FANCE: the link between Fanconi anaemia complex assembly and activity," *The EMBO Journal*, vol. 21, no. 13, pp. 3414–3423, 2002.

[46] S. M. Gordon and M. Buchwald, "Fanconi anemia protein complex: mapping protein interactions in the yeast 2- and 3-hybrid systems," *Blood*, vol. 102, no. 1, pp. 136–141, 2003.

[47] F. Léveillé, M. Ferrer, A. L. Medhurst et al., "The nuclear accumulation of the Fanconi anemia protein FANCE depends on FANCC," *DNA Repair*, vol. 5, no. 5, pp. 556–565, 2006.

[48] R. K. Nookala, S. Hussain, and L. Pellegrini, "Insights into Fanconi anaemia from the structure of human FANCE," *Nucleic Acids Research*, vol. 35, no. 5, pp. 1638–1648, 2007.

[49] S. Seki, M. Ohzeki, A. Uchida et al., "A requirement of FancL and FancD2 monoubiquitination in DNA repair," *Genes to Cells*, vol. 12, no. 3, pp. 299–310, 2007.

[50] F. A. E. Kruyt, F. Abou-Zahr, H. Mok, and H. Youssoufian, "Resistance to mitomycin C requires direct interaction between the Fanconi anemia proteins FANCA and FANCG in the nucleus through an arginine- rich domain," *The Journal of Biological Chemistry*, vol. 274, no. 48, pp. 34212–34218, 1999.

[51] Q. Waisfisz, J. P. de Winter, F. A. E. Kruyt et al., "A physical complex of the Fanconi anemia proteins FANCG/XRCC9 and FANCA," *Proceedings of the National Academy of Sciences of the United States of America*, vol. 96, no. 18, pp. 10320–10325, 1999.

[52] P. A. J. Huber, A. L. Medhurst, H. Youssoufian, and C. G. Mathew, "Investigation of Fanconi anemia protein interactions by yeast two-hybrid analysis," *Biochemical and Biophysical Research Communications*, vol. 268, no. 1, pp. 73–77, 2000.

[53] T. Reuter, S. Herterich, O. Bernhard, H. Hoehn, and H. J. Gross, "Strong FANCA/FANCG but weak FANCA/FANCC interaction in the yeast 2-hybrid system," *Blood*, vol. 95, no. 2, pp. 719–720, 2000.

[54] E. Blom, H. J. van de Vrugt, Y. De Vries, J. P. de Winter, F. Arwert, and H. Joenje, "Multiple TPR motifs characterize the Fanconi anemia FANCG protein," *DNA Repair*, vol. 3, no. 1, pp. 77–84, 2004.

[55] S. Hussain, J. B. Wilson, E. Blom et al., "Tetratricopeptide-motif-mediated interaction of FANCG with recombination proteins XRCC3 and BRCA2," *DNA Repair*, vol. 5, no. 5, pp. 629–640, 2006.

[56] J. B. Wilson, E. Blom, R. Cunningham, Y. Xiao, G. M. Kupfer, and N. J. Jones, "Several tetratricopeptide repeat (TPR) motifs of FANCG are required for assembly of the BRCA2/D1-D2-G-X3 complex, FANCD2 monoubiquitylation and phleomycin resistance," *Mutation Research/Fundamental and Molecular Mechanisms of Mutagenesis*, vol. 689, no. 1-2, pp. 12–20, 2010.

[57] D. Adachi, T. Oda, H. Yagasaki et al., "Heterogenous activation of the Fanconi anemia pathway by patient-derived FANCA mutants," *Human Molecular Genetics*, vol. 11, no. 25, pp. 3125–3134, 2002.

[58] D. Näf, G. M. Kupfer, A. Suliman, K. Lambert, and A. D. D'Andrea, "Functional activity of the Fanconi anemia protein FAA requires FAC binding and nuclear localization," *Molecular and Cellular Biology*, vol. 18, no. 10, pp. 5952–5960, 1998.

[59] F. Léveillé, E. Blom, A. L. Medhurst et al., "The Fanconi anemia gene product FANCF is a flexible adaptor protein," *The Journal of Biological Chemistry*, vol. 279, no. 38, pp. 39421–39430, 2004.

[60] P. Kowal, A. M. Gurtan, P. Stuckert, A. D. D'Andrea, and T. Ellenberger, "Structural determinants of human FANCF protein that function in the assembly of a DNA damage signaling complex," *The Journal of Biological Chemistry*, vol. 282, no. 3, pp. 2047–2055, 2007.

[61] S. M. Gordon, N. Alon, and M. Buchwald, "FANCC, FANCE, and FANCD2 form a ternary complex essential to the integrity of the Fanconi anemia DNA damage response pathway," *The Journal of Biological Chemistry*, vol. 280, no. 43, pp. 36118–36125, 2005.

[62] T. Taniguchi and A. D. D'Andrea, "The Fanconi anemia protein, FANCE, promotes the nuclear accumulation of FANCC," *Blood*, vol. 100, no. 7, pp. 2457–2462, 2002.

[63] A. L. Medhurst, E. H. Laghmani, J. Steltenpool et al., "Evidence for subcomplexes in the Fanconi anemia pathway," *Blood*, vol. 108, no. 6, pp. 2072–2080, 2006.

[64] A. Alpi, F. Langevin, G. Mosedale, Y. J. Machida, A. Dutta, and K. J. Patel, "UBE2T, the Fanconi anemia core complex, and FANCD2 are recruited independently to chromatin: a basis for the regulation of FANCD2 monoubiquitination," *Molecular and Cellular Biology*, vol. 27, no. 24, pp. 8421–8430, 2007.

[65] T. Taniguchi, I. Garcia-Higuera, P. R. Andreassen, R. C. Gregory, M. Grompe, and A. D. D'Andrea, "S-phase-specific interaction of the Fanconi anemia protein, FANCD2, with BRCA1 and RAD51," *Blood*, vol. 100, no. 7, pp. 2414–2420, 2002.

[66] X. Wang, P. R. Andreassen, and A. D. D'Andrea, "Functional interaction of monoubiquitinated FANCD2 and BRCA2/FANCD1 in chromatin," *Molecular and Cellular Biology*, vol. 24, no. 13, pp. 5850–5862, 2004.

[67] J. Wang, T. R. Sarkar, M. Zhou et al., "CCAAT/enhancer binding protein delta (C/EBPδ, CEBPD)-mediated nuclear import of FANCD2 by IPO4 augments cellular response to DNA damage," *Proceedings of the National Academy of Sciences of the United States of America*, vol. 107, no. 37, pp. 16131–16136, 2010.

[68] P. S. Rudland, A. M. Platt-Higgins, L. M. Davies et al., "Significance of the Fanconi anemia FANCD2 protein in sporadic and metastatic human breast cancer," *American Journal of Pathology*, vol. 176, no. 6, pp. 2935–2947, 2010.

[69] D. J. Ma, S. J. Li, L. S. Wang, J. Dai, S. L. Zhao, and R. Zeng, "Temporal and spatial profiling of nuclei-associated proteins upon TNF-α/NF-κB signaling," *Cell Research*, vol. 19, no. 5, pp. 651–664, 2009.

[70] A. Borriello, A. Locasciulli, A. M. Bianco et al., "A novel Leu153Ser mutation of the Fanconi anemia FANCD2 gene is associated with severe chemotherapy toxicity in a pediatric T-cell acute lymphoblastic leukemia," *Leukemia*, vol. 21, no. 1, pp. 72–78, 2007.

[71] T. Yamashita, D. L. Barber, Y. Zhu, N. Wu, and A. D. D'Andrea, "The Fanconi anemia polypeptide FACC is localized to the cytoplasm," *Proceedings of the National Academy of Sciences of the United States of America*, vol. 91, no. 14, pp. 6712–6716, 1994.

[72] A. R. Meetei, S. Sechi, M. Wallisch et al., "A multiprotein nuclear complex connects Fanconi anemia and bloom syndrome," *Molecular and Cellular Biology*, vol. 23, no. 10, pp. 3417–3426, 2003.

[73] A. Thomashevski, A. A. High, M. Drozd et al., "The Fanconi anemia core complex forms four complexes of different sizes in different subcellular compartments," *The Journal of Biological Chemistry*, vol. 279, no. 25, pp. 26201–26209, 2004.

[74] A. J. Deans and S. C. West, "FANCM connects the genome instability disorders bloom's syndrome and Fanconi anemia," *Molecular Cell*, vol. 36, no. 6, pp. 943–953, 2009.

[75] G. Mosedale, W. Niedzwiedz, A. Alpi et al., "The vertebrate Hef ortholog is a component of the Fanconi anemia tumor-suppressor pathway," *Nature Structural and Molecular Biology*, vol. 12, no. 9, pp. 763–771, 2005.

[76] Y. Xue, Y. Li, R. Guo, C. Ling, and W. Wang, "FANCM of the Fanconi anemia core complex is required for both monoubiquitination and DNA repair," *Human Molecular Genetics*, vol. 17, no. 11, pp. 1641–1652, 2008.

[77] J. M. Kim, Y. Kee, A. Gurtan, and A. D. D'Andrea, "Cell cycle-dependent chromatin loading of the Fanconi anemia core complex by FANCM/FAAP24," *Blood*, vol. 111, no. 10, pp. 5215–5222, 2008.

[78] H. Yang et al., "*Saccharomyces cerevisiae* MHF complex structurally resembles the histones (H3-H4)$_2$ heterotetramer and functions as a heterotetramer," *Structure*, vol. 20, no. 2, pp. 364–370, 2012.

[79] S. J. Collis, A. Ciccia, A. J. Deans et al., "FANCM and FAAP24 function in ATR-mediated checkpoint signaling independently of the Fanconi anemia core complex," *Molecular Cell*, vol. 32, no. 3, pp. 313–324, 2008.

20

Association of Colecalciferol, Ferritin, and Anemia among Pregnant Women: Result from Cohort Study on Vitamin D Status and Its Impact during Pregnancy and Childhood in Indonesia

Raden Tina Dewi Judistiani [ID],[1] **Lani Gumilang,**[1] **Sefita Aryuti Nirmala** [ID],[1] **Setyorini Irianti,**[2] **Deni Wirhana,**[3] **Irman Permana,**[4] **Liza Sofjan,**[4] **Hesty Duhita,**[5] **Lies Ani Tambunan,**[6] **Jeffry Iman Gurnadi,**[6] **Umar Seno,**[7] **Reni Ghrahani,**[8] **Agnes Rengga Indrati,**[9] **Yunia Sribudiani,**[10] **Tetty Yuniati,**[8] **and Budi Setiabudiawan**[8]

[1] Public Health Department, Faculty of Medicine, Universitas Padjadjaran, Sumedang, West Java, Indonesia
[2] Obstetric and Gynecology Department, Dr. Hasan Sadikin Hospital, Bandung, West Java, Indonesia
[3] Obstetric and Gynecology Department, Waled Regency Public Hospital, Cirebon, West Java, Indonesia
[4] Department of Child Health, Waled Regency Public Hospital, Cirebon, West Java, Indonesia
[5] Obstetric and Gynecology Department, Syamsudin SH Public Hospital, Sukabumi, West Java, Indonesia
[6] Obstetric and Gynecology Department, Cibabat General Hospital, Cimahi, West Java, Indonesia
[7] Obstetric and Gynecology Department, Kota Bandung General Hospital, Bandung, West Java, Indonesia
[8] Department of Child Health, Faculty of Medicine, Universitas Padjadjaran, Sumedang, West Java, Indonesia
[9] Clinical Pathology Department, Faculty of Medicine, Universitas Padjadjaran, Sumedang, West Java, Indonesia
[10] Department of Biochemistry and Molecular Biology, Faculty of Medicine, Universitas Padjadjaran, Sumedang, West Java, Indonesia

Correspondence should be addressed to Raden Tina Dewi Judistiani; judistiani@gmail.com

Academic Editor: Duran Canatan

Studies had shown that iron-cycling was disturbed by inflammatory process through the role of hepcidin. Pregnancy is characterized by shifts of interleukin. Our objective was to determine if 25(OH) vitamin D (colecalciferol) status was associated with ferritin, anemia, and its changes during pregnancy. *Method.* A cohort study was done in 4 cities in West Java, Indonesia, beginning in July 2016. Subjects were followed up until third trimester. Examinations included were maternal ferritin, colecalciferol, and haemoglobin level. *Result.* 191 (95.5%) subjects had low colecalciferol, and 151 (75.5%) among them were at deficient state. Anemia is found in 15 (7.5%) subjects, much lower than previous report. Proportion of anemia increased by trimester among women with colecalciferol deficiency. Ferritin status and prepregnancy body mass index in the first trimester were correlated with anemia ($r = 0.147$, $p = 0.038$ and $r = -0.56$, $p = 0.03$). Anemia in the second trimester was strongly correlated with anemia in the third trimester ($r = 0.676$, $p < 0.01$). *Conclusion.* Our study showed that the state of colecalciferol was not associated with either ferritin state or anemia, but proportion of anemia tends to increase by trimester in the colecalciferol deficient subjects.

1. Introduction

The emerging awareness on hypovitaminosis D as major health problem across countries and regions has driven more researches from observational studies to clinical trials.

Hypovitaminosis D, defined by serum 25-hydroxy vitamin D (colecalciferol) level below 25 nmol/L, is most common in South Asia and the Middle East [1]. Other studies classified the state as deficient, insufficient, and normal with respect to the disease of interest and also geographical area [1–8].

Certain characteristics were linked to hypovitaminosis D such as life style, less sunlight exposure, dietary habits, and not having fortified food, all included in the major factors that were significantly associated with lower colecalciferol levels [1]. The first report of colecalciferol status among pregnant women from a study in West Java, Indonesia, year 2016, stated that only 4.4% of 160 pregnant women in their first trimester had normal level of colecalciferol (>30 ng/mL), approximately 70% were insufficient (20–29 ng/mL), and the remaining 25.6% were deficient (<20 ng/mL) [9].

Anemia is also a global health problem not only for its prevalence but also for the burden caused by anemia itself. Kassebaum reported that global anemia prevalence in 2010 was 32.9%, accounted for 8.8% of the total disability from all condition; children and women were more affected [10]. Studies also reported that maternal anemia is associated with fetal and neonatal well-being [11–13]. The latest study on anemia among pregnant women in Jatinangor-West Java was as high as 21.9% [14].

Pregnancies are characterized by a shift toward proinflammatory mediators in later gestational age, while the opposite condition occurs in the earlier period to avoid pregnancy failure [15–18]. The link between anemia and inflammation was found from the study by Nicolas through the gene encoding hepcidin [19]. Later studies had proven that hepcidin was the king regulatory for iron hemostasis, allowing transfer of iron stores to blood circulation [20–23].

The clinical importance of colecalciferol deficiency with regard to anemia among pregnant women in Indonesia had never been reported until this article was written. We suspected that there might be an association of colecalciferol and haemoglobin. With iron as a crucial component for haemoglobin production, we know that the ultimate regulation of iron metabolism in human body is by the role of hepcidin, in the hepcidin-ferroportin gate system [22]. One study by Baccheta stated that hepcidin is downregulated by colecalciferol, but the study by Koenig found that different state of pregnancy may also influence the hepcidin level [21, 24]. In the iron-regulatory process ferritin has been formerly known as one of indicators for iron store besides transferrin. In absolute iron deficiency, low serum ferritin level tends to reflect low iron reserves, but other evaluations has been suggested like transferrin saturation to exclude iron depletion of other causes [25]. With its iron component, ferritin also can act as an acute phase reactant to inflammatory process so that a single measurement of normal or high ferritin may undermined the presence of actual iron deficiency [25].

The importance of assuring iron stores is mainly related to prevent of anemia, but the cause of anemia itself is rarely in isolation [26]. While clinical significance of ferritin evaluation should be the main focus for health service, knowledge development on iron metabolism is of equal importance to support treatment. Colecalciferol and the hepcidin-ferroportin iron-regulatory axis may be altered in pregnancy because pregnancy itself is a proinflammatory condition; therefore some changes in ferritin and transferrin level might occur according to the level of colecalciferol. This study aimed at finding out if colecalciferol and serum ferritin level in the first trimester would have an association with haemoglobin level or anemia in pregnancy.

The prevalence of anemia among pregnant in Indonesia has been declining over the period of 1997 to 2008, yet the last figure we found was as high as 35% or more, despite iron supplementation implementation of antenatal care policy during that period [27]. Regional areas in Indonesia had varied figures, perhaps due to chronic infection of tuberculosis, malaria endemicity, and malnutrition and it might also be due to different tools used for screening. One study which was also conducted in a small area of West Java showed approximately 65% difference in prevalence of anemia among pregnant women, using capillary finger prick test versus complete blood count from vein [14]. It was very likely that the correct prevalence of anemia among pregnant women in that study population was 21%, so we used this figure to compare our result [14].

The definition of anemia in pregnancy recommended by the Centre for Disease Control and Prevention is a haemoglobin (Hgb) or haematocrit (Hct) value less than the fifth percentile of the distribution of Hgb or Hct in a healthy reference population based on the stage of pregnancy [28]. As not every country has its own database, we refer to classification of anemia which was derived from an iron-supplemented pregnant women population, based on Hgb level and trimesters as follows: (1) Hgb levels below 11 g/dl in the first trimester; (2) Hgb below 10.5 g/dl in the second trimester; and (3) Hgb below 11 g/dl in the third trimester [28].

2. Material and Methods

This report was a part of cohort study on vitamin D status and its impact during pregnancy and childhood in Indonesia, with special interest in colecalciferol, nutrition, immunological changes and their association with both maternal and fetal outcomes. The cohort started in July 2016 in Bandung, Cimahi, Sukabumi, and Waled, West Java, Indonesia [9]. We expected to include 300 subjects to fit our budget, with approximately equal number from all cities. Our study protocol had been reviewed and ethical clearance was released from Health Research Ethical Committee of Faculty of Medicine, Universitas Padjadjaran.

2.1. Inclusion of Study Subjects. Prior to recruitment, pregnant women were given information about the study by community midwife at the primary health centres of associated sites. If they were interested, they were referred to study site hospitals, that is, Dr. Hasan Sadikin Hospital and Kota Bandung Hospital (Bandung sites), Cibabat Hospital (Cimahi site), Samsudin Hospital (Sukabumi site), and Waled Hospital (Waled site). At these hospitals complete information regarding this study was given by our trained midwives in the research team. After giving written consent, further obstetric anamnesis or confirmation and ultrasound screening were performed by our participating obstetricians. These obstetricians had followed training for standard setting in ultrasound examinations. Eligible subjects were women with singleton pregnancy between 10 and 14 weeks, fetus was normal, and subjects would comply with our study procedures. Recruitment was conducted consecutively until the expected numbers 70–75 were met at each site.

2.2. Steps after Recruitment. Each pregnant woman was interviewed for personal data, obstetric history, and knowledge on nutrition support in pregnancy by research team midwives. Pregnant women were then taught to fill in a three-day diary within the following week. The diary was about the food they consumed, how they dressed, and their activity pertaining to duration of sun exposure. We also set to repeat obstetric ultrasound examination, selected interview, and laboratory tests in the second and third trimester follow-up visits. All women were given freedom to choose their birth attendants and sites of baby deliveries and during labor they were also accompanied by our team midwives who would observe, but not interfere with, the labor process. Our team recorded any events until completion of stage 4 of labor. All records of each pregnant woman were kept as individual case report file in data storage for later entry.

2.3. Collection, Preservation, and Transfer of Blood Samples for Examination of Haemoglobin, Vitamin D, and Ferritin Level. Blood drawn from median cubital veins were directly transported to local site hospital lab for complete blood count and serum preparation. The separated serum was stored at −20 degree Celsius, before being transported to Dr. Hasan Sadikin Hospital in coolbox for colecalciferol and ferritin analysis. The longest transport time was from Waled and Sukabumi, which were up to 4 hours.

2.4. Complete Blood Count, Vitamin D, and Ferritin Assay and Interpretation. All complete blood count measurements were done using automated hematology analyzer with impedance method measurement (Sysmex XP-100, Japan). It was used to measure at least 8 parameters including Hb, mean corpuscular volume (MCV), and red blood count (RBC). Vitamin D and ferritin measurement was performed by ELISA.

Anemia was defined by Hgb level and trimesters as follows: (1) Hgb levels below 11 g/dl in the first trimester; (2) Hgb below 10.5 g/dl in the second trimester; and (3) Hgb below 11 g/dl in the third trimester. We also calculated Mentzer index to detect any pregnant women of β thalassemia trait and excluded one case.

The minimum measurable level of vitamin D in serum was 8.1 ng/mL; any level below that was reported as 8 ng/mL. Vitamin D status was defined as (1) deficient if its level was below 20 ng/mL; (2) insufficient if its level was between 20 and 29.99 ng/mL; and (3) normal if its level was 30 ng/mL or more.

Pregnant women with low iron store (hypoferritinemia) were defined if serum ferritin was below 30 ng/mL and normal if 30 ng/mL or more.

2.5. Statistical Analysis. Three members of our team performed entry and data cleaning from case report file into our customized Excel sheet (Microsoft Corp., USA). Making sure that data was cleaned, it was transferred into SPSS software. Only data on pregnant women characteristics, haemoglobin, and ferritin laboratory results were used for this article. The remaining data would be reported in our next report. Descriptive analysis on characteristics and laboratory data were done; dispersion analysis was conducted by Kolmogorov-Smirnoff and resulted in the fact that our data showed skewness (test result not shown). We therefore performed two sets of nonparametric analysis.

3. Result and Discussion

Between July 2016 and July 2017 a total of 201 pregnant women had been completely followed up until third trimester and included for this report. The others were recruited later that they had not met our minimum observation time. Only one subject had a low Mentzer index (<13) and anemia; she was excluded from analysis. The characteristics of our study subjects were as shown in Table 1.

In this study the terminology of "at risk" was chosen instead of "low risk" due to our own perspective that no single pregnancy is risk-free and that the switch from normal to pathologic conditions could happen in an instant. Our study population had high-risk cases, that is, 45 cases form age group (<20 years or >35 years) and 79 cases from parity group (parity 4 or more). The previous study had lower proportion of high-risk group on parity (11% versus 39.8%) but there were no data on maternal age and prepregnancy BMI [14].

The nutritional state was defined by prepregnancy body mass index classification from WHO [29]. The result showed that about 27% of our subjects had nutritional problem in the extremes. There were more underweight women than obese which could be a risk factor the presence of anemia.

We recruited pregnant women from first trimester, while in previous study we recruited women from both first and second trimester [14]. First trimester laboratory results from all 200 study subjects are presented in Table 2. Colecalciferol and ferritin level in the second and trimester were not available, yet by the time this article was written.

The number of study subjects who had returned for follow-up visit in the second and third trimester was lower than in first trimester for several reasons, some just failed to show up, and others were not yet due to schedule. The laboratory results from our study showed that 193 subjects (96.5%) had hypovitaminosis D (below 30 ng/mL); that is, 151 (75.5%) were deficient and 42 (21%) were insufficient in the first trimester. One study in the United States reported that their prevalence on hypovitaminosis D among pregnant women in their first trimester reached 70%, with mean serum concentration of 27.6 ng/mL and range of 13–71.6 ng/mL [30]. Mean colecalciferol from our study result was much lower, even below the cutoff for colecalciferol deficiency (Table 2). A different result came from a study in Tunisia which reported that no mother had an adequate vitamin D status during term delivery, with so much lower mean serum colecalciferol concentrations at 6.82 ± 5.14 ng/mL (range 3.60–23.77) [31].

Figure 1 showed that subjects who were deficient or insufficient of colecalciferol state in the first trimester had higher risk to develop anemia in the third trimester, RR (95% CI) = 2.96 (0.36–24.63), and that the proportion of subjects with anemia increased in every subgroup colecalciferol state.

Anemia was present in 15 (7.5%) subjects of our study. This figure was much lower compared to two previous studies in Indonesia. Susanti, whose study was more similar to ours, reported a 21% prevalence of anemia in pregnancy in 2017,

TABLE 1: Descriptive summary of study subjects' characteristic.

Characteristics group	Number (%)	Mean (+SD)	Median (IQR)
Age (years)		28.38 (±5.9)	28.0 (16–43)
At risk	155 (77.61)		
High risk	45 (22.39)		
BMI (kg/m^2)		23.27 (±5.44)	22.04 (14.67–50.89)
Underweight	32 (16.92)		
Normal	112 (56.21)		
Overweight	34 (16.91)		
Obese	21 (10.44)		
Parity		na	na
At risk	121 (60.20)		
High risk	79 (39.80)		

Note. 1 case of suspected β thalassemia trait was excluded from analysis; na = not applicable.

TABLE 2: Descriptive summary of laboratory results in trimester 1.

	Mean (+standard deviation)	Median (interquartile range)
Colecalciferol (ng/mL)	15.34 (+6.99)	14.25 (8.0–43.5)
Ferritin (ng/mL)	67.81 (+53.81)	50.22 (4.8–306)
Haemoglobin (gr/dL)	12.58 (+1.18)	12.80 (8.2–14.4)

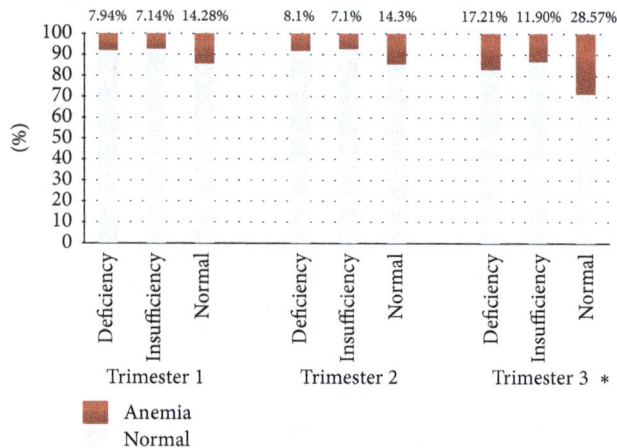

FIGURE 1: Proportion of subjects with anemia in trimesters 1, 2, and 3 by first trimester colecalciferol status. *Relative risk (95% CI) for anemia in the third trimester among subjects with calciferol deficiency and insufficiency in the first trimester, combined = 2.96 (0.36–24.63).

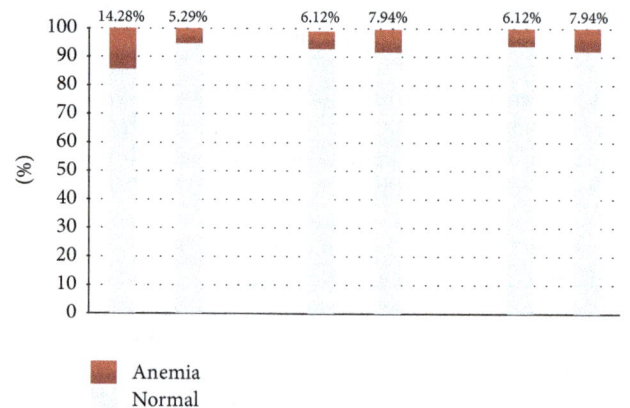

FIGURE 2: Proportion of subjects with anemia in trimesters 1, 2, and 3 by first trimester ferritin status. Correlation of first trimester ferritin level and first trimester anemia ($r = 0.147$, $p = 0.038$), no correlation found with second or third trimester anemia.

while Barkley reported that anemia in pregnant women above 15 years old was as high as 37.3% as a result from Indonesian Family Survey [14, 27]. Twenty-four point nine percent of our study subjects had hypoferritinemia (below 30 ng/mL) in the first trimester. We had not found any report which specifically reported on the actual cutoff of serum ferritin level to assess iron deficiency among pregnant women in Indonesia. A distinction between absolute and functional iron deficiency was also very important in pregnancy, even more with those who had chronic inflammation.

Figure 2 showed the comparison of anemia in trimesters 1, 2, and 3 based on the state of ferritin level in the first trimester only.

Our study showed that first trimester ferritin status was correlated positively with the presence of anemia in the first trimester, but not with the second or third trimesters. One report showed that in spite of satisfactory iron reserves with normal or even increased serum ferritin, the availability of iron for the bone marrow is limited substantially due to increased hepcidin transcription in chronic inflammation [32]. Unfortunately the examination to exclude chronic inflammation has not become a routine part in prepregnancy assessment. It is especially important as Indonesia is known to be one of the countries with highest tuberculosis burden [33]. Tuberculosis screening is not provided in routine prenatally for its high cost.

We calculated and found no correlation between age, parity, and BMI class at baseline and the state of colecalciferol and serum ferritin, so the statistical analysis results are not shown.

As we recruited pregnant women from first trimester, we observed that the number of anemia cases showed quite some changes from one trimester to another and from one state to another, especially with regard to colecalciferol deficiency. Haemodilution is known as the main factor for the presence of anemia in the second trimester, which may explain why the proportion of anemia was higher than in first trimester. Further exploration turned that haemoglobin level dropped even further among all of subjects with anemia in the second trimester, in average −1.44 gr/dL. Fifteen subjects who were normal in second trimester also had dropped in average −0.99 dr/dL. These findings needed more exploration on the iron-cycle itself during pregnancy. It was quite an important alarm as we know that the presence of anemia near parturition or at parturition also increased the risk for postpartum hemorrhage.

4. Conclusion

Our study showed that first trimester state of colecalciferol was not associated with ferritin. Subjects with vitamin D deficiency in the first trimester were more prone to develop anemia, with increasing proportion as pregnancy progressed to third trimester. First trimester ferritin state was correlated with anemia in the first trimester.

Conflicts of Interest

The authors declare that there are no conflicts of interest.

Authors' Contributions

Raden Tina Dewi Judistiani was the primary investigator who developed the idea, research design, data analysis, and manuscript writing. Budi Setiabudiawan supervised the research process and manuscript writing. Setyorini Irianti, Irman Permana, Deni Wirhana, Liza Sofjan, Hesty Duhita, Lies Ani Tambunan, Jeffry Iman Gurnadi, and Umar Seno, were involved in recruitment and performing antenatal care for all pregnant women in this study. Agnes Rengga Indrati contributed as laboratory examination coordinator. Tetty Yuniati, Yunia Sribudiani, and Reni Ghrahani contributed to discussion and grant development. Lani Gumilang and Sefita Aryuti Nirmala were involved in supervising recruitment, examination procedures, and follow-up.

Acknowledgments

The authors thank all the staff at the Bandung, Cimahi, Waled, and Sukabumi Health Office and Primary Health Centres for their contribution to enable this study in these cities. They express their greatest appreciation to all the staff, nurses, and midwives at Dr. Hasan Sadikin Hospital, Rumah Sakit Kota Bandung Hospital, Cibabat Hospital, Al Mulk Hospital, and Waled Hospital for the cooperation and hard work especially during data collection and follow-up. They thank field researchers, Bunga Mars, Putri Anisa, Devi Agustini, and Devi Yuli Agustini, for their faithful effort made for this study. Funding for this study came from Academic Leadership Grant from Universitas Padjadjaran and partial contribution came from the Government of West Java Province Indonesia.

References

[1] A. Mithal, D. A. Wahl, J. Bonjour et al., "Global vitamin D status and determinants of hypovitaminosis D," *Osteoporosis International*, vol. 20, no. 11, pp. 1821-1821, 2009.

[2] H. J. Jin, J. H. Lee, and M. K. Kim, "The prevalence of vitamin D deficiency in iron-deficient and normal children under the age of 24 months," *Blood Research*, vol. 48, no. 1, pp. 40–45, 2013.

[3] S. Finer, K. S. Khan, G. A. Hitman, C. Griffiths, A. Martineau, and C. Meads, "Inadequate vitamin D status in pregnancy: Evidence for supplementation," *Acta Obstetricia et Gynecologica Scandinavica*, vol. 91, no. 2, pp. 159–163, 2012.

[4] G. N. Society, "New Reference Values for Vitamin D," *Annals of Nutrition and Metabolism*, vol. 60, no. 4, pp. 241–246, 2012.

[5] C. E. Thomas, R. Guillet, R. A. Queenan et al., "Vitamin D status is inversely associated with anemia and serum erythropoietin during pregnancy," *American Journal of Clinical Nutrition*, vol. 102, no. 5, pp. 1088–1095, 2015.

[6] J. L. Finkelstein, C. Duggan, S. Mehta et al., "Maternal Vitamin D Status and Adverse Pregnancy and Neonatal Outcomes in India," *The FASEB Journal*, vol. 30, no. 1, article 44.6, 2016.

[7] C. K. H. Yu, R. Ertl, E. Skyfta, R. Akolekar, and K. H. Nicolaides, "Maternal serum vitamin D levels at 11-13 weeks of gestation in preeclampsia," *Journal of Human Hypertension*, vol. 27, no. 2, pp. 115–118, 2013.

[8] S.-Q. Wei, H.-P. Qi, Z.-C. Luo, and W. D. Fraser, "Maternal vitamin D status and adverse pregnancy outcomes: a systematic review and meta-analysis," *The Journal of Maternal-Fetal & Neonatal Medicine*, vol. 26, no. 9, pp. 889–899, 2013.

[9] S. Irianti, S. Rachmawaty, R. Fauziah et al., "The First Report of a Longitudinal Study in West Jawa Barat Province Indonesia: Do Pregnant Women Have the Advantage from Living in the Equator to avoid Vitamin D deficiency?" in *Proceedings of the 1st World Congress on Fetal Maternal Neonatal Medicine*, London, UK, April 2017.

[10] N. J. Kassebaum, R. Jasrasaria, M. Naghavi et al., "A systematic analysis of global anemia burden from 1990 to 2010," *Blood*, vol. 123, no. 5, pp. 615–624, 2014.

[11] J. L. Finkelstein, A. V. Kurpad, T. Thomas, K. Srinivasan, and C. Duggan, "Maternal Anemia of Inflammation and Adverse Pregnancy and Neonatal Outcomes in India," *The FASEB Journal*, vol. 30, no. 1, article 668.3, 2016.

[12] A. Alemayehu, L. Gedefaw, T. Yemane, and Y. Asres, "Prevalence, Severity, and Determinant Factors of Anemia among Pregnant Women in South Sudanese Refugees, Pugnido, Western Ethiopia," *Anemia*, vol. 2016, Article ID 9817358, 11 pages, 2016.

[13] H. Messenger and B. Lim, "The Prevalence of Anemia In Pregnancy In A Developed Country – How Well Understood Is It?" *Journal of Pregnancy and Child Health*, vol. 03, no. 02, 2016.

[14] A. I. Susanti, E. Sahiratmadja, G. Winarno, A. K. Sugianli, H. Susanto, and R. Panigoro, "Low Hemoglobin among Pregnant

Women in Midwives Practice of Primary Health Care, Jati-nangor, Indonesia: Iron Deficiency Anemia or β-Thalassemia Trait?" *Anemia*, vol. 2017, Article ID 6935648, 5 pages, 2017.

[15] T. Weissenbacher, R. P. Laubender, S. S. Witkin et al., "Diagnostic biomarkers of pro-inflammatory immune-mediated preterm birth," *Archives of Gynecology and Obstetrics*, vol. 287, no. 4, pp. 673–685, 2013.

[16] M.-T. Gervasi, R. Romero, G. Bracalente et al., "Midtrimester amniotic fluid concentrations of interleukin-6 and interferon-gamma-inducible protein-10: evidence for heterogeneity of intra-amniotic inflammation and associations with spontaneous early (<32 weeks) and late (>32 weeks) preterm delivery," *Journal of Perinatal Medicine*, vol. 40, no. 4, pp. 329–343, 2012.

[17] A. Szarka, J. Rigó Jr., L. Lázár, G. Beko, and A. Molvarec, "Circulating cytokines, chemokines and adhesion molecules in normal pregnancy and preeclampsia determined by multiplex suspension array," *BMC Immunology*, vol. 11, article 59, 2010.

[18] S. M. Keeler, D. G. Kiefer, O. A. Rust et al., "Comprehensive amniotic fluid cytokine profile evaluation in women with a short cervix: which cytokine(s) correlates best with outcome?" *American Journal of Obstetrics & Gynecology*, vol. 201, no. 3, pp. 276–e6, 2009.

[19] G. Nicolas, C. Chauvet, L. Viatte et al., "The gene encoding the iron regulatory peptide hepcidin is regulated by anemia, hypoxia, and inflammation," *The Journal of Clinical Investigation*, vol. 110, no. 7, pp. 1037–1044, 2002.

[20] P. S. Oates, *The role of hepcidin and ferroportin in iron absorption*, Histol Histopathol, 2007.

[21] M. D. Koenig, L. Tussing-Humphreys, J. Day, B. Cadwell, and E. Nemeth, "Hepcidin and iron homeostasis during pregnancy," *Nutrients*, vol. 6, no. 8, pp. 3062–3083, 2014.

[22] G. Rishi, D. F. Wallace, and V. N. Subramaniam, "Hepcidin: regulation of the master iron regulator," *Bioscience Reports*, vol. 35, no. 3, Article ID e00192, pp. 1–12, 2015.

[23] S. M. Zughaier, J. A. Alvarez, J. H. Sloan, R. J. Konrad, and V. Tangpricha, "The role of vitamin D in regulating the iron-hepcidin-ferroportin axis in monocytes," *Journal of Clinical & Translational Endocrinology*, vol. 1, no. 1, pp. e19–e25, 2014.

[24] J. Bacchetta, J. J. Zaritsky, J. L. Sea et al., "Suppression of iron-regulatory hepcidin by vitamin D," *Journal of the American Society of Nephrology*, vol. 25, no. 3, pp. 564–572, 2014.

[25] F. A. Naoum, "Adjusting thresholds of serum ferritin for iron deficiency: a moving target," *Revista Brasileira de Hematologia e Hemoterapia*, vol. 39, no. 3, pp. 189-190, 2017.

[26] WHO, *Worldwide Prevalence of Anaemia 1993–2005*, 2008.

[27] J. S. Barkley, K. L. Kendrick, K. Codling, S. Muslimatun, and H. Pachón, "Anaemia prevalence over time in Indonesia: estimates from the 1997, 2000, and 2008 Indonesia Family Life Surveys," *Asia Pacific Journal of Clinical Nutrition*, vol. 24, no. 3, pp. 452–455, 2015.

[28] WHO, *Nutritional Anaemias: Tools for Effective Prevention and Control*, 2017.

[29] BMI Classification [Internet]. World Health Organization. 2017 [cited 1 Dec 2017]. Available from: http://apps.who.int/bmi/index.jsp?introPage=intro_3.html.

[30] S. K. Flood-Nichols, D. Tinnemore, R. R. Huang, P. G. Napolitano, and D. L. Ippolito, "Vitamin D deficiency in early pregnancy," *PLoS ONE*, vol. 10, no. 4, pp. 1–15, 2015.

[31] I. D. Ayadi, E. B. H. Nouaili, E. Talbi et al., "Prevalence of vitamin D deficiency in mothers and their newborns in a Tunisian population," *International Journal of Gynecology and Obstetrics*, vol. 133, no. 2, pp. 192–195, 2016.

[32] L. T. Goodnough, E. Nemeth, and T. Ganz, "Detection, evaluation, and management of iron-restricted erythropoiesis," *Blood*, vol. 116, no. 23, pp. 4754–4761, 2010.

[33] Ministry of Health Indonesia, *Tuberkulosis Temukan Obati Sampai Sembuh*, 2016, http://www.depkes.go.id/download.php?file=download/pusdatin/infodatin/InfoDatin.

21

Malaria, Moderate to Severe Anaemia, and Malarial Anaemia in Children at Presentation to Hospital in the Mount Cameroon Area

Irene Ule Ngole Sumbele,[1] **Sharon Odmia Sama,**[1] **Helen Kuokuo Kimbi,**[1,2] **and Germain Sotoing Taiwe**[1]

[1]*Department of Zoology and Animal Physiology, University of Buea, Buea, Cameroon*
[2]*Department of Medical Laboratory Sciences, University of Bamenda, Bamenda, Cameroon*

Correspondence should be addressed to Irene Ule Ngole Sumbele; sumbelei@yahoo.co.uk

Academic Editor: Duran Canatan

Background. Malaria remains a major killer of children in Sub-Saharan Africa, while anaemia is a public health problem with significant morbidity and mortality. Examining the factors associated with moderate to severe anaemia (MdSA) and malarial anaemia as well as the haematological characteristics is essential. *Methodology.* Children (1–14 years) at presentation at the Regional Hospital Annex-Buea were examined clinically and blood samples were collected for malaria parasite detection and full blood count evaluation. *Results. Plasmodium falciparum*, anaemia, and malarial anaemia occurred in 33.8%, 62.0%, and 23.6% of the 216 children, respectively. Anaemia prevalence was significantly higher in malaria parasite positive children and those with fever than their respective counterparts. MdSA and moderate to severe malarial anaemia (MdSMA) were detected in 38.0% and 15.3% of the participants, respectively. The prevalence of MdSA was significantly higher in children whose household head had no formal education, resided in the lowland, or was febrile, while MdSMA was significantly higher in febrile children only. Children with MdSMA had significantly lower mean white blood cell, lymphocyte, and platelet counts while the mean granulocyte count was significantly higher. *Conclusion.* Being febrile was the only predictor of both MdSA and MdSMA. More haematological insult occurred in children with MdSMA compared to MdSA.

1. Background

In spite of the increase in control measures and reported 18% and 48% decline in the number of malaria cases and deaths, respectively, globally between 2000 and 2015, malaria remains a major killer of children especially in Sub-Saharan Africa, taking the life of a child every 2 minutes [1]. However, in order to properly evaluate control measures, regular updates of disease morbidities in public health services and community settings in the country are invaluable. Even though studies have been carried out on severe and uncomplicated malaria in children admitted to hospitals in different parts of the country [2, 3] as well as uncomplicated and asymptomatic malaria in the communities [4] and primary school children [5], there is a dearth of information on malaria-related morbidities at presentation in the general medical outpatient department in the country.

While malaria is one of the factors that contributes to the public health problem of anaemia in children in Cameroon [2, 6, 7], in almost all countries in Sub-Saharan Africa, anaemia is a moderate or severe public health problem causing significant morbidity and mortality [8]. Much of the burden of infections operates through the mechanism of anaemia which is characterized by a reduction in haemoglobin concentration causing impairment in meeting the oxygen demands of the body. In African children this haematological state is determined by combinations of nutritional deficiencies, infectious diseases (malaria, hookworm infections, and human immunodeficiency virus infections), and the genetic constitution of red cell haemoglobin [9–12]. However, WHO malaria report [1] stated that, in most malaria endemic areas, less than half of patients with suspected malaria infection are truly infected with a malaria parasite. Consequently, parasitological confirmation by light microscopy or rapid diagnostic tests before the commencement of treatment, in children in the outpatient department, is invaluable. Additionally, this provides an opportunity to evaluate the burden of malaria and the prevalence of anaemia and its severity in febrile children. The findings might serve as a predictor of malaria-related mortality.

Malarial anaemia (MA) is a multifactorial disease for which the complex etiological basis is only partially defined. Severe MA is one of the main clinical presentations of severe malaria caused by *P. falciparum* [2]. The aetiology of severe MA in malaria endemic areas may include a number of discrete as well as overlapping features, such as lysis of infected and uninfected RBCs [13], splenic sequestration of RBCs [14], dyserythropoiesis and bone marrow suppression [15], infectious diseases, and chronic transmission of malaria. While haematological insults resulting in moderate and severe anaemia in infection with *Plasmodium falciparum* have been established [16], the exact differences in the pathophysiology of anaemia in the various clinical settings, ages, and geographic areas are poorly defined [17].

In children presenting at a hospital in western Kenya, wasting was associated with increased presentation of MA. In addition the caretakers level of education and occupation significantly correlated with anaemia and MA [12]. On the other hand, hospital based studies in the Mount Cameroon area indicated severe MA as the main clinical presentation of severe malaria but did not examine sociodemographic or nutritional factors associated with the presentation [2]. Hence, assessing the influence of some sociodemographic and nutritional indices on the prevalence of MdSA and MA in children will provide valuable information to the health authorities. This will enable informed decision and the appropriate allocation of scarce resources for proper child health management and control of these morbidities. This study was undertaken to explore the hypothesis that sociodemographic factors and nutritional indices influence the presentation of children in the outpatient department with MdSA and MdSMA. The objectives of the study therefore were to determine the prevalence of *falciparum* malaria, MA, MdSA, and MdSMA in children at presentation for consultation in general medical outpatient department, evaluate the attributable risk of anaemia caused by malaria, and assess the variation in haematological indices in moderate to severe anaemic and malarial anaemic children.

2. Materials and Methods

2.1. Study Area. This study was carried out in the Regional Hospital Annex-Buea, Fako Division, South West Region. Buea, a town in the Mount Cameroon area, is situated at latitude $3°57'-4°27'$N and longitude $8°58'-9°25'$E, 500–4080 metres above sea level (asl) and is located on the southeast slope of Mount Cameroon. Buea has an estimated population of above 200.000 inhabitants constituting essentially of the Bakweri indigenes in the villages and a highly cosmopolitan population in the urban space with the indigenes at a minority [18]. The climate in Buea tends to be humid, with temperatures varying from 18°C to 27°C, average relative humidity of 80%, and average rainfall of 4000 mm. There are two seasons, the rainy and the dry seasons, which start from mid-March to October and November to mid-March, respectively. The prevalence of malaria parasitaemia in the Mount Cameroon area varies from 60.6%, in lowland altitude, to 7.7% in the highlands [5].

2.2. Study Population. The study population included children of both sexes aged 1–14 years, who presented themselves at the Regional Hospital Annex-Buea for consultation during the period of study. Children who participated in the study came from various localities and altitudes. The altitude was classified as lowland (0–167 m asl), middle belt (600–650 m asl), and highland (897–918 m asl) as reported by Kimbi et al. [5]. Only children whose parent/guardian signed the informed consent/assent forms following the education on the importance of the study were enrolled. For the purpose of comparability, patients with a history of antimalarial treatment in the preceding two weeks or who had a blood transfusion three months prior to the start of study or had haemoglobin genotype SS were not enrolled in the study.

2.3. Study Design. This cross-sectional hospital based study was carried out during the peak malaria transmission season from the month of May to August 2014, in the Regional Hospital Annex-Buea. Following administrative clearances and ethical approval for the study, informed consent/assent forms explaining the purpose, risks, and benefits of the study were given to parent or guardian. After obtaining consent/assent from the participant, clinical evaluation was carried out and a questionnaire was administered prior to blood sample collection. Blood sample was collected from each child for determination of malaria parasite status and full blood count evaluation. The optimum sample size was calculated using the prevalence of *P. falciparum* parasitaemia in the region of 36.6% [4] and anaemia prevalence in a hospital based studies in the Mount Cameroon area of 94.7% [2]. The sample size was determined using the formula $n = z^2 pq/d^2$ [19], where n represented the sample size required; z was 1.96, which is the standard normal deviate (for a 95% confidence interval, CI); p values were 36.6% and 94.7%, the proportion of malaria parasitaemia and anaemia prevalence, respectively; q was $1 - p$; and d was 0.05, the acceptable error willing to be committed. The optimum sample size obtained from the average of both sample sizes was 217.

2.4. Ethical Consideration. Ethical clearance document for the study was obtained from the Institutional Review Board hosted by the Faculty of Health Sciences, University of Buea (2014-04-0261/UB/FHS/IRB) following administrative clearance from the Regional Delegation of Public Health. Informed consent/assent forms were given or read and explained to parents or guardians of the study participants at presentation. The consent/assent forms stated the purpose and benefits of the study and the amount of blood to be collected from each child. Emphasis was laid on the voluntary participation of the children in the study and on the point that their refusal to participate in the study will in no way affect the treatment quality the children were to receive. Only those who signed the consent/assent forms were enrolled into the study. The parents or guardians were free at any point in time to stop the participation of the child/children in the study.

2.5. Clinical Evaluation. For each child a general clinical evaluation was carried out by the medical personnel in charge. The axillary temperature was measured using a digital thermometer and fever was classified as temperature $\geq 37.5°C$. Symptoms and the duration of the symptoms were recorded. Anthropometric parameters such as height and weight were measured using a measuring tape and a weighing scale, respectively. Height-for-age (HA), weight-for-age (WA), and weight-for-height (WH) standard deviation (SD) scores (z scores) were computed based on the National Centre for Health Statistics- (NCHS-) WHO growth reference curves using the nutrition module of the Epi Info 2000 program [20]. Underweight was defined as weight-for-age z (WAZ) score of <-2; wasting was defined as a weight-for-height z (WHZ) score of <-2; and stunting was defined as height-for-age z (HAZ) score of <-2. A child was identified as being malnourished if he or she scored <-2 in one of the anthropometric indices of HA, WA, and WH [21]. The spleen was felt at the tip by pressing the abdomen under the left costal border and splenomegaly was graded according to Hackett's classification [22].

2.6. Questionnaire. A structured questionnaire was administered to parent or guardian of the child in order to obtain information on demography, socioeconomic status (SES), type of accommodation, health-seeking behaviour, access to health facilities, malaria control measures, knowledge on the signs of anaemia, and feeding practices. The socioeconomic status was classified as poor, average, and rich as described by Kimbi et al. [5] and Sumbele et al. [23].

2.7. Laboratory Methods. Venous blood samples (about 4 mL) were collected using sterile disposable syringes from children whose parent or guardian signed the assent forms. Thin and thick blood films were prepared and the remaining blood sample dispensed into labelled ethylenediaminetetraacetate (EDTA) tubes. Labelled blood samples were transported on ice in a cool box of temperature between 8 and 10°C to the University of Buea Malaria Research Laboratory for further analyses. The thick and thin blood films prepared on glass slides at the time of blood sampling were stained with Giemsa and examined following standard protocols [24]. Parasite density was determined based on the number of parasites per 200 leukocytes on thick blood film with reference to participants' white blood cell count. If gametocytes were seen, the count was extended to 500 leukocytes [25]. Parasitaemia was categorised as low ($<1,000$ parasites/μL blood), moderate ($1,000-4,999$ parasites/μL blood), high ($5,000-99,999$ parasites/μL blood), and hyperparasitaemia ($\geq100,000$) [4, 5, 26]. A complete blood count including values for white blood cell (WBC), red blood cell (RBC) and

platelet counts, haemoglobin concentration (Hb), haematocrit (Hct), mean corpuscular volume (MCV), mean corpuscular haemoglobin (MCH), mean corpuscular haemoglobin concentration (MCHC), mean platelet volume (MPV), red cell distribution width (RDW), platelet distribution width (PDW), red blood cell distribution width coefficient of variation (RDW-CV), and red blood cell distribution width standard deviation (RDW-SD) was obtained using an autohaematology analyser, the Beckman Coulter counter (URIT 3000), following the manufacturer's instructions. Anaemia was defined as Hb < 11.0 g/dL [27] and further classified as described by Cheesbrough [24] as severe (Hb < 7.0 g/dL), moderate (Hb between 7.0 and 10.0 g/dL), and mild (>10 g/dL Hb <11 g/dL). Malarial anaemia (MA) was defined as children with a malaria-positive smear for *P. falciparum* parasitaemia (of any density) and Hb < 11 g/dL. Moderate to severe anaemia was defined as Hb < 10 g/dL and moderate to severe malarial anaemia defined as malaria parasite positive + Hb < 10 g/dL.

2.8. Statistical Analysis. Data collected was cleaned up and analysed using the IBM-Statistical Package for Social Sciences (IBM-SPSS) version 20. Continuous variables were summarized into means and standard deviations and categorical variables reported as frequencies and percentages were used to evaluate the descriptive statistics. The differences in proportions were evaluated using Pearson's Chi-Square (χ^2) and the bivariate associations between haematological values and malaria parasite density by Pearson's rank correlations (r). Group means were compared using analysis of variance (ANOVA), Student's t-test, or Kruskal Wallis test where appropriate. Parasite density was log transformed before analysis. A multinomial logistic regression model analysis was conducted to evaluate potential determinants of MdSA and MdSMA with age, sex, SES, level of education, altitude, fever, and nutritional status as independent variables. The odd ratios (OR) computed was used to evaluate the risk factors. The attributable risk (AR) of anaemia caused by malaria (AR%) was calculated accordingly [28]: $[(n_1 m_0 - n_0 m_1)/n(n_0 + m_0)] \times 100$, where n_0 = anaemic children without malaria and n_1 = anaemic children with malaria, whereby $n_0 + n_1 = n$, m_0 = nonanaemic children without malaria, and m_1 = nonanaemic children with malaria, whereby $m_0 + m_1 = m$. Significant levels were measured at 95% confidence interval (CI) with significant differences set at $P < 0.05$.

3. Results

3.1. Characteristics of Participants. The consent of 254 children at presentation to the general outpatient department in the Regional Hospital Annex-Buea was sought for their participation in the study of the burden of malaria, MdSA, and MdSMA. Complete clinical and laboratory data for a total of 216 (85%) children, with a mean age of 6.3 ± 4.1 (range = 1–14) years, were included in the cross-sectional study. Majority of the parents/guardians of the children had some knowledge about malaria (94.4%) and anaemia (75.8%) and more than half of the children ate fruits (58.3%) and vegetables (56.5%) regularly.

TABLE 1: Sociodemographic, altitude, and clinical characteristics of the participants by age and sex.

Parameters	Age groups in years			Gender		Total
	1–5	6–10	11–14	Male	Female	
% (N)	51.4 (111)	23.2 (61)	20.4 (44)	52.3 (113)	47.7 (103)	100 (216)
Mean age (SD) in years	2.8 (1.3)	7.8 (1.4)	12.7 (1.2)	6.1 (4.0)	6.5 (4.3)	6.3 (4.1)
Mean weight (SD) in Kg	14.9 (3.8)	26.0 6.1)	45.6 (11.8)	23.5 (14.8)	25.1 (14.8)	24.3 (13.6)
Mean height (SD) in cm	90.3 (15.1)	124.2 (14.0)	154 .7 (11.0)	111.5 (28.9)	114.7 (29.6)	113.0 (29.2)
SES						
Poor	31.5 (25)	34.4 (21)	31.8 (14)	30.1 (34)	35.0 (36)	32.4 (70)
Average	55.9 (62)	42.9 (30)	36.4 (16)	53.1 (60)	46.6 (48)	50 0 (108)
Rich	12.6 (14)	16.4 (10)	31.8 (14)	16.8 (19)	18.4 (19)	17.6 (38)
Education level of Parent/caregiver						
No formal (n)	2.7 (3)	3.3 (2)	0.0 (0)	2.7 (3)	1.9 (2)	2.3 (5)
Primary (n)	19.8 (22)	16.4 (10)	11.4 (5)	16.8 (19)	17.5 (18)	17.1 (37)
Secondary (n)	43.2 (48)	41.0 (25)	47.7 (21)	39.8 (45)	47.6 (49)	43.5 (94)
Tertiary (n)	34.2 (38)	39.3 (24)	40.9 (18	40.7 (46)	33.0 (34)	37.0 (80)
Altitude of residence						
Lowland (n)	7.2 (8)	9.8 (6)	11.4 (5)	7.8 (8)	10.7 (11)	8.8 (19)
Middle belt (n)	72.1 (80)	77.0 (47)	77.3 (34)	75.2 (85)	73.8 (76)	74.5 (161)
Highland (n)	20.7 (23)	13.1 (8)	11.4 (5)	17.7 (20)	15.5 (16)	16.7 (36)
MBN use (n)	58.6 (65)	50.8 (31)	43.2 (19)	52.2 (59)	54.4 (56)	53.2 (115)
Clinical						
Mean temperature (SD) in °C	37.7 (1.1)	37.4 (0.9)	37.6 (1.1)	37.6 (1.0)	37.6 (1.0)	37.6 (1.0)
Fever Prevalence (n)	52.3 (58)	50.8 (31)	40.9 (18)	48.7 (55)	50.5 (52)	49.5 (107)
Malaria prevalence (n)	29.7 (33)	34.4 (21)	43.2 (19)	29.2 (33)	38.8 (40)	33.8 (73)
GMPD/μL of blood	7091	2805	3932	5423	4109	4658
Splenomegaly prevalence (n)	16.2 (18)	27.9 (17)	29.5 (13)	21.2 (24)	23.2 (24)	22.2 (48)
Mean Hb (SD) in g/dL	10 0 (2.3)	10.3 (2.6)	10.9 (2.7)	10.5 (2.8)	10.1 (2.2)	10.3 (2.5)
Anaemia prevalence (n)	67.6 (75)*	63.9 (39)*	45.5 (20)*	60.2 (68)	64.1 (66)	62.0 (134)
Malarial anaemia prevalence (n)	21.6 (24)	24.6 (15)	27.5 (12)	19.5 (22)	28.2 (29)	23.6 (51)
Malnutrition (n)	23.4 (26)	26.2 (16)	22.7 (10)	21.2 (24)	27.2 (28)	24.1 (52)
Wasting (n)	4.5 (5)	6.6 (4)	9.1 (4)	1.8 (2)$^\delta$	10.7 (11)$^\delta$	6.0 (13)
Underweight (n)	3.6 (4)	6.6 (4)	6.8 (3)	2.7(3)	7.8 (8)	5.1 (11)
Stunting (n)	19.8 (22)	19.7 (12)	13.6 (6)	18.6 (21)	18.4 (19)	18.5 (40)

*Significantly different with age ($\chi^2 = 6.67$, $P = 0.036$).
$^\delta$Significantly different with sex ($\chi^2 = 5.21$, $P = 0.022$).
Fever = axillary temperature $\geq 37.5°$C.
Anaemia = Hb < 11 g/dL.
Malarial anaemia = MP positive + Hb < 11 g/dL.
Malnutrition = <−2 z score in one of the anthropometric indices (HA, WA, and WH).

As revealed in Table 1, 52.3% (113) of the participants were males and 47.7% (103) were females. Majority of the children resided in the middle belt (75.6%) of the Buea municipality, were from homes of average socioeconomic status (50.0%), and their parents/caregivers had at least secondary level education (43.5%). The proportion of mosquito bed net (MBN) use in the studied population was 53.2% with comparable usage amongst the different age groups and sexes.

Fever, splenomegaly, malarial anaemia, and malnutrition were observed in 49.5%, 22.2%, 23.6%, and 24.1% of the children, with no significant differences in age and sex.

The prevalence of anaemia in the studied population was 62.0%, with children of the 1–5 years age group having the highest occurrence (67.6%) compared to their counterparts. The difference was statistically significant ($P = 0.036$). Wasting occurred in 6.0% of the children. While the prevalence of wasting was significantly higher ($P = 0.02$) in females (10.7%) than males (1.8%), a comparison of the different age groups revealed no significant difference (Table 1).

3.2. Falciparum Malaria. Plasmodium falciparum occurred in 33.8% (73) of the 216 children at presentation with no

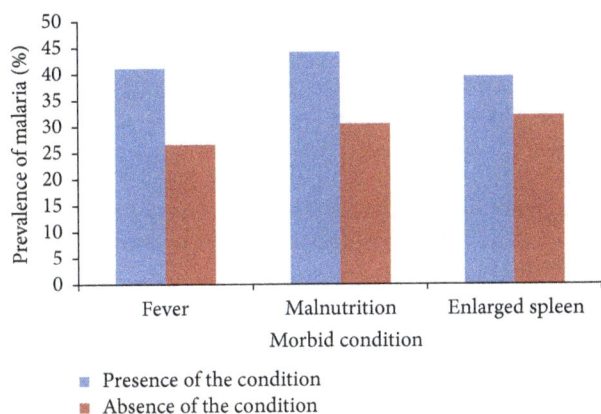

FIGURE 1: Prevalence of malaria parasite as affected by the status of fever, malnutrition, and splenomegaly. Presence of a morbid condition refers to (i) presence of fever (children with temperature $\geq 37.5°C$) and (ii) presence of malnutrition (children with $<-2\ z$ scores in one of the anthropometric indices (HA, WA, and WH)) and (iii) presence of enlarged spleen (children with enlarged spleen). Absence of a condition refers to (i) absence of fever (children with body temperature $< 37.5°C$), (ii) absence of malnutrition (well nourished children with $>-2\ z$ score in all anthropometric indices), and (iii) absence of enlarged spleen (children with normal spleen size).

significant difference in sex and age. Although not significant, children of the 1–5 years age group and males had the highest geometric mean parasite density (GMPD)/μL of blood compared to their counterparts as shown in Table 1. The prevalence of malaria was highest in patients from the lowland (47.4%, 9) compared to their counterparts from the middle belt (32.3%, 32) and highland (33.3%, 12) although the difference was not statistically significant ($\chi^2 = 1.73$, $P = 0.42$). A greater proportion of the children had high parasite densities (45.2%, 33) while low, moderate, and hyperparasitaemia occurred in 28.8% (21), 17.8% (13), and 8.2% (6) of them, respectively. In addition, the prevalence of malaria was significantly higher ($\chi^2 = 5.09$, $P = 0.024$) in children with fever (41.1%) when compared with those with no fever (26.6%) at presentation. On the other hand, the high prevalence of malaria observed in malnourished children (44.2%) and those with enlarged spleens (39.6%) compared to their counterparts was not statistically significant as shown in Figure 1.

3.3. Monthly Prevalence.

The prevalence of fever was highest in the month of July (57.1%), while malaria parasite, anaemia, and MA were highest in the month of May (43.1, 73.8, and 35.4%, resp.) as shown in Figure 2. However, only the monthly difference in prevalence of MA was statistically significant ($\chi^2 = 8.59$, $P = 0.035$).

3.4. Anaemia and Falciparum Malaria/Fever.

As shown in Figure 3, children who were malaria parasite positive had significantly higher ($\chi^2 = 3.96$, $P = 0.047$) prevalence of anaemia than those negative. Similarly, the prevalence of

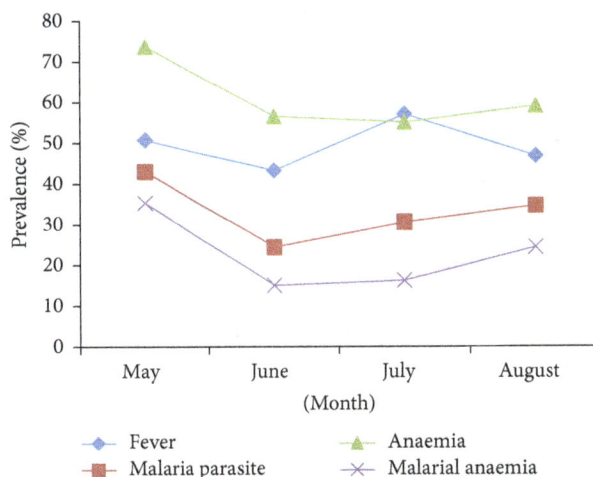

FIGURE 2: Monthly prevalence of fever, malaria parasite, anaemia, and malarial anaemia during the study period.

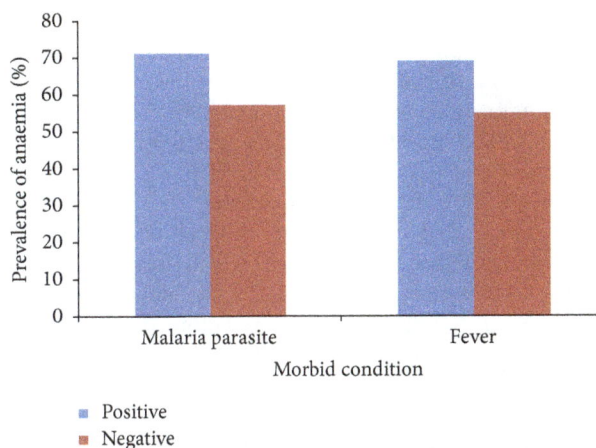

FIGURE 3: Prevalence of anaemia as affected by malaria parasite and fever status. Positive denotes (i) positive for malaria parasite (participants with positive slide for malaria parasite) and (ii) positive for fever (participants with temperature $\geq 37.5°C$). Negative denotes (i) negative for malaria parasite (participants with negative slide for malaria parasite) and (ii) negative for fever (participants with temperature $< 37.5°C$).

anaemia was significantly higher ($\chi^2 = 4.57$, $P = 0.033$) in children who presented with fever than their nonfeverish counterparts. The prevalence of anaemia as influenced by the morbid state is shown in Figure 4. Children with both fever and detectable malaria parasitaemia had a higher prevalence of anaemia (79.5%) that approached significance when compared with those with fever only (61.9%).

3.5. Moderate to Severe Anaemia and Malarial Anaemia.

Mild, moderate, and severe anaemia were prevalent in 23.6%, 29.6%, and 8.3% of the children, respectively, with no significant difference in sex and age. At presentation for consultation, MdSA and MdSMA were detected in 38.0% and 15.3% of the children, respectively. While the prevalence of MdSA and MdSMA was comparable amongst age group,

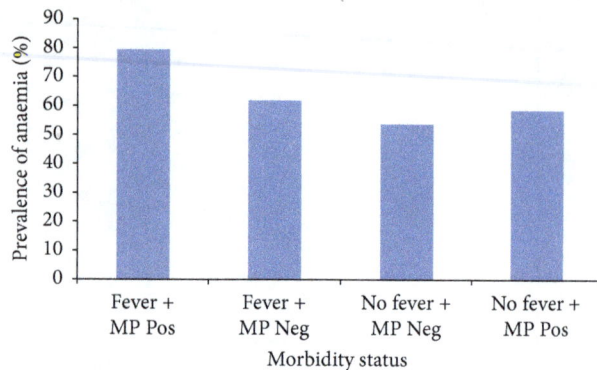

FIGURE 4: Prevalence of anaemia as influenced by morbidity status. MP Pos = malaria parasite positive. MP Neg = malaria parasite negative. Comparison of participants with fever + MP positive and those with fever and MP negative (χ^2 = 3.78, P = 0.052). Comparison of participants with no fever + MP negative versus those with no fever + MP positive (χ^2 = 0.20, P = 0.651).

gender, SES, family size, splenic, and nutritional status, and statistically significant differences were observed with the level of education of head of household (P = 0.046), altitude of residence (P = 0.012), and fever status (P = 0.019 and P = 0.012) as shown in Table 2. Explicitly, in comparison with their contemporaries, the prevalence of MdSA was significantly higher in children who came from homes where the head of household had no formal education (60.3%), resided in the lowland (63.2%), or had fever (45.8%). On the other hand, MdSMA was significantly higher in children who had fever only (21.5%) when compared with their corresponding equivalents.

The multinomial logistic regression model demonstrated that the altitude, more specifically the lowland (P = 0.02), and being febrile (P = 0.016) were significant predictors of MdSA, while being febrile (P = 0.016) was the only significant factor associated with MdSMA as shown in Table 3.

3.6. Attributable Risk of Anaemia due to Malaria. The AR of anaemia caused by malaria in the studied population was 7.6% and this was higher in females (12.0%) than males (4.4%) and in children of the 6–10 years age group (10.1%) than the 1–5 years (3.2%) and the 11–14 years age group (5.6%). On the other hand, the AR of moderate to severe anaemia caused by malaria was 9.4% with that of females (16.3%) being higher than males (2.2%). In addition, the AR of moderate to severe anaemia due to malaria was higher in children of the 11–14 years age group (36.0%) compared to the 1–5 years (7.2%) and the 6–10 years (7.2%) ones.

3.7. Haematological Indices. Correlations between haematological values and malaria parasite density revealed a significant negative association between malaria parasite density and lymphocyte count percentage (r = −0.239, P = 0.041) while a significant positive relationship was observed between granulocyte count % and malaria parasitaemia (r = 0.254, P = 0.03). A nonsignificant negative trend was observed between platelet count and malaria parasitaemia

(r = −0.133, P = 0.267). Findings from the study revealed significantly lower WBC counts (P = 0.037), lymphocyte % (P = 0.004), and platelet counts (P = 0.04) in children with MdSMA when compared with those with MdSA. On the other hand, children with MdSMA had significantly higher (P = 0.033) granulocyte % than those with MdSA (Table 4). Although not statistically significant the mean RBC, Hb, Hct, PDW, and RDW-SD were lower in those with MdSMA than those with MdSA.

4. Discussion

This cross-sectional study examines P. falciparum malaria, moderate to severe anaemia, and malarial anaemia as public health problems in children ≤14 years at presentation in the general medical outpatient department in the Regional Hospital Annex-Buea, Mount Cameroon area. The overall malaria parasite prevalence of 33.8% observed by microscopy is higher than the overall 29.8% reported for children reporting to the Mbakong Health Centre, in the North West Region of Cameroon, between 2006 and 2012 [3] and the 29% observed in febrile outpatients that visit either a public or a private health facility or medicine retail store in Bamenda and Yaoundé [29]. The equatorial climate in the Mount Cameroon area is characterized by abundant rainfall and constant humidity, all of which are factors that favour intense and perennial transmission of the malaria parasite [2], which may be a contributing factor in the higher prevalence of malaria in spite of the intensification of control measures.

Against the backdrop of a decline, the increased prevalence of malaria parasite observed with age culminating in children of the 11–14 years age group having the highest prevalence (43.2%) and a greater presence of high parasite densities (45.2%) signals a change in burden. Similar observation of a change in malaria morbidity following control measures had been reported earlier in the region [4]. While this trend may be linked to the effective use of mosquito bed nets observed in children of the 1–5 years age group when compared with the other age groups, the significantly higher prevalence of malaria in febrile children highlights fever as one of the symptoms characteristic of malaria infection. Similar significant association between malaria and fever has been reported in the same region [5, 30] even though fever may be a poor indicator of malaria where infection with other pathogens is possible [31]. Nevertheless the confirmed malaria case in febrile children (38.2%) is similar to the trend observed in Ethiopia [32].

Findings from the study revealed an anaemia prevalence of 62% with the highest prevalence in children of the 1–5 years age group. This observation is comparable to the national value of 60% reported in 2011 [33] but lower when compared with the >73.5% observed in febrile Gabonese children in a health facility based survey [34]. The significantly higher prevalence of anaemia in feverish children compared to nonfeverish ones is in line with other studies [4, 7, 34, 35]. Similarly, the significantly higher prevalence of anaemia in malaria-positive individuals is consistent with findings of several studies [34, 36, 37]. However, worthy of note,

TABLE 2: Prevalence of MdSA and MdSMA as affected by sociodemographic and clinical factors at presentation.

Characteristic	Category	N	Prevalence of MdSA (n)	χ^2 P value	Prevalence of MdSMA (n)	χ^2 P value
Age group in years	1–5	111	41.4 (46)	3.95 0.14	14.4 (16)	0.14 0.93
	6–10	61	41.0 (25)		16.4 (10)	
	11–14	44	25.0 (11)		15.9 (7)	
Gender	Male	113	36.3 (41)	0.28 0.59	11.5 (13)	2.61 0.11
	Female	103	39.8 (41)		19.4 (20)	
SES	Poor	70	42.9 (30)	4.16 0.13	14.3 (10)	0.35 0.84
	Average	108	39.8 (43)		16.7 (18)	
	Rich	38	23.7 (9)		13.2 (5)	
Family size	1–5	107	40.2 (43)	1.32 0.52	15.0 (16)	1.66 0.44
	6–10	94	34.0 (32)		13.8 (13)	
	>10	15	46.7 (7)		26.7 (4)	
Level of education of household head	Not formal	5	60.0 (3)	8.00 0.046	0	1.98 0.58
	Primary	37	35.1 (13)		16.2 (6)	
	Secondary	94	46.8 (44)		18.1 (17)	
	Tertiary	80	27.5 (22)		12.5 (10)	
Altitude of residence	Lowland	19	63.2 (12)	8.93 0.012	26.3 (5)	3.14 0.21
	Middle belt	161	38.5 (62)		15.5 (25)	
	Highland	36	22.2 (8)		8.3 (3)	
Fever status	Febrile	107	45.8 (49)	5.25 0.019	21.5 (23)	6.33 0.012
	Afebrile	109	30.3 (33)		9.2 (10)	
Splenomegaly	Enlarged	48	39.6 (19)	0.07 0.79	14.6 (7)	0.023 0.88
	Normal	168	37.5 (63)		15.5 (26)	
Nutritional status	Malnourished	52	44.2 (23)	1.14 0.29	23.1 (12)	3.22 0.07
	Normal	164	36.0 (59)		12.8 (21)	
Total		216	38.0 (82)		15.3 (33)	

the 71.2% prevalence of anaemia observed in children with malaria parasitaemia and 79.5% in children who were both febrile and malaria parasite positive is lower than 94.7% and 80.3% obtained by Achidi et al. [2] and Sumbele et al. [7], respectively, in the same region. This regional drop in prevalence of anaemia in children with malaria may be accredited to the sustained malaria control measures and its impact on the outcome measure. More so, frequent research and sensitization campaigns carried out in this study area raise awareness on the condition.

Observation from the study revealed no significant differences in the categorisation of anaemia (severe, mild, and moderate) when the various groups were compared. Hence, the moderate and severe groups of anaemia were lumped together for comparison with such other studies. However, the intention of the paper was to report on moderate to severe anaemia with or without malaria. Findings revealed a 38.0% prevalence of moderate to severe anaemia not associated with malaria and its occurrence was found to be significantly associated with fever. Furthermore, the logistic regression analysis revealed febrile children were two times at odds of being moderate to severely anaemic than their afebrile counterparts. This is not unusual as fever is not specific to

infection with malaria parasite only but could be indicative of other anaemia-causing infections [38]. As with anaemia, the significantly ($P = 0.046$) higher prevalence of MdSA in children whose parent/guardian/head of household had no formal education corroborates the findings of Oliveira et al. [39]. Lower levels of education may lead to lower paid work, hence less access to quality food, goods, and services that are beneficial to a child's health [40]. On the other hand, above secondary schooling may facilitate better feeding practices and habits gained through knowledge on nutritional composition of foods and health education.

The highest prevalence of MdSA observed in children who came from the lowland (63.2%) in contrast to the lowest prevalence observed in high altitude dwellers (22.2%) is not surprising given that haemoglobin concentration increases with altitude [27] and the lowland has favourable environmental and climatic conditions which may promote the rapid growth of the anopheline vectors and consequently a high rate of malaria transmission [5, 41] in the area. This cohort of children may have been exposed to the impact of repeated infections with malaria parasites even though they were negative at the time of examination. However, in a combination of factors in the logistic regression analysis, our

TABLE 3: Multinomial logistic regression analysis examining sociodemographic and clinical factors influencing MdSA and MdSMA.

Factors	Category	MdSA		MdSMA	
		OR (95% CI)	P value	OR (95% CI)	P value
Age group in years	1–5	0.45 (0.19–1.06)	0.07	1.08 (0.39–2.99)	0.889
	6–10	0.48 (0.19–0.122)	0.12	0.94 (0.31–2.86)	0.913
	11–14	Reference		Reference	
Gender	Male	1.07 (0.59–1.95)	0.82	1.77 (0.80–3.88)	0.16
	Female	Reference		Reference	
SES	Poor	1.32 (0.48–3.63)	0.59		
	Average	0.88 (0.43–1.78)	0.72		
	Rich	Reference		Reference	
Level of education	Not formal	3.16 (0.45–22.19)	0.22225		
	Primary	1.29 (0.19–8.74)	0.80		
	Secondary	2.26 (0.31–16.60)	0.42		
	Tertiary	Reference			
Altitude	Lowland	0.13 (0.04–0.49)	0.002	0.24 (0.05–1.21)	0.08
	Middle belt	0.38 (0.18–1.09)	0.08	0.51 (0.14–1.86)	0.31
	Highland	Reference		Reference	
Fever	Febrile	2.11 (1.45–3.87)	0.02	2.73 (1.20–6.21)	0.02
	Afebrile	Reference		Reference	
Nutritional status	Malnourished	0.76 (0.39–1.51)	0.44	0.57 (0.25–1.30)	0.18
	Normal	Reference			

findings revealed to a certain extent a significant protection against moderate to severe anaemia in children from the lowland.

The prevalence of MdSMA (15.3%) is comparable to the 13% recorded in Mozambican children [42]. In the context of a decline in the prevalence of malaria in the region, the moderate prevalence of malarial anaemia (23.6%) and the low occurrence of MdSMA at presentation probably suggest that malaria is not the major contributing factor to the public health problem of anaemia. Even though the study had as limitation the length of the period in which the investigation was carried out and the number of children examined, that notwithstanding, the investigation was carried out during the peak season of malaria transmission to ensure probability of encountering malaria parasite positive cases. However, the contribution of malaria to the public health problem of anaemia should be interpreted with caution and further study in different ecological settings and a larger population should be carried out.

In conformity with Leite et al. [43] who stated that children in household with four to five children and nine or more total residents were prone to anaemia, children who lived in homes with >10 persons had a higher prevalence of MdSA and MdSMA than their counterparts. The constraints of large family size may not only be the number of individuals to provide adequate diet in terms of nutrients and proportions, but the lack of resources to provide adequate health care such as providing appropriate malaria treatment. Delayed treatment-seeking and inappropriate medication, both of which are common among people in the Mount Cameroon area, have been reported earlier as risk factors of anaemia [7].

The low estimate of the risk of anaemia (7.6%) and moderate to severe anaemia (9.4%) that may be attributed to malaria in the children at presentation clearly indicate the important contribution of other inflammatory infections or diseases. Why females had a higher attributable risk of anaemia and moderate to severe anaemia due to malaria is unclear as no significant gender differences were observed in prevalence and density. Even though studies on the attributable risk of anaemia and moderate to severe anaemia due to *falciparum* malaria have seldom been carried out in Cameroon, previous studies in the Mount Cameroon area, in apparently healthy children, revealed a moderate (24.5%) contribution of *falciparum* malaria to anaemia [23]. Inferences from both studies most likely indicate the notion that of greater importance is the contribution of asymptomatic *P. falciparum* infection to the public health problem of anaemia compared to falciparum infection in febrile children. However, out of the ordinary is the major contribution of *falciparum* malaria to moderate to severe anaemia (36.0%) in children of the 11–14 years group which cannot be ignored.

The significant negative correlation observed between parasite density and lymphocyte percentage as well as the significantly lower lymphocyte counts in children with MdSMA is not unusual. Previous studies have reported a decrease in lymphocyte counts in malaria infection [36, 44]. On the other hand, in line with Lucien et al. [45], findings from this study revealed a significantly higher mean granulocyte counts in children with MdSMA with a significant positive relationship between parasite density and the percentage of granulocytes ($P = 0.02$). Although lymphocytosis has been reported elsewhere [46] the negative relationship observed

TABLE 4: Variation in mean haematological values in children with MdSA and MdSMA.

Variable	Category	Number examined	Mean (SD)	t-test P value	Mean difference (95% confidence interval)
WBC $\times 10^9/\mu$L	MdSA	49	11.1 (7.2)	2.12	2.9 (0.2–5.7)
	MdSMA	33	8.1 (4.1)	0.037	
Lymphocyte%	MdSA	49	37.0 (14.3)	2.94	8.9 (2.9–14.9)
	MdSMA	33	28.1 (11.9)	0.004	
Granulocyte%	MdSA	49	50.9 (16.0)	−2.17	−7.7 (−14.7−−0.6)
	MdSMA	33	58.6 (15.3)	0.033	
RBC $\times 10^{12}/\mu$L	MdSA	49	3.9 (1.7)	0.78	0.3 (−0.4–0.8)
	MdSMA	33	3.6 (0.8)	0.44	
Hb (g/dL)	MdSA	49	8.1 (2.0)	0.37	0.2 (−0.7–1.0)
	MdSMA	33	7.9 (1.8)	0.71	
Hct (%)	MdSA	49	26.9 (7.1)	0.43	0.6 (−2.3–3.6)
	MdSMA	33	26.2 (5.8)	0.67	
MCV (fl)	MdSA	49	74.3 (10.1)	−0.11	−0.2 (−4.5–4.0)
	MdSMA	33	74.5 (8.2)	0.91	
MCH (pg)	MdSA	49	21.7 (5.1)	−1.25	−1.2 (−3.2–0.7)
	MdSMA	33	22.9 (3.1)	0.22	
MCHC (g/dL)	MdSA	49	31.1 (2.1)	0.58	0.32 (−0.8–1.4)
	MdSMA	33	30.8 (2.8)	0.56	
Platelet $\times 10^9$/L	MdSA	49	233.5 (133.8)	3.37	89.9 (36.7–142.9)
	MdSMA	33	143.7 (86.2)	0.001	
MPV (fl)	MdSA	49	9.7 (1.5)	−0.97	−0.3 (−1.0–0.3)
	MdSMA	33	9.9 (1.4)	0.34	
PDW	MdSA	49	13.0 (2.9)	1.55	1.1 (−0.3–2.5)
	MdSMA	33	11.9 (3.0)	0.13	
RDW-CV (%)	MdSA	49	15.8 (3.0)	−0.80	−1.99 (−6.9–2.9)
	MdSMA	33	17.8 (17.0)	0.43	
RDW-SD (fl)	MdSA	49	43.9 (7.2)	0.77	1.1 (−1.7–3.8)
	MdSMA	33	42.9 (4.1)	0.44	

may be attributed to the role lymphocytes, particularly T cells, play in malaria immunity and probably reflect redistribution of lymphocytes with sequestration in the spleen [47, 48].

The nonsignificant lower values of RBC, Hb, and Hct observed in children with MdSMA compared to MdSA reflect the haematological abnormalities which is a hallmark of *falciparum* malaria earlier reported by several studies [16, 36]. However, the lack of any significant differences in red cell indices probably indicates that the erythropoietic response to infection between those with MdSMA and MdSA may not have been different. This may be apparent in the similarities in values of markers (RDW-SD and RDW-CV) of ineffective erythropoiesis of bone marrow [49] and inflammation [50] which were within the normal range.

The association between platelet counts and malaria parasite has been reported by several studies [5, 16]. The lower than normal mean platelet counts observed in children with MdSMA (143.7 $\times 10^9/\mu$L as against 233.5 $\times 10^9/\mu$L) clearly highlight the common occurrence of thrombocytopenia (57.6%) in this cohort of children. The high presence of

thrombocytopenia may be considered as a marker of disease severity as indicated by Maina et al. [16] and not parasite burden as no association was observed between platelet counts and parasite density. Albeit studies in Nigeria [51] revealed children with low platelet counts were likely to have anaemia, findings from this study reveal no significant association between platelet counts and Hb or parasite density. While observations from the study showed similarities in MPV in children with MdSMA and MdSA, the reason why the negative correlations between MPV and platelet counts in children with MdSMA was not significant ($r = -0.116$, $P = 0.528$) while that of MdSA was significant ($r = -0.240$, $P = 0.031$) requires further investigation to explain the difference.

Although hospital based survey is a limitation of the representation in the general population, these findings represents an approximation of the morbidity and factors related to moderate to severe anaemia and malarial anaemia which can be applicable in a wider population with different settings although with caution. There was a limitation in the diagnostic facilities of other causes of anaemia such as bacterial or viral infections and inherited haemoglobinopathies such as thalassemias, which are known to cause or are contributing factors in the aetiology of anaemia. Hence their confounding influence could not be ascertained.

5. Conclusions

Even with the decline, *falciparum* malaria is a public health problem with higher occurrence in children presenting with fever and those of the 11–14 years age group. The prevalence of anaemia is high in febrile and malaria parasite positive children with moderate to severe anaemia being a moderate public health problem. The factors significantly associated with M*d*SA include residing in the lowland and being febrile at presentation while being febrile was the only factor significantly associated with M*d*SMA. The AR of anaemia due to malaria was low; however, children of the 11–14 years age group had the highest risk of moderate to severe anaemia attributable to malaria. Haematological insult with a significant reduction in WBC, lymphocyte, and platelet counts occurred in children with M*d*SMA. To assert these findings the cross-sectional study needs to be extended in period and facilities to draw broad base conclusions.

Competing Interests

The authors declare that they have no competing interests.

Authors' Contributions

Irene Ule Ngole Sumbele was involved in all phases of the study, including literature search, study design, and data collection, analysis, and interpretation, and wrote the manuscript; Sharon Odmia Sama was involved in literature search, collection, and laboratory examination of samples; Helen Kuokuo Kimbi and Germain Sotoing Taiwe supervised the study and revised the manuscript. All authors read and approved the final manuscript.

Acknowledgments

The authors are grateful to the children who took part in the study as well as the support and cooperation received from the parents, guardians, and medical staff of the Regional Hospital Annex-Buea.

References

[1] WHO, *World Malaria Report 2015*, World Health Organization Publication, Geneva, Switzerland, 2015, http://www.who.int.

[2] E. A. Achidi, T. O. Apinjoh, J. K. Anchang-Kimbi, R. N. Mugri, A. N. Ngwai, and C. N. Yafi, "Severe and uncomplicated falciparum malaria in children from three regions and three ethnic groups in Cameroon: prospective study," *Malaria Journal*, vol. 11, article 215, 2012.

[3] I. C. Ndong, M. Van Reenen, D. A. Boakye, W. F. Mbacham, and A. F. Grobler, "Trends in malaria admissions at the Mbakong Health Centre of the North West Region of Cameroon: A

Retrospective Study," *Malaria Journal*, vol. 13, no. 1, article 328, 2014.

[4] I. U. N. Sumbele, T. R. Ning, O. S. M. Bopda, and T. Nkuo-Akenji, "Variation in malariometric and red cell indices in children in the Mount Cameroon area following enhanced malaria control measures: evidence from a repeated cross-sectional study," *Malaria Journal*, vol. 13, no. 1, article 334, 2014.

[5] H. K. Kimbi, I. U. Sumbele, M. Nweboh et al., "Malaria and haematologic parameters of pupils at different altitudes along the slope of Mount Cameroon: a cross-sectional study," *Malaria Journal*, vol. 12, no. 1, article 193, 2013.

[6] T. K. Nkuo-Akenji, P. C. Chi, J. F. Cho, K. K. J. Ndamukong, and I. Sumbele, "Malaria and helminth co-infection in children living in a malaria endemic setting of mount Cameroon and predictors of anemia," *Journal of Parasitology*, vol. 92, no. 6, pp. 1191–1195, 2006.

[7] I. U. Sumbele, M. Samje, and T. Nkuo-Akenji, "A longitudinal study on anaemia in children with *Plasmodium falciparum* infection in the Mount Cameroon region: prevalence, risk factors and perceptions by caregivers," *BMC Infectious Diseases*, vol. 13, article 123, 2013.

[8] M. B. van Hensbroek, F. Jonker, and I. Bates, "Severe acquired anaemia in Africa: new concepts," *British Journal of Haematology*, vol. 154, no. 6, pp. 690–695, 2011.

[9] C. Menendez, A. F. Fleming, and P. L. Alonso, "Malaria-related anaemia," *Parasitology Today*, vol. 16, no. 11, pp. 469–476, 2000.

[10] A. M. van Eijk, J. G. Ayisi, F. O. ter Kuile et al., "Malaria and human immunodeficiency virus infection as risk factors for anemia in infants in Kisumu, Western Kenya," *The American Journal of Tropical Medicine and Hygiene*, vol. 67, no. 1, pp. 44–53, 2002.

[11] A. Koukounari, B. B. A. Estambale, J. Kiambo Njagi et al., "Relationships between anaemia and parasitic infections in Kenyan schoolchildren: a Bayesian hierarchical modelling approach," *International Journal for Parasitology*, vol. 38, no. 14, pp. 1663–1671, 2008.

[12] J. M. Ong'echa, C. C. Keller, T. Were et al., "Parasitemia, anemia, and malarial anemia in infants and young children in a rural holoendemic *Plasmodium falciparum* transmission area," *American Journal of Tropical Medicine and Hygiene*, vol. 74, no. 3, pp. 376–385, 2006.

[13] R. N. Price, J. A. Simpson, F. Nosten et al., "Factors contributing to anemia after uncom-plicated falciparum malaria," *American Journal of Tropical Medicine and Hygiene*, vol. 65, no. 5, pp. 614–622, 2001.

[14] P. A. Buffet, I. Safeukui, G. Milon, O. Mercereau-Puijalon, and P. H. David, "Retention of erythrocytes in the spleen: a double-edged process in human malaria," *Current Opinion in Hematology*, vol. 16, no. 3, pp. 157–164, 2009.

[15] R. E. Phillips, S. Looareesuwan, D. A. Warrell et al., "The importance of anaemia in cerebral and uncomplicated falciparum malaria: role of complications, dyserythropoiesis and iron sequestration," *The Quarterly Journal of Medicine*, vol. 58, no. 227, pp. 305–323, 1986.

[16] R. N. Maina, D. Walsh, C. Gaddy et al., "Impact of *Plasmodium falciparum* infection on haematological parameters in children living in Western Kenya," *Malaria Journal*, vol. 9, supplement 3, article S4, 2010.

[17] A. A. Lamikanra, D. Brown, A. Potocnik, C. Casals-Pascual, J. Langhorne, and D. J. Roberts, "Malarial anemia: of mice and men," *Blood*, vol. 110, no. 1, pp. 18–28, 2007.

[18] United Councils and Cities of Cameroon (UCCC), 2014, http://cvuc.cm/national/index.php/fr/carte-communale/region-du-sud/142.

[19] F. J. Bryan, *The Design and Analysis of Research Studies*, University of Otago, Dunedin, New Zealand; Cambridge University Press, Cambridge, UK, 1992.

[20] WHO, *WHO Child Growth Standards: Length/Height-for-Age, Weight-for-Age, Weight-for-Length, Weight-for-Height and Body Mass Index-for-Age*, vol. 15, World Health Organization, Geneva, Switzerland, 2006, http://www.who.int/childgrowth/standards/technical_report/en/.

[21] J. C. J. Calis, K. S. Phiri, E. B. Faragher et al., "Severe anemia in Malawian children," *The New England Journal of Medicine*, vol. 358, no. 9, pp. 888–899, 2008.

[22] H. M. Gilles, *Pathology of Malaria: Handbook of Malaria Infection in the Tropics*, Italian Association, Amicidi Raoul Follerau (AIFO), Bologna, Italy, 1997.

[23] I. U. N. Sumbele, H. K. Kimbi, J. L. Ndamukong-Nyanga et al., "Malarial anaemia and anaemia severity in apparently healthy primary school children in urban and rural settings in the Mount Cameroon area: cross sectional survey," *PLoS ONE*, vol. 10, no. 4, article e0123549, 2015.

[24] M. Cheesbrough, *District Laboratory Practice in Tropical Countries*, vol. 1 2, part 1-2, Cambridge University Press, Edinburg Building, UK, 2009.

[25] J. F. Trape, "Rapid evaluation of malaria parasite density and standardization of thick smear examination for epidemiological investigations," *Transactions of the Royal Society of Tropical Medicine and Hygiene*, vol. 79, no. 2, pp. 181–184, 1985.

[26] K. A. Koram, S. Owusu-Agyei, G. Utz et al., "Severe anemia in young children after high and low malaria transmission seasons in the Kassena-Nankana district of northern Ghana," *American Journal of Tropical Medicine and Hygiene*, vol. 62, no. 6, pp. 670–674, 2000.

[27] WHO, *Iron Deficiency Anaemia: Assessment, Prevention and Control: A Guide for Programme Managers*, World Health Organization, Geneva, Switzerland, 2001, http://www.who.int/nutrition/publications/micronutrients/anaemia_iron_deficiency/WHO_NHD_01.3/en/index.html.

[28] J. Benichou, "A review of adjusted estimators of attributable risk," *Statistical Methods in Medical Research*, vol. 10, no. 3, pp. 195–216, 2001.

[29] L. J. Mangham, B. Cundill, O. A. Achonduh et al., "Malaria prevalence and treatment of febrile patients at health facilities and medicine retailers in Cameroon," *Tropical Medicine and International Health*, vol. 17, no. 3, pp. 330–342, 2012.

[30] J. Ndamukong-Nyanga, "Socio-demographic and environmental factors influencing asymptomatic Malaria and Anaemia Incidence among School Children in Fako Division, South West Cameroon," *British Journal of Medicine & Medical Research*, vol. 4, no. 20, pp. 3814–3827, 2014.

[31] E. A. Okiro and R. W. Snow, "The relationship between reported fever and *Plasmodium falciparum* infection in African children," *Malaria Journal*, vol. 9, article 99, 2010.

[32] A. Alemu, D. Muluye, M. Mihret, M. Adugna, and M. Gebeyaw, "Ten year trend analysis of malaria prevalence in Kola Diba, North Gondar, Northwest Ethiopia," *Parasites & Vectors*, vol. 5, no. 1, article 173, 2012.

[33] National Institute of Statistics Cameroon Demographic and health survey and multiple indicators cluster survey (DHS-MICS) 2011, preliminary report, 2012, http://www.statistics-cameroon.org/.

[34] M. K. Bouyou-Akotet, D. P. Mawili-Mboumba, E. Kendjo et al., "Anaemia and severe malarial anaemia burden in febrile Gabonese children: a nine-year health facility based survey," *Journal of Infection in Developing Countries*, vol. 7, no. 12, pp. 983–989, 2013.

[35] M. K. Bouyou-Akotet, A. Dzeing-Ella, E. Kendjo et al., "Impact of *Plasmodium falciparum* infection on the frequency of moderate to severe anaemia in children below 10 years of age in Gabon," *Malaria Journal*, vol. 8, no. 1, article 166, 2009.

[36] I. U. N. Sumbele, T. Nkuo-Akenji, M. Samje, T. Ndzeidze, E. M. Ngwa, and V. P. K. Titanji, "Haematological changes and recovery associated with treated and untreated *Plasmodium falciparum* infection in children in the Mount Cameroon Region," *Journal of Clinical Medicine and Research*, vol. 2, no. 9, pp. 143–151, 2010.

[37] E. M. Foote, K. M. Sullivan, L. J. Ruth et al., "Determinants of anemia among preschool children in rural, western Kenya," *American Journal of Tropical Medicine and Hygiene*, vol. 88, no. 4, pp. 757–764, 2013.

[38] I. Ngnie-Teta, O. Receveur, and B. Kuate-Defo, "Risk factors for moderate to severe anemia among children in Benin and Mali: insights from a multilevel analysis," *Food and Nutrition Bulletin*, vol. 28, no. 1, pp. 76–89, 2007.

[39] M. A. A. Oliveira, M. M. Osório, and M. C. F. Raposo, "Socioeconomic and dietary risk factors for anemia in children aged 6 to 59 months," *Jornal de Pediatria*, vol. 83, no. 1, pp. 39–46, 2007.

[40] M. M. Osório, "Determinant factors of anaemia in children," *Journal de Pediatria*, vol. 78, no. 4, pp. 269–278, 2002.

[41] E. A. Achidi, T. O. Apinjoh, E. Mbunwe et al., "Febrile status, malarial parasitaemia and gastro-intestinal helminthiases in school children resident at different altitudes, in south-western Cameroon," *Annals of Tropical Medicine and Parasitology*, vol. 102, no. 2, pp. 103–118, 2008.

[42] C. Guinovart, Q. Bassat, B. Sigaúque et al., "Malaria in rural Mozambique. Part I: children attending the outpatient clinic," *Malaria Journal*, vol. 7, article 36, 2008.

[43] M. S. Leite, A. M. Cardoso, C. E. Coimbra et al., "Prevalence of anemia and associated factors among indigenous children in Brazil: results from the first National Survey of Indigenous People's Health and Nutrition," *Nutrition Journal*, vol. 12, no. 1, article 69, 2013.

[44] M. Kotepui, B. Phunphuech, N. Phiwklam, C. Chupeerach, and S. Duangmano, "Effect of malarial infection on haematological parameters in population near Thailand-Myanmar border," *Malaria Journal*, vol. 13, article 218, 2014.

[45] K. F. H. Lucien, S. A. Atah, and A. N. Longdoh, "Relationships between blood cell counts and the density of malaria parasites among patients at the regional hospital, Limbe, Cameroon," *African Journal of Clinical and Experimental Microbiology*, vol. 11, no. 2, pp. 120–137, 2010.

[46] S. Ladhani, B. Lowe, A. O. Cole, K. Kowuondo, and C. R. J. C. Newton, "Changes in white blood cells and platelets in children with falciparum malaria: relationship to disease outcome," *British Journal of Haematology*, vol. 119, no. 3, pp. 839–847, 2002.

[47] S. N. Wickramasinghe and S. H. Abdalla, "Blood and bone marrow changes in malaria," *Best Practice & Research Clinical Haematology*, vol. 13, no. 2, pp. 277–299, 2000.

[48] L. M. Erhart, K. Yingyuen, N. Chuanak et al., "Hematologic and clinical indices of malaria in a semi-immune population of Western Thailand," *The American Journal of Tropical Medicine and Hygiene*, vol. 70, no. 1, pp. 8–14, 2004.

[49] D. L. Simel, E. R. DeLong, J. R. Feussner, J. B. Weinberg, and J. Crawford, "Erythrocyte anisocytosis. Visual inspection of blood films vs automated analysis of red blood cell distribution width," *Archives of Internal Medicine*, vol. 148, no. 4, pp. 822–824, 1988.

[50] H. S. Bazick, D. Chang, K. Mahadevappa, F. K. Gibbons, and K. B. Christopher, "Red cell distribution width and all-cause mortality in critically ill patients," *Critical Care Medicine*, vol. 39, no. 8, pp. 1913–1921, 2011.

[51] A. D. Adedapo, C. O. Falade, R. T. Kotila, and G. O. Ademowo, "Age as a risk factor for thrombocytopenia and anaemia in children treated for acute uncomplicated falciparum malaria," *Journal of Vector Borne Diseases*, vol. 44, no. 4, pp. 266–271, 2007.

22

Hyperglycaemic Environment: Contribution to the Anaemia Associated with Diabetes Mellitus in Rats Experimentally Induced with Alloxan

Oseni Bashiru Shola and Fakoya Olatunde Olugbenga

Department of Biomedical Sciences, Faculty of Basic Medical Sciences, College of Health Sciences, Ladoke Akintola University of Technology, Ogbomosho 210214, Oyo State, Nigeria

Correspondence should be addressed to Fakoya Olatunde Olugbenga; dantuned85@yahoo.com

Academic Editor: Aurelio Maggio

Background. Diabetes mellitus characterized by hyperglycaemia presents with various complications amongst which anaemia is common particularly in those with overt nephropathy or renal impairment. The present study has examined the contribution of the hyperglycaemic environment in diabetic rats to the anaemia associated with diabetes mellitus. Method. Sixty male albino rats weighing 175–250 g were selected for this study and divided equally into control and test groups. Hyperglycaemia was induced with 170 kgbwt^{-1} alloxan intraperitoneally in the test group while control group received sterile normal saline. Blood samples obtained from the control and test rats were assayed for packed cell volume (PCV), haemoglobin (Hb), red blood cell count (RBC), reticulocyte count, glucose, plasma haemoglobin, potassium, and bilirubin. *Result*. Significant reduction ($P < 0.01$) in PCV (24.40 ± 3.87 versus 40.45 ± 3.93) and haemoglobin (7.81 ± 1.45 versus 13.39 ± 0.40) with significant increase ($P < 0.01$) in reticulocyte count (12.4 ± 1.87 versus 3.69 ± 0.47), plasma haemoglobin (67.50 ± 10.85 versus 34.20 ± 3.83), and potassium (7.04 ± 0.75 versus 4.52 ± 0.63) was obtained in the test while plasma bilirubin showed nonsignificant increase (0.41 ± 0.04 versus 0.24 ± 0.06). *Conclusion*. The increased plasma haemoglobin and potassium levels indicate an intravascular haemolytic event while the nonsignificant increased bilirubin showed extravascular haemolysis. These play contributory roles in the anaemia associated with diabetes mellitus.

1. Introduction

Diabetes mellitus is a disorder of impaired carbohydrate metabolism resulting from a relative or an absolute deficiency of the hormone insulin. It is documented to have a global prevalence, ranking among the top causes of death in the Western world [1].

Without preference to classification, diabetes mellitus generally presents with hyperglycaemia. Hyperglycaemia is referred to as blood sugar greater than the upper reference limit for age, sex, and environmental and physiological condition [2]. In hyperglycaemic state, glucose supplies to metabolizing cells are usually impaired but not to the red blood cell. The glucose transporter on the red cell membrane, *glucose-permease*, is non-insulin-dependent; hence an excessively high concentration of red cell intracellular glucose in hyperglycaemic state is imminent [3].

Studies have shown that accumulation of intracellular glucose may increase peroxidation of red cell membrane predisposing to cell membrane defects [4]. This may influence deformability [5] as observed in the red cells of patients with diabetic retinopathy [6, 7] and also contribute to reduced blood flow in the capillaries and microcirculation as hypothesized by other research workers [8–10]. It has also been reported that effective erythropoietin synthesis may be impaired following pathologic conditions of the kidneys, contributing to the anaemia observed in diabetes mellitus [11]. These factors and several others play a role in the anaemia associated with diabetes; the effect of the hyperglycaemic environment on the red cell survival is therefore investigated by this study.

2. Materials and Methods

The experimental study was conducted at the Mercyland Campus of Ladoke Akintola University of Technology (LAUTECH), Osogbo. Sixty (60) white male albino rats weighing 175–250 g were acclimated for 14 days to the animal house of the Mercyland Campus of Ladoke Akintola University, Osogbo. The selected animals were housed in wire mesh, well aerated cages at normal atmospheric temperature (25 ± 5°C) and normal 12-hour light/dark cycle. They had free access to water and supplied daily with standard diet of known composition *ad libitum*. All animal procedures were in accordance with the standard recommendations for care and use of laboratory animals [12].

2.1. Chemicals, Reagent, and Equipment. Alloxan monohydrate was purchased from Sigma-Aldrich Chemicals Co. (St. Louis, MO, USA), protected from direct light exposure, and stored at 2–4°C. All other chemicals including stains (Leishman) were of analytical grade and obtained from licensed laboratory reagent suppliers. Machines and equipment used were properly calibrated and quality-controlled before respective analyses.

2.2. Induction of Diabetes. Rats were weighed and blood samples collected from the tail vein for baseline plasma glucose (glucose oxidase method) estimation using Randox glucose kit (Randox Laboratories Ltd., BT29 QY, United Kingdom). Subsequently, the animals were divided equally into two (2) groups.

Group 1 (control group) were injected with freshly prepared sterile saline. Group 2 (test group) received 170 kgbwt^{-1} alloxan preparation (2,4,5,6-tetraoxypyrimidine; 2,4,5,6-pyrimidinetetrone). All injections were done through single intraperitoneal administration using a total volume of 0.5 mL after estimating the effective dose and administered volume with respect to their weights [13].

2.3. Experimental Design. On days 3, 6, and 9 after injection, rats were reweighed and glucose estimation was done in all the two (2) groups described above. On day 10, twenty-four (24) rats had very high plasma glucose level greater than 250 mg/dL and were included for group 2 while four (4) lower responsive rats were excluded. Animals were sacrificed by exposure to chloroform within a closed system and blood samples were collected for the various investigations into appropriate specimen bottles. The following investigations were carried out in the course of the study: haematocrit (HCT), haemoglobin (Hb), and red blood cell count (RBC), extracted from a complete blood count analysis using SYS-MEX Automated Hematology Analyzer (KX-21N, Sysmex Corporation, Chuo-ku, Kobe 651-0073, Japan); peripheral blood for reticulocyte count incubated with new methylene blue at 37°C, smeared, and estimated manually; serum total

TABLE 1: The effect of alloxan on plasma glucose level.

| Control (n = 30) | | Test (n = 28) | |
| Saline injection | | Alloxan injection | |
Days	Average plasma glucose (mg/dL)	Days	Average plasma glucose (mg/dL)
0	79	0	79
3	82	3	102
6	80	6	207
9	80	9	267
12	79	12	308

bilirubin estimated using Randox kit (Randox Laboratories Ltd., BT29 QY, United Kingdom); calorimetric method on BSA 3000 Semiautometed Biochemistry Analyser (SFRI San, Lieu dit Berganton, 33127 Saint Jean d'Illac, France); and Plasma haemoglobin according to Dacie and Lewis [14]. Plasma potassium was estimated using ISE 6000 electrolyte analyzer (SFRI San, Lieu dit Berganton, 33127 Saint Jean d'Illac, France).

2.4. Statistical Analysis. Data obtained were analyzed using statistical package for social sciences version 15 (SPSS Inc., Chicago, IL) for windows and expressed as mean ± 1standard deviation. Test of significance comparing control and test was done using Student's t-test and defined as $P < 0.01$.

3. Results

A total of fifty-four (54) rats, 30 controls and 24 (80%) alloxan induced hyperglycaemic tests rats, were used for this study. Two (6.6%) of the test rats were lost to death on days 2 and 3 after induction. In Table 1 we summarize the effect of alloxan administration on plasma glucose level. On day 9 after induction, significant hyperglycaemia ($\geq$250 mg/dL) was observed in 24 (80%) rats. Four (13.3%) test rats showed no significant increase in plasma glucose after alloxan induction; there was no significant difference between the baseline glucose and glucose concentration after alloxan induction in these rats. Average plasma glucose level on day 9 after induction was significantly higher ($P < 0.01$) than the control (267 mg/dL versus 80 mg/dL). Since significant hyperglycaemia was not established in four (13.3%) of the rats, they were excluded from further studies. Data comparing the average mean values and standard deviations between parameters of the test and control group were summarized in Tables 2 and 3. In Table 2, we compare the results of plasma haemoglobin, plasma potassium, and total bilirubin concentration between the two groups. There was a significant increase ($P < 0.01$) in plasma haemoglobin and potassium concentration in hyperglycaemic rats; total bilirubin, however, was not significantly increased between the two groups although average mean was increased in the test group. Table 3 showed the relationship between the haematocrit, haemoglobin, total red blood cell count, and reticulocyte count in the two groups. We observed a statistically significant reduction ($P < 0.01$) in haematocrit, haemoglobin, and red blood cell count among

TABLE 2: Table of significance comparing test and control plasma haemoglobin, potassium, and bilirubin concentration.

Subject	Plasma Hb (mg/L)	Plasma K$^+$ (mmol/L)	Plasma total bilirubin (mg/dL)
Test mean ($n = 24$)	67.50 ± 10.85	7.04 ± 0.75	0.41 ± 0.04
Control mean ($n = 30$)	34.20 ± 3.83	4.52 ± 0.63	0.24 ± 0.06
t-test	26.4	11.52	0.28
P value	<0.01	<0.01	>0.01

TABLE 3: The test of significance of hyperglycaemia on PCV, Hb, RBC, and reticulocyte count.

Subject	PCV (%)	Hb (g/dL)	RBC ($\times 10^{12}$/L)	Retics. count (%)
Test mean ($n = 24$)	24.40 ± 3.87	7.81 ± 1.45	3.47 ± 0.29	12.4 ± 1.87
Control mean ($n = 30$)	40.45 ± 3.93	13.39 ± 0.40	7.16 ± 0.25	3.69 ± 0.47
t-test	-13.04	-16.61	-42.77	-20.19
P value	<0.01	<0.01	<0.01	<0.01

the hyperglycaemic rats; reticulocyte count was statistically higher in this group also. The red cell parameters (HCT, Hb, and RBC) were higher and stable in the control sets and reticulocyte count remained within normal limits.

4. Discussion

Induction of diabetes experimentally by alloxan (2,4,5,6-tetraoxypyrimidine; 2,4,5,6-pyrimidineterione) remains one of the most effective methods of establishing experimental diabetes. It is a well-known diabetogenic agent and has been widely reported to generate stable hyperglycaemia for prolong period [15]. In our study as summarized in Table 1, there was progressive induction of hyperglycaemia following alloxan administration and a stable hyperglycaemic state in 24(80%) of the alloxan induced rats. This is in consonance with several research studies that induced hyperglycaemia using alloxan [13, 16]. Misra and Aiman [17] in their study observed alloxan induced diabetes in 60% of rats using the same dosage as in our study; however they reported a dose-dependent mortality in 40% of the rats in this group. They hypothesized that susceptibility to diabetogenic and toxic effects of alloxan differs among animals of the same species. Alloxan has a narrow diabetogenic range of 160-180 kgbwt^{-1} [13]; induction therefore with a lower dose may autorevert the hyperglycaemic state following a regeneration of the pancreatic beta cells [18] while a higher dose may be cytotoxic, damaging not only the pancreatic cells but other important organs [19].

Hyperglycaemia was established on the sixth day of our study. This showed that the onset of alloxan action may be delayed [18]. Optimization of the diabetogenic agent is dependent on the dose range, route of administration, rate of injection, and age and species of experimental animal used [13, 17–20]. A study on the pharmacokinetic and pharmacodynamic profile of alloxan hypothesized unpredictable diabetes inducing alloxan effect except when administered by rapid intravenous injection [18]. Hyperglycaemic response and stability were monitored in the animals throughout

the experimental process to rule out autoreversion (Table 1). Significant increase in plasma potassium and haemoglobin in the test group as depicted in Table 2 suggests episodes of intravascular red cell destruction (haemolysis within the peripheral circulation). This may be attributable to fragmentation of the red blood cells in the peripheral circulation as a result of the glucose *permease* enabled accumulated red cell intracellular glucose and generation of reactive substances, distorting the well programmed structural and functional character of the cell [3]. In addition, some red cells withstanding breakage in the circulation getting to the spleen lose deformability and are phagocytosed by the reticuloendothelial macrophages, releasing bilirubin [21]. We posit that this incidence must have informed the nonsignificant increase in total bilirubin seen in this study.

The red blood cells are clinically important haematologic cells and uniquely identified as one of the early cells affected in diabetes [22], before development of other diabetic complications. Carroll and colleagues recorded that the red cells play important role in the onset and development of several diabetic complications [23]. The mechanism underlying red cell destruction in hyperglycaemia is complex. Normal erythrocytes are biconcave shaped cells, measuring about 8 μm in diameter, with an average volume of 90fL and surface area of 140 μm^2. According to Mohandas and Gallagher, red blood cell has a membrane which is highly elastic, rapidly responds to applied fluid stress, and is stronger than steel in terms of structural resistance [24]. Despite this unique feature, a slight alteration in structural composition, small increased surface area, haemoglobin hyperviscosity, and autooxidation, amongst others, poses a challenge to the oxygen transporting cell and results in cell lysis [25, 26]. In the process of performing oxygen transport function, RBCs are exposed to high level of endogenous and exogenous oxidative metabolites [27]. These accumulating reactive substances potentiate complex oxidative processes with severe damaging consequence on the cell membrane, structure, and function. However, to optimize their exclusive role as well as to survive the rigors of circulation, the highly specialized blood cells have evolved an extensive array of enzymatic and nonenzymatic antioxidants systems, including membrane oxidoreductases, cellular antioxidants such as catalase and superoxide dismutase (SOD), and enzymes that continuously produce reducing agents through the glutathione (GSH) system [28]. In hyperglycaemic state, generation of reactive oxidative substances is markedly increased creating a redox imbalance within the red cell environment and limiting the cell antioxidative potential [22, 29]. Tiwari and Ndisang reported that glucose mediated increase in reactive oxygen species is one of the biochemical changes associated with type 1 diabetes (enhanced hyperglycaemia-mediated oxidative stress) [30]; other biochemical reactions associated with hyperglycaemia are diacylglycerol production and subsequent activation of the protein kinase C pathway, flux through the polyol metabolic pathway, secretion of cytokines, and modification of proteins and lipids that becomes nonenzymatically glycated forming Schiff bases and amadori products with resultant, irreversible generation and accumulation of glycated end products [31–35]. The red cells demonstrating an unregulated access to glucose uptake are in this state exposed to high glucose concentration both intracellularly and within the vascular environment [35]; this increases glucose oxidation and accumulates glucose metabolites, including NADPH which promotes susceptibility to lipid peroxidation, membrane damage, and intravascular cell death [4]. One of the greatest challenges to the well-equipped red cell antioxidant system as documented by Mohanty and colleagues is the increased autoxidation of haemoglobin (Hb) bound to the membrane in hyperglycaemic state which is relatively inaccessible to the antioxidant system [36]. Besides haemoglobin, ROS also critically affects other proteins in the red cell since they are easy target of ROS, majorly the spectrin, ankyrin, actin, and protein 4.1 [37]. Oxidation of biomolecules at amino acid active sites can also trigger rapid deactivation of enzyme and shut down the antioxidant system [22]. RBCs thus become highly susceptible to oxidative damage from accumulated reactive substance generation. A number of *in vitro/in vivo* studies have shown that several RBCs parameters are negatively affected by increased oxidative stress as observed in diabetes [38–41]. One of these is an assessment of heme degradation products (HDP) to determine the red cell oxidative status which was increased in older RBC as they tend to senescence [36]; this was also observed in RBC of diabetics [42] suggesting reduced membrane deformability [23]. In addition, oxidative stress also inhibits Ca-ATPase, responsible for regulating the intracellular concentration of calcium [43, 44]. With increased intracellular calcium, the Gardos channel is activated causing leakage of intracellular potassium; this alters cation homeostasis resulting in cell shrinking and lysis [45] as described in our study. Besides the red cell are the vascular endothelial cells with high amount of glucose transporter and also an unrestricted access to glucose in-flow [35]. Vascular complications in diabetes are associated with formation of cross-links between key molecules in the basement membrane of ECM and eruption of basement membrane lesions; this results in thickening of the blood vessels subjecting the already weakened red blood cells to fragmentation and contributing to premature destruction of the red cell in circulation [46]. Hence, red

cell fragmentation and intravascular haemolysis are common events associated with damaged blood vessels, especially within the microvascular environment (microangiopathy).

Despite the undoubted fact that hyperglycaemia battles all the tissues in the body, it is established that diabetic complications are observed in a subset of cell types; capillary endothelial cells in the retina, mesangial cells in the renal glomerulus, and neurons and Schwann cells in peripheral nerves. Brownlee explained that, in hyperglycaemic state, most cells reduce transport of glucose inside the cell so that their internal glucose concentration stays constant. However, the cells damaged by hyperglycemia, including the red blood cells, are those that cannot do this efficiently because glucose transport rate does not decline rapidly, leading to high glucose inside the cell [35]. In view of this we propose that oxidative stress distorted biochemical processes and impaired deformability and cell membrane weakness, fragmentation, and intravascular and extravascular destructions; as observed in our study are the features characterizing the onset of anaemia associated with type 1 diabetes.

Anaemia stimulated hypoxia has been shown to increase hypoxia-inducible factor 1 which promotes synthesis of erythropoietin, inducing reticulocytosis [47]. The bone marrow responsiveness to the haemolysis through significant reticulocytosis indicates that alloxan toxicity has no destructive effect on the bone marrow at dosage used. It is further established that anaemia observed in earlier diabetes is contributed to by intravascular and extravascular haemolysis while anaemia of chronic long standing diabetics is caused by renal pathology [48].

In conclusion, we infer from our study that red cell destruction due to hyperglycaemic environment is predominantly intravascular with minor contribution from the extravascular environment and the presenting anaemia is a responsive type differing from the nonresponsive chronic anaemia associated with diabetic nephropathy documented by other workers.

Conflict of Interests

The authors declare that there is no conflict of interests regarding the publication of this paper.

Acknowledgment

The authors are grateful to the technical staff of Mercyland, Animal House, Osogbo, for helping out with care of animals and scientists of LAUTECH Teaching Hospital.

References

[1] A. C. Guyton and J. E. Hall, *A TextBook of Medical Physiology*, W.B. Saunders Company, Philadelphia, Pa, USA, 12th edition, 2012.

[2] O. J. Ochei and A. A. Kolhatkar, *Medical Laboratory Science Theory and Practice*, Tata McGraw-Hill, New Delhi, India, 1st edition, 2001.

[3] R. K. Murray, D. K. Granner, P. A. Mayes, and V. W. Rodwell, *Harper's Iluustrated Biochemistry*, McGraw-Hill, New Delhi, India, 26th edition, 2003.

[4] S. K. Jain, "Hyperglycemia can cause membrane lipid peroxidation and osmotic fragility in human red blood cells," *The Journal of Biological Chemistry*, vol. 264, no. 35, pp. 21340–21345, 1989.

[5] C. D. Brown, H. S. Ghali, Z. Zhao, L. L. Thomas, and E. A. Friedman, "Association of reduced red blood cell deformability and diabetic nephropathy," *Kidney International*, vol. 67, no. 1, pp. 295–300, 2005.

[6] R. Agrawal, R. Bhatnagar, T. Smart et al., "Assessment of red blood cell deformability by optical tweezers in diabetic retinopathy," *Investigative Ophthalmology & Visual Science*, vol. 56, no. 7, p. 5183, 2015.

[7] T. Rimmer, J. Fleming, and E. M. Kohner, "Hypoxic viscosity and diabetic retinopathy," *British Journal of Ophthalmology*, vol. 74, no. 7, pp. 400–404, 1990.

[8] Y. I. Cho, M. P. Mooney, and D. J. Cho, "Hemorheological disorders in diabetes mellitus," *Journal of Diabetes Science and Technology*, vol. 2, no. 6, pp. 1130–1138, 2008.

[9] S. Shin, Y. Ku, M.-S. Park, J.-H. Jang, and J.-S. Suh, "Rapid cell-deformability sensing system based on slit-flow laser diffractometry with decreasing pressure differential," *Biosensors and Bioelectronics*, vol. 20, no. 7, pp. 1291–1297, 2005.

[10] S. Chien, "Red cell deformability and its relevance to blood flow," *Annual Review of Physiology*, vol. 49, pp. 177–192, 1987.

[11] C. Hasslacher, "Anaemia in patients with diabetic nephropathy—prevalence, causes and clinical consequences," *European Cardiology Review*, vol. 3, no. 1, pp. 80–82, 2007.

[12] Committee for the Update of the Care and Use of Laboratory Animals, *Guide for the Care and Use of Laboratory Animals*, Committee for the Update of the Care and Use of Laboratory Animals, Washington, DC, USA, 2001, http://grants.nih.gov/grants/olaw/guide-for-the-care-and-use-of-laboratory-animals.pdf.

[13] D. C. Ashok, N. P. Shrimant, M. G. Pradeep, and U. A. Akalpita, "Optimization of Alloxan dose is essential to induce stable diabetes for prolonged period," *Asian Journal of Biochemistry*, vol. 2, no. 6, pp. 402–408, 2007.

[14] J. Babara and B. Imelda, "Basic haematological techniques," in *Practical Hematology*, S. M. Lewis, B. J. Bain, and I. Bates, Eds., pp. 139–140, Edinburgh ChurchHill LivingStone, Edinburgh, UK, 2004.

[15] R. Ankur and A. Shahjad, "Alloxan induced diabetes: mechanisms and effects," *International Journal of Research in Pharmaceutical and Biomedical Sciences*, vol. 3, pp. 819–823, 2012.

[16] T. Szkudelski, "The mechanism of alloxan and streptozotocin action in B cells of the rat pancreas," *Physiological Research*, vol. 50, no. 6, pp. 537–546, 2001.

[17] M. Misra and U. Aiman, "Alloxan: an unpredictable drug for diabetes induction," *Indian Journal of Pharmacology*, vol. 44, no. 4, pp. 538–539, 2012.

[18] D. K. Jain and R. K. Arya, "Anomalies in alloxan-induced diabetic model: it is better to standardize it first," *Indian Journal of Pharmacology*, vol. 43, article 91, 2011.

[19] I. J. Pincus, J. J. Hurwitz, and M. E. Scott, "Effect of rate of injection of alloxan on development of diabetes in," *Proceedings of the Society for Experimental Biology and Medicine.*, vol. 86, no. 3, pp. 553–554, 1954.

[20] C. C. Rerup, "Drugs producing diabetes through damage of the insulin secreting cells," *Pharmacological Reviews*, vol. 22, no. 4, pp. 485–518, 1970.

[21] A. W. Harman and L. J. Fischer, "Alloxan toxicity in isolated rat hepatocytes and protection by sugars," *Biochemical Pharmacology*, vol. 31, no. 23, pp. 3731–3736, 1982.

[22] K. B. Pandey and S. I. Rizvi, "Biomarkers of oxidative stress in red blood cells," *Biomedical Papers of the Medical Faculty of the University Palacký, Olomouc, Czech Republic*, vol. 155, no. 2, pp. 131–136, 2011.

[23] J. Carroll, M. Raththagala, W. Subasinghe et al., "An altered oxidant defense system in red blood cells affects their ability to release nitric oxide-stimulating ATP," *Molecular BioSystems*, vol. 2, no. 6, pp. 305–311, 2006.

[24] N. Mohandas and P. G. Gallagher, "Red cell membrane: past, present, and future," *Blood*, vol. 112, no. 10, pp. 3939–3948, 2008.

[25] E. Evans, N. Mohandas, and A. Leung, "Static and dynamic rigidities of normal and sickle erythrocytes. Major influence of cell hemoglobin concentration," *The Journal of Clinical Investigation*, vol. 73, no. 2, pp. 477–488, 1984.

[26] G. S. Redding, D. M. Record, and B. U. Raess, "Calcium-stressed erythrocyte membrane structure and function for assessing glipizide effects on transglutaminase activation," *Proceedings of the Society for Experimental Biology and Medicine*, vol. 196, no. 1, pp. 76–82, 1991.

[27] J. P. Fruehauf and F. L. Meyskens Jr., "Reactive oxygen species: a breath of life or death?" *Clinical Cancer Research*, vol. 13, no. 3, pp. 789–794, 2007.

[28] M. F. McMullin, "The molecular basis of disorders of red cell enzymes," *Journal of Clinical Pathology*, vol. 52, no. 4, pp. 241–244, 1999.

[29] M. Maurizio, A. Luciano, and M. Walter, "The microenvironment can shift erythrocytes from a friendly to a harmful behavior: pathogenetic implications for vascular diseases," *Cardiores*, vol. 75, no. 1, pp. 21–28, 2007.

[30] S. Tiwari and J. F. Ndisang, "The heme oxygenase system and type-1 diabetes," *Current Pharmaceutical Design*, vol. 20, no. 9, pp. 1328–1337, 2014.

[31] P. Xia, T. Inoguchi, T. S. Kern, R. L. Engerman, P. J. Oates, and G. L. King, "Characterization of the mechanism for the chronic activation of diacylglycerol-protein kinase C pathway in diabetes and hypergalactosemia," *Diabetes*, vol. 43, no. 9, pp. 1122–1129, 1994.

[32] E. P. Feener, P. Xia, T. Inoguchi, T. Shiba, M. Kunisaki, and G. L. King, "Role of protein kinase C in glucose- and angiotensin II-induced plasminogen activator inhibitor expression," *Contributions to Nephrology*, vol. 118, pp. 180–187, 1996.

[33] A. Y. W. Lee and S. S. M. Chung, "Contributions of polyol pathway to oxidative stress in diabetic cataract," *The FASEB Journal*, vol. 13, no. 1, pp. 23–30, 1999.

[34] A. Goldin, J. A. Beckman, A. M. Schmidt, and M. A. Creager, "Advanced glycation end products: sparking the development of diabetic vascular injury," *Circulation*, vol. 114, no. 6, pp. 597–605, 2006.

[35] M. Brownlee, "The pathobiology of diabetic complications: a unifying mechanism," *Diabetes*, vol. 54, no. 6, pp. 1615–1625, 2005.

[36] J. G. Mohanty, E. Nagababu, and J. M. Rifkind, "Red blood cell oxidative stress impairs oxygen delivery and induces red blood cell aging," *Frontiers in Physiology*, vol. 5, article 84, 2014.

[37] M. Bryszewska, I. B. Zavodnik, A. Niekurzak, and K. Szosland, "Oxidative processes in red blood cells from normal and diabetic individuals," *Biochemistry and Molecular Biology International*, vol. 37, no. 2, pp. 345–354, 1995.

[38] B. Halliwell and J. M. C. Gutteridge, "Cellular responses to oxidative stress: adaptation, damage, repair, senescence and death," in *Free Radicals in Biology and Medicine*, pp. 187–267, Oxford University Press, New York, NY, USA, 4th edition, 2007.

[39] I. Maridonneau, P. Barquet, and R. P. Garay, "Na$^+$/K$^+$ transport damage induced by oxygen free radicals in human red cell membranes," *The Journal of Biological Chemistry*, vol. 258, pp. 3107–3117, 1983.

[40] K. B. Pandey and S. I. Rizvi, "Protective effect of resveratrol on markers of oxidative stress in human erythrocytes subjected to in vitro oxidative insult," *Phytotherapy Research*, vol. 24, no. 1, pp. S11–S14, 2010.

[41] K. B. Pandey and S. I. Rizvi, "Protective effect of resveratrol on formation of membrane protein carbonyls and lipid peroxidation in erythrocytes subjected to oxidative stress," *Applied Physiology, Nutrition and Metabolism*, vol. 34, no. 6, pp. 1093–1097, 2009.

[42] M. Goodarzi, A. A. Moosavi-Movahedi, M. Habibi-Rezaei et al., "Hemoglobin fructation promotes heme degradation through the generation of endogenous reactive oxygen species," *Spectrochimica Acta Part A: Molecular and Biomolecular Spectroscopy*, vol. 130, pp. 561–567, 2014.

[43] M. Samaja, A. Rubinacci, R. Motterlini, A. De Ponti, and N. Portinaro, "Red cell aging and active calcium transport," *Experimental Gerontology*, vol. 25, no. 3-4, pp. 279–286, 1990.

[44] C. R. Kiefer and L. M. Snyder, "Oxidation and erythrocyte senescence," *Current Opinion in Hematology*, vol. 7, no. 2, pp. 113–116, 2000.

[45] P. A. Ney, M. M. Christopher, and R. P. Hebbel, "Synergistic effects of oxidation and deformation on erythrocyte monovalent cation leak," *Blood*, vol. 75, no. 5, pp. 1192–1198, 1990.

[46] A. V. Hoffbrand, S. M. Lewis, and E. G. D. Tuddenham, *Postgraduate Haematology*, Arnold Medical Books, London, UK, 4th edition, 2001.

[47] N. Bersch, J. E. Groopman, and D. W. Golde, "Natural and biosynthetic insulin stimulates the growth of human erythroid progenitors in vitro," *Journal of Clinical Endocrinology and Metabolism*, vol. 55, no. 6, pp. 1209–1211, 1982.

[48] E. Ritz and V. Haxsen, "Diabetic nephropathy and anaemia," *European Journal of Clinical Investigation, Supplement*, vol. 35, no. 3, pp. 66–74, 2005.

23

Magnitude of Anemia and Associated Factors among Pregnant Women Attending Antenatal Care in Public Hospitals of Ilu Abba Bora Zone, South West Ethiopia

Adamu Kenea,[1] **Efrem Negash,**[1] **Lemi Bacha,**[1] **and Negash Wakgari** ⓘ[2]

[1]*Faculty of Public Health and Medical Sciences, Mettu University, Mettu, Ethiopia*
[2]*Department of Midwifery, College of Medicine and Health Sciences, Hawassa University, Hawassa, Ethiopia*

Correspondence should be addressed to Negash Wakgari; negashwakgari@yahoo.com

Academic Editor: Duran Canatan

Background. Anemia is a global public health problem affecting all population particularly pregnant women. Hence, this study assessed the magnitude of anemia and associated factors among pregnant. *Methods*. Institution based cross-sectional study was conducted among 416 pregnant women attending antenatal clinic in three public hospitals of Ilu Aba Bora zone. The study participants were selected by proportional allocation based on the number of pregnant women that the respective health facilities contain. Semistructured questionnaire was used for data collection. Midupper arm circumference was employed to assess the nutritional status and standard mood depression assessment tool was used to assess depression. Data were centered and analyzed using SPSS version 20.0. Logistic regression analyses were used to see the association of different variables. *Results*. In this study, 31.5% of pregnant women were anemic. In addition, having family size five and above [AOR = 2.97, 95% CI (1.69, 5.27)], being rural resident [AOR=2.74, (95%CI) (2.11, 5.06)], had a higher odds of anemia. Similarly, having soil transmitted helminthes infection [AOR= 3.19, 95% CI (1.5, 6.65)] and history of malaria infection in the last one year [AOR= 3.10, 95% CI (2.10, 5.06)] had also a higher odds anemia during pregnancy. Moreover, being undernourished [AOR= 2.74 95% CI (1.34, 5.57)] was negatively associated with magnitude of anemia. *Conclusions*. The magnitude of anemia among pregnant women was found to be significant. Residence, family sizes, history of malaria infection during the last one year, and undernourishment were significantly associated with anemia during pregnancy.

1. Introduction

Anemia is global public health problem affecting people of different age groups. However, it is more prominent in pregnant women and young children and other reproductive age [1, 2]. According to the 2008 World Health Organization (WHO) report, anemia affected 1.62 billion (24.8%) people globally [3]. It had an estimated global prevalence of 42% in pregnant women and is a major cause of maternal mortality [4, 5] Sub-Saharan Africa is the most affected region, with anemia prevalence estimated to be 17.2 million among pregnant women, which corresponds to approximately 30% of total global cases [6].

Ethiopia is among countries where there is a high level of anemia among women of reproductive age (15-49years) and

pregnant women. Seventeen percent of Ethiopian women age 15-49 are anemic, with thirteen percent having mild anemia, three percent having moderate anemia, and one percent having severe anemia [7]. A higher proportion of pregnant women are anemic (22%) than women who are breast feeding (19%) and women who are neither pregnant nor breastfeeding (15%) [8]. There is an increased iron requirement during pregnancy due to greater expansion in plasma volume that results in a decrease in hemoglobin (Hgb) level to 11g/dl [7]. Therefore, any Hgb level below 11g/dl in pregnancy is considered as anemia [7, 8]. Anemia could be classified as mild, moderate, and severe. The Hgb levels for each class of anemia in pregnancy are 10.0–10.9g/dl (mild), 7–9.9g/dl (moderate), and <7g/dl (severe) [9].

The main risk factors for anemia are low intake of iron, poor absorption, high phytate, or phenolic compounds or increased requirements during childhood and pregnancy as well as infection with malaria, HIV, and hookworm [10–12]. The effect of anemia during pregnancy on maternal and neonatal life ranges from varying degrees of morbidity to mortality. As many studies reported, severe anemia (Hg < 7g/L) during pregnancy has been associated with major maternal and fetal complications. It increases the risk of preterm delivery [13, 14], low birth weight [13–16], intrauterine fetal death [16], neonatal death [17], maternal mortality [18], and infant mortality [19] associated with child hood intellectual disability [20, 21].

The availability of local information on the magnitude and related risk factors has a major role in the management and control of anemia in pregnancy. Even though the global and national prevalence of anemia among pregnant women and its associated factors were identified, it is not well determined in the study area. Therefore, this study intended to provide information about magnitude and factors that influenced anemia among pregnant women in south west Ethiopia and also used to assist: program planners and service providers in the study area to reduce maternal morbidity, mortality and serious complication of pregnancy or childbirth related to anemia.

2. Materials and Methods

2.1. Study Design, Setting and Population. Institution based quantitative cross-sectional study design was employed in public hospitals of Ilu Abba Bora zone. Ilu Abba Bora zone is found in south west Ethiopia. The zone is 600 km far away from Addis Ababa, capital of Ethiopia. The study conducted in three hospitals found in the zone; namely Mettu, Bedele and Darimu hospitals from January to July 2016. All pregnant women who were attending antenatal care in Ilu Abba Bora zone hospitals' ANC care unit were considered as source population. Those who are critically ill and unable to hear and/or speak are not long-term residents of the study area was excluded from the study.

2.2. Sample Size and Sampling Procedures. The sample size was calculated by using 56.7% prevalence of anemia among pregnant women attending antenatal clinic from a local study done in eastern Ethiopia [22]. Accordingly, the sample size for the study was calculated by using single proportion formula:

$$n = \frac{(Z\alpha/2)^2 \times p\,(1-p)}{w^2} \qquad (1)$$

where n= sample size, p= prevalence of anemia, W = maximum allowable error = 0.05, and Z = value of standard normal distribution (Z-statistic) at 95% confidence level which is 1.96.Thus the computed sample size with 10% nonresponse rate became 416. The study subjects was selected by proportional allocation based on the number of pregnant women that the respective health facilities contain in their antenatal clinic and all pregnant women attending antenatal clinic during study period were included. Accordingly, from

Mettu Karhl Hospital 176, Bedele Hospital 141, and Darimu Hospital 199 pregnant women were included.

2.3. Data Collection Instruments and Procedures. Semistructured interviewer administered questionnaire was employed to obtain data about sociodemographic characteristics, dietary intake and habit, gynecological factors, and patient-health care provider relationship. Document review was used to obtain medical condition of the mother (HIV and hemorrhoids). Midupper arm circumference measurement was used to assess the nutritional status of pregnant women while standard mood/depression assessment questionnaire was used to screen for depression. In addition, hemoglobin level was measured on site, using capillary blood samples collected using aseptic techniques, and intestinal parasites was checked by taking a single stool sample from each participant and history of malaria infection over the past one year was interviewed.

2.4. Data Quality Control. To ensure data quality, a pretested semistructured questionnaire and midupper arm circumference measuring instrument were used. Training about purpose of the study, how to approach study subjects, and how to use the questionnaire was given for three days for the data collectors and supervisors. The sample collections and laboratory procedure were done by senior experienced professionals. The collected data was checked for the completeness, accuracy, and clarity by the principal investigator and supervisors. This quality checking was done daily after data collection and correction was made before the next data collection measure. Data clean up and cross-checking were done before analysis.

2.5. Data Processing and Analysis. Data collected through a semistructured interviewer administered questionnaire was cleaned, coded, and entered into SPSS version 20.0 for analysis. Both bivariate and multivariate logistic regression analyses were used to determine the association of each independent variable with the dependent variable. Variables significant in bivariate analysis (p-value less than or equal to 0.2) were entered into a multivariate logistic regression model to adjust the effects of confounders on the outcome variable. Odds ratio with their 95% confidence intervals was computed to identify the presence and strength of association, and statistical significance was declared if $p < 0.05$.

2.6. Ethical Considerations. Ethical approval was obtained from the Research Ethical Review Committee at the Mettu University, Faculty of Public Health and Medical Sciences. Next, official letters were submitted to Oromia Regional Health Bureau. Then written permission was obtained from Oromia Regional Health Bureau and finally from Zonal Health office and respective health institution in the study area. During data collection process the data collectors informed each study participant about the purpose and anticipated benefits of the research project and the study participants. In addition they were informed about their full right to refuse, withdraw, or completely reject part or all

TABLE 1: Socio demographic characteristics of pregnant women attended antenatal clinic in public hospitals of Ilu Aba Bora zone, south west Ethiopia, 2016 (n=416).

Variables	Yes[%]	No[%]	Total[%]
Age (years)			
18-24	33[18.7]	143[81.25%]	176[42.3]
25-31	67[16.1]	143[68.1]	210[50.5]
32-38	10[35.7]	18[64.3]	28[6.7]
39-45	1[50]	1[50]	2[0.5]
Educational status			
No formal education	47[43.5]	61[56.5]	108[25.0]
Primary	20[27.7]	52[72.3]	72[17.3]
Secondary	32[22.2]	112[77.8]	144[34.6]
Higher education	13[14.1]	79[85.9]	92[22.1]
Occupation			
Farmer	41[51.3]	39[48.7]	80[19.2]
House wife	35[30.7]	79[69.3]	114[27.4]
Employee	28[16.4]	143[83.6]	171[41.1]
Others*	9[17.6]	42[82.4]	51[12.3]
Religion			
Orthodox	39[31.7]	84[68.3]	123[29.6]
Muslim	17[28.8]	42[71.2]	59[14.2]
Protestant	55[24.8]	167[75.2]	222[53.4]
Catholic	2[16.7]	10[83.3]	12[2.9]
Ethnicity			
Amhara	4[50]	4[50]	9[1.9]
Tigre	7[28]	18[72]	25[6]
Oromo	101[26.4]	282[73.6]	383[92.1]
Marital status			
Married	100[25.2]	297[74.8]	397[95.4]
Others**	12[41.4]	7[1.7]	19[4.6]
Monthly income			
<500	65[65]	35[35]	100[24]
500-1000	35[23.6]	113[76.4]	148[35.6]
>1000	12[7.1]	156[92.9]	168[40.4]
Family size			
≤2	26[18.8]	112[81.2]	138[33.2]
3-4	44[25.7]	127[74.3]	171[41.1]
≥5	42[39.3]	65[60.7]	107[27.7]

*=Merchant, daily laborer **=single, divorced, widowed

of their part in the study and they were assured that their treatment and other benefits they gain from the hospitals will not be influenced by their participation in the study. Finally, they were asked for their informed written consent to participate or not to participate in the study and for their willingness on use of their files and records for the study.

3. Results

3.1. Sociodemographic Characteristics of the Respondents. A total of 416 pregnant women were involved in the study with a response rate of 100%. The mean age of the respondents was 25.15 (±4.29 years). Majority, 298 (71.7%), of them were urban dwellers while 118 (28.4%) of them were urban residents.

More than two-thirds 144 (77.8%) of them had attended secondary education and more than half 223 (53.5%) of them were protestant religion followers. One hundred sixty-eight (40.4%) study participants have more than 1000 Ethiopian birr monthly income. The family sizes of the study participant were between 3 and 4 for 171 (41.1%) (Table 1).

3.2. Magnitude of Anemia. In this study the magnitude of anemia among pregnant women was found to be 31.5% [CI: 28.6-34.8]. The magnitude of anemia was high among respondents who were age between 39 and 45 (50%) and live in rural area 51(43.2%). Similarly, it was high among those with no formal education 47 (43.5%) and with family size five and above 42(39.3%). Moreover 28 (19.2%) of primi gravida

TABLE 2: The magnitude of anemia among pregnant women attended antenatal clinic in public hospitals of Ilu Aba Bora zone, south west Ethiopia, 2016 (n=416).

Variables	Anemia		Total[%]
	Yes[%]	No[%]	
Gestational age			
First trimester	12[32.4]	25[67.6]	37[8.9]
Second trimester	48[21.3]	177[78.7]	225[54.1]
Third trimester	52[33.8]	102[66.2]	154[37]
Last delivery			
Health institution	34[20.1]	135[79.9]	169[62.4]
Home	49[48.0]	53[52]	102[37.6]
Birth interval			
<2years	52[47.7]	57[52.2]	109[38.7]
>2years	36[20.8]	137[79.2]	173[61.3]
Blood loss in last delivery			
Yes	41[41.4]	58[58.6]	99[36]
No	44[25]	132[75]	176[64]
History of abortion			
Yes	38[49.4]	39[50.6]	77[18.5]
No	74[21.8]	265[78.2]	339[81.5]
Use of contraceptive			
Yes	48[22.1]	169[77.9]	217[52.2]
No	64[32.2]	135[67.8]	199[47.8]
Malaria infection in the last one year			
Yes	26[36.6]	45[63.4]	71[17.1]
No	86[24.9]	259[75.1]	345[82.9]
STH infection∗			
Yes	22[68.8]	10[31.2]	32[7.7]
No	90[23.4]	294[76.6]	384[92.3]
HIV status			
Positive	7[70]	3[30]	10[2.4]
Negative	105[25.9]	301[74.1]	406[97.6]
Body mass index			
Under weight	29[60.4]	19[39.6]	48[11.5]
Normal weight	77[25.3]	227[74.7]	304[73.1]
Over weight	6[9.4]	58[90.6]	64[15.4]

∗= Soil transmitted helminthes

and 84 (31.1%) of multi gravida women were anemic (Table 2). Among anemic pregnant women 69 (61.61%) of them had mild anemia, while 40 (35.7%) and 3(2.68%) of them had moderate and severe anemia, respectively.

3.3. Factors Associated with Magnitude of Anemia.
In bivariate analysis the factors found to be significantly associated with magnitude of anaemia were age, residence, educational status, income, ethnicity, religion, marital status, delivery site, number of pregnancy, history of abortion, use of contraceptive, blood loss in the last delivery, malaria infection in the last one year, soil transmitted helminthes infection, HIV status, and nutritional status. However, residence, family size, soil transmitted helminthes infection, history of malaria infection in the last one year, and nutritional status remain significantly associated with magnitude of anaemia in the multivariate

logistic regression. The odds of anemia among pregnant mothers who live in the rural area were 2.37 times higher than the odds of anemia among pregnant mothers who lives in the urban area [AOR=2.37, 95% CI (2.11, 5.06)]. Pregnant mothers with five and above family size were 2.97 times more likely to develop anemia as compared to pregnant mothers with less than five family sizes. Soil transmitted helminthes infection was significantly associated with anemia; pregnant mothers with soil transmitted helminthes infection were 3.19 times more likely to develop anemia than pregnant mothers without soil transmitted helminthes infection. In addition, history of malaria infection in the last one year [AOR= 3.10, 95% CI (2.10, 5.06)] had also a higher odds of anemia compared to their counterparts. Furthermore being undernourished had a higher odds of anemia compared well-nourished pregnant mothers [AOR= 2.74 95% CI (1.34, 5.57)] (Table 3).

TABLE 3: Factors associated with the magnitude of anemia among pregnant women visited antenatal clinic of public hospitals in Ilu Aba Bora zone, south west Ethiopia, 2016 (n=416).

Variables	Anemia		OR(95% CI)	
	Yes[%]	No[%]	Crude OR	Adjusted OR
Residence				
Urban	61[20.5]	237[39.5]		
Rural	51[43.2]	67[56.8]	2.96(1.62,6.92)	2.37(2.11,5.06)*
Marital status				
Married	100[25.2]	297[74.8]	5.09(1.56,7.89)	1.03(0.87,1.76)
Others**	12[41.4]	7[1.7]		
Family size				
≤2	26[18.8]	112[81.2]		
3-4	44[25.7]	127[74.3]	1.49(0.46,7.65)	1.03(0.06,3.76)
≥5	42[39.3]	65[60.7]	2.78(1.07,4.56)	2.97(1.69,5.27)*
Parity				
Primi gravida	28[19.2]	118[80.8]		
Multi gravida	84[31.1]	186[68.9]	1.90(1.06,2.03)	1.61(0.54,2.43)
Last delivery				
Health institution	34[20.1]	135[79.9]	1.61(0.86,3.02)	1.28(0.54,3.01)
Home	49[48.0]	53[52]		
Birth interval				
<2years	52[47.7]	57[52.2]	1.15(0.56,2.38)	0.75(0.29,1.95)
>2years	36[20.8]	137[79.2]		
Blood loss in last delivery				
Yes	41[41.4]	58[58.6]	0.46(0.20,0.83)	0.45(.15, 1.29)
No	44[25]	132[75]		
History of abortion				
Yes	38[49.4]	39[50.6]		
No	74[21.8]	265[78.2]	0.41(0.20,0.83)	0.45(.15, 1.29)
Use of contractive				
Yes	48[22.1]	169[77.9]		0.58(0.251.365)
No	64[32.2]	135[67.8]		
Malaria infection in the last 1 year				
Yes	26[36.6]	45[63.4]	3.35(1.62,6.92)	3.1(2.1; 5.06)*
No	86[24.9]	259[75.1]		
Soil transmitted helminthes infection				
Yes	22[68.8]	10[31.2]	3.2(1.6,6.32)*	3.19(1.5,6.65)*
No	90[23.4]	294[76.6]		
HIV status				
Positive	7[70]	3[30]	1.37(0.65,2.88)	1.15(0.47,2.83)
Negative	105[25.9]	301[74.1]		
Body mass index				
Under weight	29[60.4]	19[39.6]	4.49(1.56,5.63)*	2.74(1.34,5.57)*
Over weight	6[9.4]	58[90.6]	0.30(0.04,0.82)	0.96 (0.44,5.00)
Normal weight	77[25.3]	227[74.7]		

*=significant in backward stepwise logistic regression and **= single, divorced, and widowed.

4. Discussion

This study attempted to identify magnitude of anaemia among pregnant women attending antenatal clinic and associated factors in Ilu Aba Bora Zone, south west Ethiopia. The magnitude of anemia among pregnant women was found to be 31.5% [CI: 26.5-36.5]. With the reference to the WHO cutoff points [3], the present finding indicates moderate public health significance of anemia in the study area. This finding is higher than the studies conducted in other parts of Ethiopia, Awassa (15.3%) [23] and Gondar town (22%) [24]. Moreover, this finding is lower than the studies done in Gilegle Gibe (53.9%) [22] and west Arsi (36.6%) [25]. The possible reason for the observed difference might be due to difference in sociodemographic characteristics and geographical variation of the study participants which could be explained by the possible presence of food taboos during pregnancy in certain community in Ethiopia. For instance, the study conducted in southern Ethiopia indicated 65% of women avoided at least one food type during their recent pregnancy [26].

The presence of soil transmitted parasite infections was significantly associated with anemia in pregnant women (AOR=3.19, 95% CI = 1.50-6.65). This is consistent with study conducted in Jimma [27] and Gondar town [24]. This is because adult hookworm parasites attach and injure upper intestinal mucosa and also ingest blood. This brings about gastrointestinal blood loss and induces depletion of iron, folic acid, and vitamin B12 that ultimately lead to anemia [6]. Similarly, having history of malaria infection during the last one year also significantly associated with the magnitude of anemia during pregnancy (AOR= 3.10 95% CI (2.10, 5.06). This finding is consistent with other studies [13-15]. Malaria in pregnancy has been a cause of severe anemia. In areas with high prevalence of malaria, prevalence of anemia among pregnant women with malaria was up to 68.75% as compared to those without malaria infection (42.31%) [13]. Malaria causes hemolytic anemia and in severe cases it could also a risk factor for stillbirths, low birth weight, and fetal anemia [14, 15].

Place of residence become a factor for magnitude of anaemia during pregnancy. Pregnant mothers who lives in the rural area was 2.37 times more likely to develop anemia compared to who lives in the urban area [AOR=2.37, 95% CI (2.11, 5.06)]. This is in line with the study conducted in Sidama zone, southern Ethiopia [16]. In addition, those who have family size of five and above were 2.97 times likely to develop anemia as compared to pregnant mothers with less than five family sizes. Furthermore, this study revealed that anemia is 2.74 times more likely among under nourished pregnant women compared to well-nourished pregnant women [AOR=2.74, 95% CI (1.34, 5.57)]. This finding is consistent with the study done in Nigeria [18].

5. Conclusion

The magnitude of anemia among pregnant women was found to be significant among pregnant women. Rural residence, family size five and above, soil transmitted helminthes infection, and history of malaria infection during the last one year and the undernourished were significantly associated with anemia during pregnancy. To reduce the prevalence of anemia during pregnancy, there is a need to improve the frequency of dietary level, avoiding bare foot walk, constant use of insecticide treated bed net, and strength health care seeking behavior of women to ensure early diagnosis and management of soil transmitted helminthes and malaria, especially in rural areas.

Since information about factors associated with magnitude of anemia was obtained from respondents through interviewer administered questionnaires, rather than follow-up, response, recall, and social desirability bias are the potential limitations of this study. However, numerous scientific procedures have been employed to minimize the possible effects. For instance, procedures such as supervision, pretest of data collection tool, and adequate training of data collectors and supervisors were utilized.

Conflicts of Interest

The authors declare that they have no conflicts of interest.

Acknowledgments

The authors are grateful to the Mettu University for technical and financial support. They would also like to thank the staff at Karhl, Bedele, and Darimu hospital for their guidance and support during data collection process.

References

[1] E. McLean, M. Cogswell, I. Egli, D. Wojdyla, and B. De Benoist, "Worldwide prevalence of anaemia, WHO Vitamin and Mineral Nutrition Information System, 1993–2005," *Public Health Nutrition*, vol. 12, no. 4, pp. 444–454, 2009.

[2] A. G. Ma, E. Schouten, Y. Wang et al., "Anemia prevalence among pregnant women and birth weight in five areas in China," *Medical Principles and Practice*, vol. 18, no. 5, pp. 368–372, 2009.

[3] WHO, *Worldwide Prevalence of Anaemia 1993-2005: WHO Global Database on Anaemia*, World Health Organization, Geneva, 2008, http://whqlibdoc.who.int/publications/2008/9789241596657_eng.pdf.

[4] Y. Balarajan, U. Ramakrishnan, E. Özaltin, A. H. Shankar, and S. V. Subramanian, "Anaemia in low-income and middle-income countries," *The Lancet*, vol. 378, no. 9809, pp. 2123–2135, 2011.

[5] UNICEF WHO, *Maternal Mortality in 2005: Estimates Developed by WHO, UNICEF, UNFPA and World Bank, WHO*, Geneva, Switzerland.

[6] T. Susan and D. O. Blackburn, "Maternal, Fetal, & Neonatal Physiology," *Clinical Perspective. Qualitative Health Research*, vol. 11, no. 6, pp. 780–794, 2007.

[7] Central Statistical Agency, *Preliminary report of Ethiopia Demographic and Health Survey 2011. Addis Ababa, Ethiopia*, ICF International Calverton, Maryland, USA, 2012.

[8] K. M. Sullivan, Z. Mei, L. Grummer-Strawn, and I. Parvanta, "Haemoglobin adjustments to define anaemia," *Tropical Medicine & International Health*, vol. 13, no. 10, pp. 1267–1271, 2008.

[9] C. E. Shulman, M. Levene, L. Morison, E. Dorman, N. Peshu, and K. Marsh, "Screening for severe anaemia in pregnancy in Kenya, using pallor examination and self-reported morbidity," *Transactions of the Royal Society of Tropical Medicine and Hygiene*, vol. 95, no. 3, pp. 250–255, 2001.

[10] J. Waweru, O. Mugenda, and E. Kuria, "Anaemia in the context of pregnancy and HIV/AIDS: A case of Pumwani Maternity

Hospital in Nairobi, Kenya," *African Journal of Food, Agriculture, Nutrition and Development*, vol. 9, no. 2, 2009.

[11] WHO, *Preventing and Controlling Iron Deficiency Anemia through Primary Health Care*, WHO, Geneva, 1989.

[12] A. Petros, *Assessment of Anemia and its associated factors among pregnant Women attending Antenatal care in Karamara Hospital, Jigjiga Town, Eastern Ethiopia*, 2013.

[13] T. H. Bothwell, "Overview and Mechanisms of Iron Regulation," *Nutrition Reviews*, vol. 53, no. 9, pp. 237–245, 1995.

[14] W. A. Johan, L. Dan, and S. Lang, "Anemia," in *Harrison principle of internal medicine*, p. 332, 14th edition, 1998.

[15] H. S. J. Ras, "The economics of deficiency available bank bray resources," *Journals Food policy*, vol. 28, pp. 51–75, 2003.

[16] F. W. Lone, R. N. Qureshi, and F. Emanuel, "Maternal anaemia and its impact on perinatal outcome," *Tropical Medicine & International Health*, vol. 9, no. 4, pp. 486–490, 2004.

[17] F. W. Lone, R. N. Qureshi, and F. Emmanuel, "Maternal anaemia and its impact on perinatal outcome in a tertiary care hospital in Pakistan," *Eastern Mediterranean Health Journal*, vol. 10, no. 6, pp. 801–807, 2004.

[18] H. S. Lee, M. S. Kim, M. H. Kim, Y. J. Kim, and W. Y. Kim, "Iron status and its association with pregnancy outcome in Korean pregnant women," *European Journal of Clinical Nutrition*, vol. 60, no. 9, pp. 1130–1135, 2006.

[19] F. Bodeau-Livinec, V. Briand, J. Berger et al., "Maternal anemia in Benin: Prevalence, risk factors, and association with low birth weight," *The American Journal of Tropical Medicine and Hygiene*, vol. 85, no. 3, pp. 414–420, 2011.

[20] T. Kousar, Y. Memon, S. Sheikh, S. Memon, and R. Sehto, "Risk factors and causes of death in Neonates," *Rawal Medical Journal*, vol. 35, no. 2, pp. 205–208, 2010.

[21] B. J. Brabin, M. Hakimi, and D. Pelletier, "An analysis of anemia and pregnancy-related maternal mortality," *Journal of Nutrition*, vol. 131, no. 2, 2001.

[22] G. Million, Y. Delenesaw, T. Ketema, G. Yehenew, and Z. Ahmed, "Anemia and associated risk factors among pregnant women in Gilgel Gibe dam area, Southwest Ethiopia," *Parasites & Vectors*, vol. 5, p. 296, 2012.

[23] S. Gies, B. J. Brabin, M. A. Yassin, and L. E. Cuevas, "Comparison of screening methods for anaemia in pregnant women in Awassa, Ethiopia," *Tropical Medicine & International Health*, vol. 8, no. 4, pp. 301–309, 2003.

[24] M. Alem, B. Enawgaw, A. Gelaw, T. Kenaw, M. Seid, and Y. Olkeba, "Prevalence of anemia and associated risk factors among pregnant women attending antenatal care in Azezo Health Center Gondar town, Northwest Ethiopia," *Journal of Interdisciplinary Histopathology*, vol. 1, no. 3, pp. 137–144, 2013.

[25] N. Obse, A. Mossie, and T. Gobena, "Magnitude of anemia and associated risk factors among pregnant women attending antenatal care in Shalla Woreda, West Arsi Zone, Oromia Region, Ethiopia," *Ethiopian Journal of Health Sciences*, vol. 23, no. 2, pp. 165–173, 2013.

[26] N. Baig-Ansari, S. H. Badruddin, R. Karmaliani et al., "Anemia prevalence and risk factors in pregnant women in an urban area of Pakistan," *Food and Nutrition Bulletin*, vol. 29, no. 2, pp. 132–139, 2008.

[27] J. A. Haidar and R. S. Pobocik, "Iron deficiency anemia is not a rare problem among women of reproductive ages in Ethiopia: A community based cross sectional study," *BMC Blood Disorders*, vol. 9, p. 7, 2009.

24

Multilevel Analysis of Determinants of Anemia Prevalence among Children Aged 6–59 Months in Ethiopia: Classical and Bayesian Approaches

Kemal N. Kawo,[1] **Zeytu G. Asfaw (D),**[2] **and Negusse Yohannes**[3]

[1]*Department of Statistics, Madda Walabu University, Robe, Ethiopia*
[2]*School of Mathematical and Statistical Sciences, Hawassa University, Hawassa, Ethiopia*
[3]*Department of Statistics, Dilla University, Dilla, Ethiopia*

Correspondence should be addressed to Zeytu G. Asfaw; zeytugashaw@yahoo.com

Academic Editor: Duran Canatan

Background. Anemia is a widely spread public health problem and affects individuals at all levels. However, there is a considerable regional variation in its distribution. *Objective.* Thus, this study aimed to assess and model the determinants of prevalence of anemia among children aged 6–59 months in Ethiopia. *Data.* Cross-sectional data from Ethiopian Demographic and Health Survey was used for the analysis. It was implemented by the Central Statistical Agency from 27 December 2010 through June 2011 and the sampling technique employed was multistage. *Method.* The statistical models that suit the hierarchical data such as variance components model, random intercept model, and random coefficients model were used to analyze the data. Likelihood and Bayesian approaches were used to estimate both fixed effects and random effects in multilevel analysis. *Result.* This study revealed that the prevalence of anemia among children aged between 6 and 59 months in the country was around 42.8%. The multilevel binary logistic regression analysis was performed to investigate the variation of predictor variables of the prevalence of anemia among children aged between 6 and 59 months. Accordingly, it has been identified that the number of children under five in the household, wealth index, age of children, mothers' current working status, education level, given iron pills, size of child at birth, and source of drinking water have a significant effect on prevalence of anemia. It is found that variances related to the random term were statistically significant implying that there is variation in prevalence of anemia across regions. From the methodological aspect, it was found that random intercept model is better compared to the other two models in fitting the data well. Bayesian analysis gave consistent estimates with the respective multilevel models and additional solutions as posterior distribution of the parameters. *Conclusion.* The current study confirmed that prevalence of anemia among children aged 6–59 months in Ethiopia was severe public health problem, where 42.8% of them are anemic. Thus, stakeholders should pay attention to all significant factors mentioned in the analysis of this study but wealth index/improving household income and availability of pure drinking water are the most influential factors that should be improved anyway.

1. Introduction

Anemia is a condition characterized by a low level of hemoglobin in the blood [1]. Anemia is a widespread public health problem, and severe anemia is a significant cause of childhood mortality [2]. The World Health Organization (WHO) considers anemia prevalence over 40% as a major public health problem, between 20 and 40% as a medium-level public health problem, and between 5% and 20% as a mild public health problem [1]. High prevalence of anemia and its consequences on children's health, especially for their growth and development, have made anemia an important public health problem, given the difficulty in implementing effective measures for controlling it [3]. Therefore, it is important to understand the scope and strength of individual risk factors for anemia in populations where anemia is common to design more effective interventions [3].

According to [4] above 1.62 billion people were anemic worldwide, and approximately two-thirds of preschool children in Africa and South East Asia were anemic. According to the WHO report, more than half of the world's preschool-age children (56.3%) reside in countries where anemia is a major public health problem [5]. In Sub-Saharan Africa, much of the national prevalence is estimated to be above 40% among this group [6]. In Ethiopia, more than four out of ten children under five (44%) were anemic [7]. From these, about 21% of children were mildly anemic, 20% were moderately anemic, and 3% were severely anemic. Even if the national anemia prevalence estimate has dropped by 19 percent, from 54 percent in 2005 to 44 percent in 2011, it was a major public health problem according to the WHO criteria.

Discussion about model comparison of multilevel model by using classical and Bayesian approaches is rare in literature. However, [8] examined the distribution of weighted anemia prevalence across different groups and performed logistic regression to assess the association of anemia with different factors based on BDHS (2011) data on hemoglobin (Hb) concentration among the children aged 6–59 months. Also [9] conducted a study on the determinants of anemia among children aged 6–59 months living in Kilte Awulaelo Woreda, Northern Ethiopia. Bivariate and multivariate logistic regression analyses were performed to identify factors related to anemia. In this paper we shall consider multilevel analysis of determinants of anemia prevalence among children aged 6–59 months in Ethiopia using classical and Bayesian approaches.

The main concerns of authors were to identify the major determinants and assess the prevalence of anemia among children aged 6–59 months in Ethiopia using classical and Bayesian approaches, that is,

(i) to identify significant predictors of having high prevalence of anemia among children aged 6–59 months in Ethiopia through classical and Bayesian approach,

(ii) to analyze the within- and between-regions variation of prevalence of anemia among children aged 6–59 months in Ethiopia,

(iii) to make model comparison and suggest an appropriate model for analyzing anemia prevalence in Ethiopia.

2. Materials and Methods

2.1. Data. This study used the data collected in the Ethiopian Demographic and Health Survey [7]. The Ethiopia Demographic and Health Survey was conducted by the Central Statistical Agency (CSA) under the auspices of the support of the Ministry of Health from 27 December 2010 through June 2011 with a nationally representative sample of nearly 17,817 households. The sampling frame used for the EDHS was the Population and Housing Census conducted by the Central Statistical Authority (CSA) in 2007; during the 2007 Population and Housing Census, each of the kebeles was subdivided into convenient areas called census enumeration areas (EAs). The EDHS sample was selected using a stratified, two-stage cluster design and EAs were the sampling units for the first stage. For the 2011 EDHS, a representative sample of approximately 17,817 households from 624 clusters was

selected. In the first stage, 624 clusters, 187 urban and 437 rural, were selected from the list of enumeration areas based on sampling frame. In the second stage, a complete listing of households was carried out in each selected cluster. For this study 5,507 children were included in the analysis after all incomplete observations have been deleted from the data among 9,157 total children held with hemoglobin (Hb) data.

2.2. Ethical Approval. Our study was wholly based on an analysis of existing public domain health survey data sets obtained from EDHS 2011, which is freely available online with all identifier information removed. The EDHS 2011 was reviewed and approved by the ICF Macro Institutional Review Board and the National Research Ethics Committee of the Ethiopian Medical Research Council.

2.3. Variables in the Study. Variables considered in this study were selected based on literatures which have been conducted at the global level. Potential determinant factors expected to be correlated with anemia status were included as variables of the study.

2.4. Response Variable. Hemoglobin is necessary for transporting oxygen to tissues and organs in the body. Hemoglobin analysis was carried out onsite using a battery-operated portable HemoCue analyzer. Parents of children with a hemoglobin level under 11 g/dl were instructed to take the child to a health facility for follow-up care. Unadjusted hemoglobin values are obtained using the HemoCue instrument. Given that hemoglobin requirements differ substantially depending on altitude, an adjustment to sea-level equivalents has been made before classifying children by level of anemia. Prevalence of anemia, based on hemoglobin levels is adjusted for altitude by hemoglobin in grams per decilitre (g/dl) [7]. The response variable of this study was anemia status of children aged 6–59 months in Ethiopia. For the current analysis, response variable (anemia status) was dichotomized indicating whether one is anemic or not.

$$Y_{ij} = \left\{ \begin{array}{l} \text{Not anemic} = 0 \\ \text{Anemic} = 1 \end{array} \right\} \tag{1}$$

2.5. Explanatory Variables. The explanatory variables which might determine the status of anemia of children among 6–59 months were socioeconomic, demographic, health, and environmental factors. From the source of data we considered the following variables region, place of residence, number of children under 5 in the household, wealth index, marital status, child's age in months, sex of children, husband/partner's education level, given iron pills/syrup, source of drinking water, mother's current working status, and child's size at birth.

2.6. Common Techniques for Dealing with Missing Data. Missing data is a common problem for almost every health survey data. Missing data presents a problem in statistical analyses. The first issue in dealing with the problem of missing data is determining the missing data mechanism. The work in [10] distinguishes between three types of missing data mechanism; among them we apply missing completely at random (MCAR), which means that missingness is not related to the variables under study. To handle missing value we used listwise deletion which is a common approach and easy to perform by deleting all incomplete observations from the analysis. The results can be unbiased when data are MCAR. Even so, the disadvantage for this method is reduction of sample size.

3. Methods of Statistical Analysis

Multilevel models allow the relationship between the explanatory variables at different level and dependent variables at lower level to be estimated, enabling the extent of variation in the outcome of interest to be measured at each level assumed in the model both before and after the inclusion of the explanatory variables in the model.

Two levels of data hierarchy were stated (for instance, individual children of households and regions) in a multilevel logistic regression model. Units at one level are nested within units at the next higher level. In this study the basic data structure of the two-level logistic regression is a collection of N groups (regions) and within group j (j = 1, 2, ... N) a random sample n_j of level one units (individual children of households). The response variable is denoted by

$$
Y_{ij} = \begin{cases} 1 & \text{for children having anemia} \\ 0 & \text{for normal (not anemic) children} \end{cases} \tag{2}
$$

with probability $P_{ij} = P(Y_{ij} = 1/X_{ij}, u_j)$ being the probability of children with any anemia for the ith household in the jth region and the probability $1 - P_{ij} = P(Y_{ij} = 0/X_{ij},)$ being the probability of nonanemic (normal) i^{th} children for the households in the jth regions. Here, Y_{ij} follows a Bernoulli distribution.

3.1. The Variance Components Model. The variance component two-level model for a dichotomous outcome variable refers to a population of groups (level-two units (regions)) and specifies the probability distribution for group-dependent probabilities P_j in $Y_{ij} = P_j + \epsilon_{ij}$ without taking further explanatory variables into account. We focus on the model that specifies the transformed probabilities $f(P_j)$ to have a normal distribution. This is expressed, for a general link function $f(P_j)$, by the formula

$$
\log \left[\frac{P_{ij}}{1 - P_{ij}} \right] = \beta_{0j} + U_{0j}, \tag{3}
$$

where β_0 is the population average of the transformed probabilities and U_{0j} the random deviation from this average for group j. Intraclass correlation coefficient (ICC) represents the proportion of the total variance that is attributable to between-group differences and it provides an assessment of whether or not significant between-groups variation exists.

Then the intraclass correlation coefficient (ICC) at regions level is given by

$$
ICC = \rho = \frac{\sigma_u^2}{\sigma_u^2 + \sigma_e^2} \tag{4}
$$

where σ_u^2 is the between-groups variance which can be estimated by U_{0j} and σ_e^2 is within-group variance [11].

3.2. The Random Intercept Model. The random intercept model is used to model unobserved heterogeneity in the overall response by introducing random effects. In the random intercept model the intercept is the only random effect meaning that the groups differ with respect to the average value of the response variable, but the relation between explanatory and response variables cannot differ between groups. The random intercept model expresses the log odds, i.e., the logit of P_{ij}, as a sum of linear functions of the explanatory variables. That is,

$$
logit\left(P_{ij}\right) = \log \left[\frac{P_{ij}}{1 - P_{ij}} \right] = \beta_{0j} + \sum_{h=1}^{k} \beta_h x_{hij}, \tag{5}
$$

$$
i = 1, 2, \ldots n_j, \quad j = 1, 2, \ldots 11
$$

where the intercept term β_{0j} is assumed to vary randomly and is given by the sum of an average intercept β_0 and group-dependent deviations U_{0j}; that is, $\beta_{0j} = \beta_0 + U_{0j}$.

As a result we have

$$
logit\left(P_{ij}\right) = \beta_0 + \sum_{h=1}^{k} \beta_h x_{hij} + U_{0j} \tag{6}
$$

Solving for P_{ij},

$$
P_{ij} = \frac{e^{\beta_0 + \sum_{h=1}^{k} \beta_h x_{hij} + U_{0j}}}{1 + e^{\beta_0 + \sum_{h=1}^{k} \beta_h x_{hij} + U_{0j}}} \tag{7}
$$

Equation (6) does not include a level one residual because it is an equation for the probability P_{ij} rather than for the outcome Y_{ij}, where $\beta_{0j} + \sum_{h=1}^{k} \beta_h x_{hij}$ is the fixed part of the model. The remaining U_{0j} is called the random or the stochastic part of the model. It is assumed that the residual U_{0j} is mutually independent and normally distributed with mean zero and variance σ_u^2 [12].

3.3. The Random Coefficients Model. In the random coefficient model both the intercepts and slopes are allowed to differ across the region. Suppose that there are k level one explanatory variables $X_1, X_2, \ldots, X_k$, and consider the model where all X-variables have varying slopes and random intercept. That is,

$$
logit\left(P_{ij}\right) = \log \left[\frac{P_{ij}}{1 - P_{ij}} \right]
$$

$$
= \beta_0 + \sum_{h=1}^{k} \beta_{hj} x_{hij} + U_{0j} + \sum_{h=1}^{k} U_{1j} X_{1ij} \tag{8}
$$

where $\beta_{0j} = \beta_0 + U_{0j}$ and $\beta_{hj} = \beta_h + U_{hj}$, h-1,2,...,k.

Here the first part of (8), $\beta_0 + \sum_{h=1}^{k} \beta_{hj} x_{hij}$, is called the fixed part of the model and the second part $U_{0j} + \sum_{h=1}^{k} U_{1j} X_{1ij}$ is called the random part of the model.

3.4. Parameter Estimation of Multilevel Model

3.4.1. Likelihood Method. The maximum likelihood (ML) method is a general estimation procedure, which produces estimates for the population parameters that maximize the probability of observing the data that are actually observed. Assuming that the conditional distributions of Y_{ij} given the random effect U_j are independent of each other, the conditional density of Y_{ij} is given by P_{ij}:

$$Y_{y_{ij}/u_j} = \binom{y_{ij}}{u_{ij}} \sim Bernoulli \tag{9}$$

For two-level logistic Bernoulli response model, where random effects are assumed to be multivariate normal and independent across units, the marginal likelihood function is given by

$$l(\beta, \Omega) = \prod_i f \prod_i \left[(\pi_{ij})^{y_{ij}} (1 - \pi_{ij})^{1-y_{ij}} \right] \tag{10}$$

where Ω is variance covariance matrix.

$$\pi_{ij} = \left[1 + exp(-x_{ij}\beta_j) \right], \quad \beta_j = \beta + U_j \tag{11}$$

$f(U_{ij}, \Omega)$ is typically assumed to be the multivariate normal density and can be written in the form $\int p(U_j) f(U_j) du_j$.

3.5. Bayesian Modeling.
Bayesian inference involves creating a complete probability model over all data and parameters of interest, fitting the model to observed data, and then reasoning about either the fitted parameters or about new data taking into account the uncertainty in the fitted parameters. In a Bayesian formulation the uncertainty about the value of each parameter can be represented by a probability distribution, if prior knowledge can be quantified [13]. In Bayesian approach, either mean or median of the posterior samples for each parameter of interest is reported as a point estimate. 2.5% and 97.5% percentiles of the posterior samples for each parameter give a 95% posterior credible interval (interval within which the parameter lies with probability 0.95).

3.6. The Likelihood Function.
The key ingredients to a Bayesian analysis are the likelihood function, which reflects information about the parameters contained in the data, and the prior distribution, which quantifies what is known about the parameters before observing data. The prior distribution and likelihood can be easily combined to form the posterior distribution, which represents total knowledge about the parameters after the data have been observed. Bayesian multilevel logistic analysis specifies a dichotomous dependent variable as a function of a set of explanatory variables. The

likelihood contribution from the ith subject in the jth group is Bernoulli:

$$Bernoulli(p_{ij}) = p_{ij}^{y_{ij}} (1 - p_{ij})^{1-y_{ij}}, \tag{12}$$

where p_{ij} represents the probability of the event for subject i in j group that has covariate vector x_{ij} and y_{ij} indicates the presence ($y_{ij} = 1$) or absence ($y_{ij} = 0$) of the event for that subject. In multilevel logistic regression, we know that

$$p_{ij} = \frac{e^{\beta_0 + \beta_1 x_{1ij} + \beta_2 x_{2ij} + \cdots + \beta_k x_{kij} + U_{0j}}}{1 + e^{\beta_0 + \beta_1 x_{1ij} + \beta_2 x_{2ij} + \cdots + \beta_k x_{kij} + U_{0j}}} \tag{13}$$

where $\beta_0 + \beta_1 x_{1ij} + \beta_2 x_{2ij} + \cdots + \beta_k x_{kij}$ is fixed part of the model and U_{0j} is random part of the model and $U_{0j} \sim N(0, \sigma_u^2)$.

p_{ij} is the probability of ith child in j^{th} group (region) being anemic, so that the likelihood contribution for the ith subject in the jth region is

$$L(y \mid \beta_i, \sigma_u^2) = \left(\frac{e^{\beta_0 + \beta_1 x_{1ij} + \beta_2 x_{2ij} + \cdots + \beta_k x_{kij} + U_{0j}}}{1 + e^{\beta_0 + \beta_1 x_{1ij} + \beta_2 x_{2ij} + \cdots + \beta_k x_{kij} + U_{0j}}} \right)^{y_{ij}}$$
$$\cdot \left(1 - \frac{e^{\beta_0 + \beta_1 x_{1ij} + \beta_2 x_{2ij} + \cdots + \beta_k x_{kij} + U_{0j}}}{1 + e^{\beta_0 + \beta_1 x_{1ij} + \beta_2 x_{2ij} + \cdots + \beta_k x_{kij} + U_{0j}}} \right)^{1-y_{ij}} \tag{14}$$

Since individual subjects in the group are assumed to be independent of each other, the likelihood function over a data set of n subjects in the 11 region is then

$$L(y \mid \beta_i, \sigma_u^2) = \tag{15}$$

$$\prod_{i=1}^{n} \prod_{j=1}^{11} \left[\left(\frac{e^{\beta_0 + \beta_1 x_{1ij} + \beta_2 x_{2ij} + \cdots + \beta_k x_{kij} + U_{0j}}}{1 + e^{\beta_0 + \beta_1 x_{1ij} + \beta_2 x_{2ij} + \cdots + \beta_k x_{kij} + U_{0j}}} \right)^{y_{ij}} \right.$$
$$\left. \cdot \left(1 - \frac{e^{\beta_0 + \beta_1 x_{1ij} + \beta_2 x_{2ij} + \cdots + \beta_k x_{kij} + U_{0j}}}{1 + e^{\beta_0 + \beta_1 x_{1ij} + \beta_2 x_{2ij} + \cdots + \beta_k x_{kij} + U_{0j}}} \right)^{1-y_{ij}} \right] \tag{16}$$

3.7. Prior Distribution.
The prior distribution is a probability distribution that represents the prior information associated with the parameters of interest. There are two types of prior distribution: informative priors and noninformative priors.

3.8. Model Comparison.
In this study Akaike information criterion (AIC) and Bayesian information criterion (BIC) were used for model comparison. A model with a lower AIC and BIC is preferred over a model with a larger AIC and BIC.

3.9. Software Used.
The statistical software types used in this study were SPSS version 20 (StataCorp, Texas 77845, USA) and WinBUGS14. SPSS was used for the descriptive analysis, STATA was used for multilevel analysis part, and WinBUGS14 was used for Bayesian analysis.

4. Results and Discussions

The results of the analysis are divided into descriptive analysis and multilevel binary logistic models from categorical data. Results and their discussions are presented in the following sections.

4.1. Descriptive Analysis. Descriptive statistics are a set of brief descriptive figures that summarizes a given data set, which can be a representation of entire sample. A total sample of 5,507 children aged between 6 and 59 months was included in this study. Among these, 2358 (42.8%) were anemic (Hb < 11.0 g/dl) while 3149 (57.2%) were not anemic at the date of the survey.

4.2. Bivariate Analysis between Response and Predictors. This section reports the association between the response variable and each predictor variable. The bivariate analysis, based on Pearson's chi-square statistic, provides a preliminary insight into the association/relationship between all selected independent variables and dependent variable. High values of Pearson chi-square for a given independent variable indicate that there is strong association between each of the given independent variables and the dependent variable keeping the effect of the other factors constant. That is, testing the hypotheses are as follows:

H_o = there is no association between the dependent and independent variables.

H_1 = there is association between the dependent and the particular independent variable.

The decision was based on the chi-square value and p value at 0.05 level of significance.

Basic descriptive information that summarizes the association between predictors and response variable is presented in Table 1. The results in Table 1 show the row percentage and count of anemic/not anemic status of children aged 6–59 months with respect to the categorical covariates.

The bivariate association between anemia status of children aged 6–59 months and predictors shown in Table 1 indicates that anemia status was strongly associated with region, place of residence, number of children under 5 in the household, wealth index, mother's marital status, child's age in months, husband/partner's education level, given iron pills/syrup, source of drinking water, mother's current working status, and child's size at birth. Sex of the children was the only explanatory variable that had no significant association with anemia status among children aged 6–59 months. The prevalence of anemia among children aged between 6 and 59 months varied from one region to another in Ethiopia. The highest proportion of anemia status among children aged 6–59 months was observed in Afar (67.2%) followed by Somali (61.8%) and Dire Dawa (50.5%) as opposed to the lowest percentage that was recorded in Addis Ababa (28.4%) followed by SNNP (35.1%) and Tigray (35.8). The regional variation of anemia prevalence among children ranges from low (Addis Ababa) to high (Afar).

This regional variation is very realistic and expected based on living conditions of people within and between regions. People who are living in Afar and Somalia are nomadic and the main daily meal of thus people is milk. A number of previous studies documented that the effect of milk can be a cause of anemia.

The prevalence of anemia among children aged 6–59 months also differs by type of place of residence. Accordingly, higher numbers of anemic children (44.4%) resided in rural areas, and relatively small number of anemic children (38.3%t) resided in urban areas. This is quite consistent with other similar studies conducted in Ghana, where prevalence of anemia among rural children is 17% higher than that of urban children [13]. Moreover, there is a significant variation within and between the continents. Even prevalence of anemia reported from several developing countries varied. It is about 16.1% in Philippines and 87% in Tanzania [14, 15]. The result presented in Table 1 also reveals that the prevalence of anemia among children aged between 6 and 59 months varied by families educational level. The highest percentage of anemia was observed in children whose families have no education (48.1%) as opposed to the lowest percentage of anemia which was recorded for children whose families have secondary education and above (28%) followed by primary education level (39.4%). It indicates that children of more educated families were less exposed to anemia compared to children of uneducated families.

The total number of children under five in the household is also another important variable. The prevalence of anemia among children aged between 6 and 59 months was 36.5% for children under five with total number of 0-3 in the household, 45.8% for children under five with total number of 4-6 in the household, and 46.9% for children under five with total number above 6 in the household. Hence, as the number of children under five in the household increases the prevalence of anemia among children aged between 6 and 59 months in Ethiopia was increased. The wealth index is a composite measure of the cumulative living standard of a household used as a proxy for socioeconomic status. It was calculated using household's ownership of selected assets by CSA. The result in Table 1 indicates that wealth index was found to have a significant association with anemia status among children aged between 6 and 59 months at 5% level of significance and 49.5%, 40.9%, and 35.6% of children aged between 6 and 59 months from poor, middle, and rich households were anemic, respectively. It indicates that children from rich families were less exposed to anemia compared to children from poor families. With regard to marital status, the higher percentage of anemia among children aged between 6 and 59 months was observed among children whose families were married (43.5%) followed by children whose families were widowed (40.7%) and lower proportion of anemia was observed for children whose families were divorced/separated (35.5%).

The proportion of anemia among children aged between 6 and 59 months, observed in Table 1, also differs with their age groups. For instance, higher proportion of anemia was observed for children under 6–23 months of age (50.5%) and the lowest proportion of anemia was found in the age group between 42 and 59 months (36.7%) followed by children under 24–41 months (42.7%). This finding is similar to study in Brazil, Bangladesh, and Northern Ethiopia [9, 16, 17]. Hence, as age increased the prevalence of anemia among children aged between 6 and 59 months in Ethiopia was decreased. Given iron pills/syrup is another important variable that was strongly associated with anemia status among children aged between 6 and 59 months. The proportion of anemia status was also high for children who

TABLE 1: Cross tabulation of anemia status versus predictor variables.

Variables	Anemic N	Anemic %	Not anemic N	Not anemic %	Total	DF	Chi-square	P-value
Region (RGN)					5507			
Addis Ababa	55	28.4%	139	71.6%	194			
Afar	357	67.2%	174	32.8%	531			
Amhara	244	37.2%	412	62.8%	656			
Oromiya	354	40.5%	519	59.5%	873			
Somali	261	61.8%	161	38.2%	422			
Benishangul-Gumuz	181	37.8%	298	62.2%	479	10	267.04	0.001
SNNPR	279	35.1%	516	64.9%	795			
Gambela	132	37.5%	220	62.5%	352			
Harari	117	41.8%	163	58.2%	280			
Dire Dawa	162	50.5%	159	49.5	321			
Tigray	216	35.8%	388	64.2%	604			
Place of Residence (POR					5507			
Urban	534	38.3%	862	61.7%	1396	1	15.92	0.001
Rural	1824	44.4%	2287	55.6%	4111			
Sex of child (SEX)					5507			
Male	1237	44.5%	1608	56.5%	2845	1	1.05	0.318
Female	1121	42.1%	1541	57.9%	2662			
No of children u5 in the household (NOCH)					5507			
0-3	682	36.5%	1187	63.5%	1869			
4-6	1258	45.8%	1489	54.2%	2747	2	46.62	0.001
above 6	418	46.9%	473	53.1%	891			
Wealth index (WI)					5507			
Poor	1078	49.5%	1099	50.5%	2177			
Middle	719	40.9%	1037	59.1%	1756	2	75.53	0.001
Rich	561	35.6%	1013	64.6%	1574			
Marital status (MS)					5507			
Married	2100	43.5%	2724	56.5%	4824			
Widowed	122	40.7%	178	59.3	300	2	9.93	0.001
Divorced/separated	136	35.5%	247	64.5	383			
Child's age in month (AGE)					5507			
6-23	794	50.5%	779	49.5%	1573			
24-41	859	42.7%	1152	57.3%	2011	2	67.46	0.001
42-59	705	36.7%	1218	63.3%	1923			
Mother's working status (MWS)					5507			
Not working	1559	44.4%	1953	55.6%	3512	1	9.61	0.002
Working	799	40.1%	1196	59.9%	1995			
Education level (PEL)					5507			
No education	1404	48.1%	1517	51.9%	2921			
Primary	795	39.4%	1224	60.6%	2019	2	93.18	0.001
Secondary & above	159	28.0%	408	72.0%	567			
Given iron pills (GIP)					5507			
No	1980	44.4%	2479	55.6%	4459	1	24.08	0.001
Yes	378	36.1%	670	63.9%	1048			
Size of child at birth (SIZE)					5507			
Smaller than average	684	42.4%	929	57.6%	1613			
Average	863	39.2%	1341	60.8%	2204	2	30.63	0.001
Larger than average	811	48.0%	879	52.0%	1690			
Source of drinking water (SDW)					5507			
Not improved	1861	44.3%	2339	55.7%	4200	1	15.92	0.001
Improved	498	38.1%	809	61.9%	1307			

did not receive iron pills/syrup. Children, who received iron pills/syrup, had lower risk of anemia (36.1%) than children who did not receive iron pills/syrup (44.4%). The result in Table 1 indicates that size of child at birth was found to have significant association with anemia status among children aged between 6 and 59 months at 5% level of significance and 48.0%, 39.2%, and 42,4% of children with size larger than average, equal to average, smaller than average were anemic, respectively. This indicates the prevalence of anemia among children aged between 6 and 59 months was higher for children with size smaller than average and larger than average compared to children with average size at birth.

From result presented in Table 1, source of drinking water had significant association with anemia status among children aged between 6 and 59 months in Ethiopia. The proportion of anemia status was also high for children who did not use improved water. Children, who used improved water, had lower risk of anemia (38.1%) than children who did not use improved water (44.3%). This finding supported by the study conducted in the Philippines shows association between anemia and water supply [14]. Mother's current working status also had significant association with anemia status among children aged between 6 and 59 months in Ethiopia.

The main problem with the bivariate approach is that it ignores the possibility that a collection of variables, each of which could be weakly associated with the outcome, can become an important predictor of the outcome when taken together [18]. Hence, logistic regression approach that takes into account the drawback mentioned by the bivariate technique is considered in this analysis.

Thus, authors considered multilevel logistic regression in both approaches, classical and Bayesian perspectives.

4.3. Results of Multilevel Models.

Before directly going to the analysis of multilevel models the first important step is variable selection. For this study we have used stepwise variable selection technique to determine the variables to be included in the multilevel models. Accordingly, of the total variables considered, twelve variables (region, place of residence, number of children under 5 in the household, wealth index, marital status, child's age in months, sex of children, husband/partner's education level, given iron pills/syrup, source of drinking water, mother's current working status, and child's size at birth) are selected to be included in the multilevel model.

4.3.1. Variance Components Model.

We first fitted a simple model with no predictors, i.e., variance components model that predicts the probability of anemia status.

The variance components model results in Table 2 revealed the information of the fixed effect; authors can say that the estimated average log odds of anemia status among children aged between 6 and 59 months across regions of the country are $\beta_0 = -0.2849$. Authors can convert this back to a probability 0.428; this is the overall proportion of prevalence of anemia among children aged between 6 and 59 months in Ethiopia without accounting for other sources of variation.

TABLE 2: Estimates for variance components model (EDHS, 2011).

Fixed effects	Estimate	S. error	z value	p-value
β_0 = intercept	−0.2849	0.1425	−2	0.046*
Random effect				
$\hat{\sigma}_u^2$	0.2126	0.0477	4.457	0.001
ICC(ρ)	0.0608			

The intercept for region j is $-0.2849 + U_{0j}$, where the variance of U_0 between regions in region average log odds of being anemic is estimated as $\hat{\sigma}_u^2 = 0.2126$.

We reject null hypothesis which states that the variation across region was zero. So this result suggests that the variation of prevalence of anemia among children aged between 6 and 59 months due regional difference was nonzero. Hence, we conclude that the regional difference contributed to the variation in prevalence of anemia among children aged between 6 and 59 months in Ethiopia. The variances $(\pi^2/3)$ (3.29) and 0.2126 estimate the variation among individual children in the household and regions of the country. In variance components model it is possible to decompose variance into regional level (higher level) and individual level. Individual (level 1) variance was to assess how many variations are due to individuals themselves and how many variations are due to regional level. According to [19] the individual (level 1) variance was fixed to $(\pi^2/3)$ (3.29) for logit model.

In order to get an idea of how many variations in prevalence of anemia among children aged between 6 and 59 months were attributable to the region level factors, it is useful to see the intraregional correlation coefficient. The intraregional correlation coefficient (ICC) in variance components model is ICC = 0.0607, meaning that roughly 6.07% of the total variability in prevalence of anemia among children aged between 6 and 59 months is significantly attributable to the regional level, whereas the remaining 93.03% is attributable to individual level (i.e., within-region differences).

4.3.2. Random Intercept Model.

To identify the effect of explanatory variables a multilevel binary logistic model with random intercept and fixed explanatory variables was estimated. The deviance-based chi-square for significance overall goodness fit model (χ^2 = −2log (likelihood of variance component model)-(−2log (likelihood of random intercept model)) is 224.11, P < 0.05) indicates that the random intercept model with the fixed explanatory variables is found to be a better fit as compared to the variance component model discussed in the previous section. Note that there is change (decrease) in the estimate of the between-region variance from variance component model 0.2126 to random intercept model 0.1698, suggesting that the distribution of fixed explanatory variables is somewhat different across regions of the country.

The results from the random intercept model in Table 3 showed that the random intercept (β_0) is significant implying that the average proportion of anemia among children aged between 6 and 59 months differs from region to region.

TABLE 3: Estimates of random intercept model (EDHS, 2011).

Fixed effects	Categories	coefficients	SE	z-value	p-value	$\exp(\hat{\beta})$	95% C.I for $\exp(\hat{\beta})$	
							lower	upper
β_0-intercept		0.3536	0.1733	2.04	0.041		0.0139	0.6933
Place of Residence	Urban (ref)							
	Rural	0.0773	0.07535	1.03	0.305	1.0804	0.9320	1.252
Sex of child	Male (ref)							
	Female	−0.0355	0.05755	−0.62	0.537	0.9651	0.8622	1.080
Number of children under 5 in household	0-3 (ref)							
	4-6	0.2624	0.066	3.99	0.001	1.3	1.1427	1.479
	above 6	0.1718	0.089	1.92	0.054	1.187	0.9968	1.415
Wealth index	Poor (ref)							
	Middle	−0.1876	0.0699	−2.68	0.007	0.829	0.7228	0.9508
	Rich	−0.3296	0.0788	−4.18	0.001	0.7192	0.6163	0.8393
Marital status	Married (ref)							
	Widowed	0.0654	0.1276	0.51	0.608	1.0676	0.8314	1.371
	Divorced/Separated	−0.0624	0.1177	−0.53	0.596	0.9395	0.7460	1.1833
Child's age in month	6-23 (ref)							
	24-41	−0.3111	0.0714	−4.36	0.001	0.7326	0.6370	0.8426
	42-59	−0.5876	0.0728	−8.08	0.001	0.5556	0.4818	0.6408
Mother's current working status	Not working (ref)							
	Working	−0.1540	.0615	−2.50	0.012	0.8572	0.7599	0.9671
Husband/partner's education level	No education (ref)							
	Primary	−0.1493	0.0646	−2.31	0.021	0.8613	0.7588	0.9776
	Secondary & above	−0.7062	0.1129	−6.25	0.001	0.4935	0.3955	0.6158
Given iron pills/syrup	No (ref)							
	Yes	−0.2993	0.0795	−3.76	0.001	0.7414	0.6344	0.8664
Size of child at birth	Larger than average (ref)							
	Average	−0.1530	0.0701	−2.18	0.029	0.8581	0.7480	0.9845
	Smaller than average	0.1123	0.0747	1.50	0.132	1.1189	0.9666	1.2952
source of drinking water	Not improved (ref)							
	Improved	−0.2685	0.0679	−3.96	0.001	0.7645	0.6693	0.8733
Random effect								
$\hat{\sigma}_u^2 = \text{var}(u_{0j})$		0.1698	0.0768	2.21			0.2645	0.6420
ICC(ρ)		0.0491						

The intercept estimation is random at the regional level, $\text{var}(U_{0j})$. Thus, the value of $\text{var}(U_{0j}) = \sigma_u^2 = 0.1698$ is the estimated variance of the intercept. The multilevel logistic regression analysis result displayed in Table 3 confirmed the significance of regional difference in prevalence of anemia among children aged between 6 and 59 months in Ethiopia. The deviance-based chi-square = 224.11, p value < 0.001 for random effects in random intercept model, suggesting that children with the same characteristics in different regions have different anemia status in Ethiopia; that is, there is a clear regional effect.

The results displayed in Table 3 showed that the intraregional correlation coefficient (ICC) is estimated as $\hat{\rho} = 0.0491$, meaning that roughly 4.91% of the total variability

in prevalence of anemia among children aged between 6 and 59 months is attributable to the regional level, with the remaining unexplained 95.09% being due to individual differences. From Table 3, the analysis of multilevel binary logistic regression revealed that the prevalence of anemia among children aged between 6 and 59 months varied among regions. In addition, the number of children under five in the household, wealth index, child's age in month, mother's current working status, husband/partner's education level, given iron pills/syrup, size of child at birth, and source of drinking water were also found to be significant determinants of variation in prevalence of anemia among children aged between 6 and 59 months, whereas sex of children, place of residence, and marital status were insignificant predictors of variation in prevalence of anemia among children aged between 6 and 59 months. From the random part variance component of the random intercept model σ_u^2 was found to be significant, which implies that regions difference contributes to the variation of prevalence of anemia among children from the random intercept and fixed explanatory model. Accordingly, the test statistics explored that marital status and sex of the children are the only explanatory variables that are found to be insignificant (p > 0.05) factors of the dependent variables (anemia status) among the considered explanatory variables. There was no statistically significant difference of the sex in terms of prevalence. This result maintains what is stated with studies done in [19, 20].

The prevalence of anemia among children aged between 6 and 59 months, those from middle and rich families, decreased by 17% and 28%, respectively, as compared to those from poor families (ref) controlling for other variables in the model. This could be because families with middle and rich economic level can afford basic requirements such as clear water, medical care, and sufficient food/nutritional requirements needed for proper children health compared to those families with poor economic level who are unable to provide the basic needs. This finding is consistent with a previous study conducted in Bangladesh [8].

This study also revealed that the values 0.2645 and 0.1735 are increasing in log odds of anemia status among children aged 6–59 months in the household with total number of children under five being 4-6 and above six, respectively; the odds ratio being exp(0.2645) = 1.30 and exp(0.1735) = 1.19, respectively, means that odds of anemic children in the household with total number of children being 4-6 and above six were 1.30 times and 1.19 times higher compared to children in the household in group with total number of 0-3 (ref) keeping other variables in the model constant. It is implied that the prevalence of anemia among children aged between 6–59 months in Ethiopia was higher in the households with more number of children under five relative to households with lower number of children under five. This result maintains what is stated by studies done by [21].

The odds of prevalence of anemia among children aged between 6 and 59 months whose families have primary and secondary/above level of education reduced by 13.78% and 50.62%, respectively, as compared to children of uneducated family (ref) controlling for other variables in the model. This implies that families education is an important socioeconomic characteristic of anemia status; that is, the prevalence of anemia among children aged between 6 and 59 months in the country decreases as family's education level increases, because educated families give attention to their status. They also provide clear environment to children, are more likely to have more knowledge about care taking, and have higher demands. This finding is consistent with the previous studies done in Ethiopia [22].

Likewise, the odds of anemia status among children aged between 6 and 59 months of children who had been given iron pills/syrup were significantly different from children who had not been given iron pills/syrup (ref). A child who had been given iron pills/syrup was 0.7324 times less [OR: 0.7324; 95% CI: 0.6352, 0.8674] likely to have anemia compared with children who had not been given iron pills/syrup (ref). Or from the multilevel binary logistic regression analysis the value –0.2981 ($\hat{\beta}$) decreases log odds of anemia status among children aged between 6 and 59 months who had been given iron pills/syrup [OR: 0.7324, 95% CI: (0.6352, 0.8674)]. It means that odds of the prevalence of anemia among children aged between 6 and 59 months had statistically decreased by 26.76% for children who had been given iron pills/syrup. Iron deficiency is the main factor for the prevalence of anemia. This finding is consistent with the previous studies done by [23].

The current study found that the prevalence of anemia among children aged between 6 and 59 months is significantly associated with age of children. For a one-step increase in age category (to age group 24-41), the log odds of prevalence of anemia in children aged 6–59 months were decreased by 26.73% when compared with age group of 6–23 (ref). For a one-step increase in age category (to 42-59), the log odds of prevalence of anemia in children aged 6–59 months were decreased by 44.54% compared with age group of 6–23 (ref). Therefore, children are more likely to be anemic in age category of 6–23 as compared to other age categories. This indicates that the prevalence of anemia among children aged between 6 and 59 months in Ethiopia is more likely in their early ages of 6–23 (ref). This result maintains what is stated with studies done by [21, 24].

4.3.3. Results of Random Coefficients Model. It is possible to generalize the model so that the effect of level 1 covariates is different in each region. This can be done by adding random coefficients in front of some of the individual-level covariates of the model. This model contains a random slope for source of drinking water and family education level, which means that it allows the effect of the coefficient of the explanatory variable to vary from region to region.

By adding level 1 predictors, the ICC increased and is estimated as $\hat{\rho}$ = 0.075, meaning that roughly 7.5% of the total variability in prevalence of anemia among children aged between 6 and 59 months is attributable to the random factor and region in random coefficient multilevel binary logistic model. From Table 4 the random coefficient estimates for intercepts and the slopes vary significantly at 5% significance level, which implies that there is a considerable variation in the effects of family education level and source of drinking water; these variables differ significantly across the regions. The variance of intercept in the random slope model is 0.2303, which is still large, relative to its standard error of 0.1070. Thus there remains some regional level variance unaccounted for in the model. The variance corresponding to the slope of source of drinking water is 0.0066, which is relatively small with respect to its standard error; this suggests that the effect of source of drinking water may be justified in constraining the effect to be fixed. The effect of improved source of drinking water as log odds of prevalence of anemia in region j is estimated as $-0.2776 + \widehat{U}_{1j}$, and the between-regions variance in the effect of source of drinking water is estimated as 0.0066. Likewise, the variance corresponding to the slope of family education level is 0.0282, which is

TABLE 4: Estimates of random coefficients model (EDHS, 2011).

Fixed effects	Categories	coefficients	SE	z-value	p-value	$\exp(\widehat{\beta})$	95% C.I for $\exp(\widehat{\beta})$ lower	upper
Wealth index	Poor (ref)							
	Middle	−0.18087	0.07025	−2.58	0.010	0.8346	0.7273	0.9577
	Rich	−0.3187	0.0792	−4.02	0.001	0.7271	0.6225	0.8492
Number of children under 5	0-3 (ref)							
	4-6	0.2620	0.0659	3.97	0.001	1.2995	1.1420	1.4788
	above 6	0.1656	0.0896	1.85	0.065	1.1800	0.9899	1.4067
Place of Residence	Urban (ref)							
	Rural	0.0732	0.0757	0.97	0.334	1.0759	0.9276	1.2480
Marital status	Married (ref)							
	Widowed	0.0816	0.1281	0.64	0.524	1.0850	0.8441	1.3950
	Divorced/Separated	−0.0619	0.11767	−0.526	0.599	0.9410	0.7470	1.1855
Child's age in month	6-23 (ref)							
	24-41	−0.3061	0.0715	−4.28	0.001	0.7363	0.6401	0.8471
	42-59	−0.5852	0.0729	−8.03	0.001	0.5570	0.4829	0.6425
Mother's current working status	Not working (ref)							
	Working	−0.1542	0.0616	−2.50	0.012	0.8571	0.7596	0.9671
Husband/partner's education level	No education (ref)							
	Primary	−0.1578	0.0844	−1.87	0.061	0.8540	0.7238	1.0076
	Secondary & above	−0.7413	0.1548	−4.79	0.001	0.4765	0.3518	0.6454
Given iron pills/syrup	No (ref)							
	Yes	−0.2943	0.0796	−3.70	0.001	0.7450	0.6374	0.8708
Size of child at birth	Larger than average (ref)							
	Average	−0.1561	0.0702	−2.22	0.026	0.8555	0.7455	0.9816
	Smaller than average	0.1044	0.0744	1.40	0.161	1.1100	0.9594	1.2844
source of drinking water	Not improved (ref)							
	Improved	−.2776	.0736	−3.77	0.001	0.7576	0.6558	0.8752
β_0-intercept		0.3431	0.1651	2.08	0.038		0.0196	0.667
Random effect								
$\sigma_0^2 = \text{var}(U_{0j})$	0.2303	0.1070					0.0927	0.573
$\sigma_1^2 = \text{var}(U_{1j})$	0.0282	0.0228					0.0058	0.1380
$\sigma_2^2 = \text{var}(U_{2j})$	0.0066	0.027					2.10e − 06	21.043
$\sigma_{12} = \text{cov}(U_{1j}, U_{2j})$	0.0075	0.0192					−0.0302	0.0452
$\sigma_{10} = \text{cov}(U_{1j}, U_{0j})$	−0.0571	0.0415					−0.1384	0.0242
$\sigma_{20} = \text{cov}(U_{2j}, U_{0j})$	−0.0267	0.0397					−0.1046	0.0512
ICC(ρ)	0.075							

relatively large with respect to its standard error (SE = 0.0228); thus, this suggests that the effect of family education may be justified in constructing the effect to be random. The effect of secondary education and above as log odds of prevalence of anemia in region j is estimated as $-0.7413 + \widehat{U}_{1j}$, and the

between-regions variance in the effect of secondary education/above was estimated as 0.0282.

The significance of this difference further indicates that a model with a random coefficient is more appropriate to explain regional variation than a model with fixed

TABLE 5: Model comparison.

Fitted model	Variance component model	Random intercept model	Random coefficients model
−log likelihood	−3650.20	−3530.50	−3527.18
Deviance-based chi-square	220.49	224.11	187.5
P-value	0.001	0.001	0.001
AIC	7304.4	7098.61	7100.36
BIC	7317.63	7224.27	7252.48

coefficients. The correlation between the intercept and random slope of source of drinking water is −0.0267. This implies that the prevalence of anemia among children aged between 6 and 59 months who have used improved water was less than among those who have not used improved water by a larger factor at regions with higher intercepts compared to regions with lower intercepts.

4.3.4. Model Comparison.
The choice of relevant multilevel model is an important step, and it should be based on the necessity of parsimony in the model. Parsimony means that models should be as simple as possible [25].

As shown in Table 5 the deviance-based chi-square value ($\chi^2 = 220.49$, p value < 0.001) is significant for the variance components model. The deviance-based chi-square value ($\chi^2 = 224.11$, p value < 0.001) is significant for random intercept model which implies that the random intercept model fits better as compared to variance components model. Also the deviance-based chi-square value for random effects ($\chi^2 = 187.5$, p value < 0.001) for multilevel random slope model (random coefficient model) is also statistically significant. Both models seem to be better for the data compared to variance component model. However, based on deviance, AIC and BIC, authors can see that model fit statistic values (AIC = 7098.61 and BIC = 7224.27) for random intercept model were the smallest among models considered. Therefore, the random intercept model better fits the data to predict prevalence of anemia among children aged between 6 and 59 months in Ethiopia.

Comparison between the two prominent statistical thoughts, classical and Bayesian approaches, and then sound conclusion should be made on the best one for having realistic implementation.

4.4. Bayesian Multilevel Analysis.
The Gibbs sampler algorithm was implemented with 30,000 iterations in three different chains, 10,000 burn-in terms discarded, to obtain 60,003 samples from the full posterior distribution for the multilevel model. We used noninformative normal prior distribution with mean = 0 and precision = 0.001 for the fixed effect and inverse gamma distribution for sigma with *scale* = 0.1, *shape* = 0.1 for the random effect. This implies that the parameters of the covariates were estimated by 60,003 Markov chain sample values, simply using the Markov chain samples after the burn-in state. Assessment of model convergence also was checked through time series plot, kernel density, and Gelman-Rubin statistics. All were confirmed as the model successfully converged.

4.4.1. Results of Bayesian Analysis.
The Bayesian parameter estimation method is explored for the selected model and the random intercept model. The results are displayed in Table 6.

From Table 6, the sample obtained from posterior distribution, summary statistics of all parameters for posterior distribution are presented and the predictor variables like age of children, husband/partners' education level, wealth index, number of children under five in the household, mothers' current working status, size of child at birth, given iron pills/syrup, place of residence, and source of drinking water were also found to be significant determinants of anemia among children aged between 6 and 59 months at 5% level of significance (since the credible intervals of these variables do not contain zero (at least for one category)).

The Bayesian multilevel logistic regression analysis result displayed in Table 5 also estimates the random effect at the regional level, var(u_{0j}). Thus, the value of var(u_{0j}) = σ_u^2 = 0.2658 and since 95% credible confident interval does not contain zero it is significant at 5%. This confirmed the significance of regional difference in prevalence of anemia. That is, there is a clear regional effect. The fixed effect parametric multilevel random intercept models in classical approach and in Bayesian approach were fitted. Both methods give almost consistent results, but most of the parameters in Bayesian analysis had smaller standard error than the corresponding classical multilevel random intercept model. Therefore, Bayesian multilevel random intercept model gives better fit than the classical multilevel random intercept models. In the estimation of random effects, there is a difference between the estimation of likelihood and Bayesian approaches, that is, 0.1698 and 0.2658, respectively, and the Bayesian approach estimates more than the likelihood approach in explaining the variation of prevalence of anemia across the region of the country. Bayesian analysis gave consistent estimates with the respective multilevel models and additional solutions as posterior distribution of the parameters convergence.

The results displayed in Table 6 also showed that the intraregional correlation coefficient (ICC) is estimated as $\hat{\rho}$ = 0.074. This means that about 7.4% of the total variability in prevalence of anemia is due to differences across regions, with the remaining unexplained 92.6% attributable to individual differences.

5. Conclusions

The current study confirmed that prevalence of anemia among children aged 6–59 months in Ethiopia was severe public health problem, where 42.8% of them anemic and

TABLE 6: Bayesian estimates for random intercept model.

Fixed part	categories (level)	node	mean	Sd	MC error	2.5%	median	97.5%
Intercept		alpha	0.3487	0.1735	0.006318	0.1714	0.349	0.5245
Sex of child	Male (ref)							
	Female	beta[1]	−0.03455	0.05672	3.674E − 4	−0.1483	−0.03459	0.07822
Child's age in month	6-23 (ref)							
	24-41	beta[2]	−0.2962	0.07136	6.348E − 4	−0.4352	−0.2965	−0.1557
	42-59	beta[3]	−0.5756	0.07284	6.278E − 4	−0.7187	−0.5759	−0.4328
Place of Residence	Urban (ref)							
	Rural	beta[4]	0.1743	0.07371	9.129E − 4	0.03031	0.1742	0.3196
No of children u5	0-3 (ref)							
	4-6	beta[5]	0.2947	0.06551	6.801E − 4	0.158	0.2946	0.4308
	above 6	beta[6]	0.2098	0.08454	7.711E − 4	0.02496	0.2096	0.3946
Wealth index	Poor (ref)							
	Middle	beta[7]	−0.218	0.06826	5.559E − 4	−0.355	−0.2182	−0.08018
	Rich	beta[8]	−0.4143	0.07668	7.599E − 4	−0.566	−0.4138	−0.2648
Marital status	Married (ref)							
	Widowed	beta[9]	0.04532	0.128	5.975E − 4	−0.2066	0.04626	0.2932
	Divorced/Separated	beta[10]	−0.09123	0.1178	5.506E − 4	−0.3231	−0.0906	0.1392
Education level	No education (ref)							
	Primary	beta[11]	−0.07366	0.08864	0.001167	−0.09975	−0.07367	−0.03468
	Secondary	beta[12]	−0.1211	0.08781	0.001177	−0.05145	−0.1212	−0.02918
Mother's current working status	Not working (ref)							
	Working	beta[13]	−0.2006	0.07009	7.051E − 4	−0.3391	−0.2001	−0.06329
Given iron pills/syrup	No (ref)							
	Yes	beta[14]	−0.2927	0.07935	4.086E − 4	−0.4492	−0.2926	−0.138
Size of child at birth	Larger than average (ref. cat)							
	Average	beta[15]	−0.1473	0.07012	6.419E − 4	−0.2848	−0.1474	−0.01014
	Smaller than average	beta[16]	0.1308	0.07479	6.401E − 4	−0.01628	0.1311	0.2775
source of drinking water	Not improved (ref)							
	Improved	beta[17]	−0.2641	0.06788	3.453E − 4	−0.3978	−0.2639	−0.1319
Random effects								
sigma		σ_u^2	0.2658	0.1566	0.0016	0.09924	0.2266	0.6693

based on WHO criteria greater than 40% are categorized under severe public health problem. Thus, stakeholders should pay attention to all significant factors mentioned in the analysis of this study but wealth index/improving household income and availability of pure drinking water are the most influential factors that should be improved anyway. Regional variation is the sole finding of this paper and hence potential stakeholders have to give special consideration for children who are living in the highest anemic prevalence regions. Moreover, those households who are living in nomadic region like Afar and Somalia should be trained on the cause of anemia and its consequences.

From the methodological aspect, it was found that multilevel random intercept model is better compared to variance components model and random coefficients model in fitting the data. Bayesian analysis gave consistent estimates with the respective multilevel models and additional solutions as posterior distribution of the parameters.

Conflicts of Interest

The authors declare that they have no conflicts of interest.

Authors' Contributions

Kemal N. Kawo, Zeytu G. Asfaw, and Negusse Yohannes generated the idea; the corresponding author Kemal N. Kawo contributed to the data analysis and interpretation; Zeytu G. Asfaw and Negusse Yohannes contributed as advisors; Kemal N. Kawo is equal contributor.

Acknowledgments

The authors acknowledge School of Mathematical and Statistical Sciences, Hawassa University, Hawassa, Ethiopia, for financial support.

References

[1] WHO, *Iron Deciency Anemia, Assessment, Prevention, and Control: A Guide for Program Managers*, WHO, Geneva, Switzerland, 2001.

[2] B. J. Brabin, M. Hakimi, and D. Pelletier, "Iron-deciency anemia: reexamining the nature and magnitude of the public health problem," *Journal of Nutrition*, pp. 604S–615S, 2001.

[3] R. J. Stoltzfus, "Defining iron-deficiency anemia in public health terms: a time for reflection," *Journal of Nutrition*, vol. 131, supplement 2, pp. 565S–567S, 2001.

[4] WHO, *Worldwide Prevalence of Anemia 1993-2005: WHO Global Database on Anemia*, WHO, Geneva, Switzerland, 2008.

[5] E. McLean, M. Cogswell, I. Egli, D. Wojdyla, and B. De Benoist, "Worldwide prevalence of anaemia, WHO vitamin and mineral nutrition information system, 1993-2005," *Public Health Nutrition*, vol. 12, no. 4, pp. 444–454, 2009.

[6] R. J. S. Magalhaes and C. A. Archie, "Clements: spatial variation in childhood anemia in Africa," *Bulletin of the World Health Organization*, vol. 89, pp. 459–468, 2011.

[7] Central Statistical Agency and ORC Macro, *Ethiopia Demographic and Health Survey*, Central Statistical Agency, Addis Ababa, Ethiopia; ORC Macro, Calverton, Md, USA, 2011.

[8] J. R. Khan, N. Awan, and F. Misu, "Determinants of anemia among 6-59 months aged children in Bangladesh: evidence from nationally representative data," *BMC Pediatrics*, vol. 16, no. 1, article 3, 2016.

[9] G. Gebreegziabiher, B. Etana, and D. Niggusie, "Determinants of anemia among children aged 6-59 months living in Kilte Awulaelo Woreda, Northern Ethiopia," *Anemia*, vol. 2014, Article ID 245870, 9 pages, 2014.

[10] R. J. Little and D. B. Rubin, in *Statistical Analysis with Missing Data*, vol. 88, pp. 125–134, John Wiley, New York, NY, USA, 1987.

[11] D. John, Multilevel analysis in the study of Crime and justice. The most pervasive Fallacy of philosophic goes back to neglect of context, 2009.

[12] T. A. B. Snijders and R. J. Bosker, *An Introduction to Basic and Advanced Multilevel Modeling*, Department of Statistics, University of Poone, 1st edition, 1999.

[13] M. Kynn, Eliciting Expert Knowledge for Bayesian Logistic Regression in Species Habitat Modeling, 2005.

[14] L. W. Tengco, P. Rayco-Solon, J. A. Solon, J. N. Sarol Jr., and F. S. Solon, "Determinants of anemia among preschool children in the Philippines," *Journal of the American College of Nutrition*, vol. 27, no. 2, pp. 229–243, 2008.

[15] J. E. Ewusie, C. Ahiadeke, J. Beyene, and J. S. Hamid, "Prevalence of anemia among under-5 children in the Ghanaian population: estimates from the Ghana demographic and health survey," *BMC Public Health*, vol. 14, no. 1, article 626, 2014.

[16] M. De Novaes Oliveira, R. Martorell, and P. Nguyen, "Risk factors associated with hemoglobin levels and nutritional status among Brazilian children attending daycare centers in Sao Paulo city, Brazil," *Archivos Latinoamericanos de Nutrición*, vol. 60, no. 1, pp. 23–29, 2010.

[17] R. D. Merrill, A. A. Shamim, H. Ali et al., "High prevalence of anemia with lack of iron deficiency among women in rural Bangladesh: a role for thalassemia and iron in groundwater," *Asia Pacific Journal of Clinical Nutrition*, vol. 21, no. 3, pp. 416–424, 2012.

[18] D. W. Hosmer and S. Lemeshow, *Applied Logistic Regression*, John and Sons, Inc, 1989.

[19] B. Entwisle, W. M. Mason, and A. I. Hermalin, "The multilevel dependence of contraceptive use on socioeconomic development and family planning program strength," *Demography*, vol. 23, no. 2, pp. 199–216, 1986.

[20] M. M. Osório, P. I. C. Lira, M. Batista-Filho, and A. Ashworth, "Prevalence of anemia in children 6–59 months old in the state of Pernambuco, Brazil," *Revista Panamericana de Salud Pública*, vol. 10, no. 2, pp. 101–107, 2001.

[21] L. P. Leal, M. B. Filho, P. I. C. de Lira, J. N. Figueiroa, and M. M. Osório, "Prevalence of anemia and associated factors in children aged 6–59 months in Pernambuco, Northeastern Brazil," *Revista de Saúde Pública*, vol. 45, no. 3, pp. 457–466, 2011.

[22] D. Habte, K. Asrat, M. G. M. D. Magafu et al., "Maternal risk factors for childhood anaemia in Ethiopia," *African Journal of Reproductive Health*, vol. 17, no. 3, pp. 110–118, 2013.

[23] J. K. Kikafunda, "Anemia and associated factors under five children and their mothers in Bushenyi District western Uganda," 2009.

[24] H. N. Giebel, D. Suleymanova, and G. W. Evans, "Anemia in young children of the Muynak District of Karakalpakistan, Uzbekistan: prevalence, type, and correlates," *American Journal of Public Healthy*, vol. 88, no. 5, pp. 805–807, 1998.

[25] J. Hox, *Multilevel Analysis: Techniques and Applications*, Lawrence Erlbaum, Mahwah, NJ, USA, 2000.

Erythropoiesis in Malaria Infections and Factors Modifying the Erythropoietic Response

Vrushali A. Pathak[1] and Kanjaksha Ghosh[2]

[1]Department of Haematogenetics, National Institute of Immunohaematology (ICMR), KEM Hospital, Parel, Mumbai 400012, India
[2]Surat Raktadan Kendra & Research Centre, Udhna Khatodara Urban Health Centre, Udhna Magdalla Road, Surat, Gujrat 395002, India

Correspondence should be addressed to Kanjaksha Ghosh; kanjakshaghosh@hotmail.com

Academic Editor: Maria Stella Figueiredo

Anemia is the primary clinical manifestation of malarial infections and is responsible for the substantial rate of morbidity. The pathophysiology discussed till now catalogued several causes for malarial anemia among which ineffective erythropoiesis being remarkable one occurs silently in the bone marrow. A systematic literature search was performed and summarized information on erythropoietic response upon malaria infection and the factors responsible for the same. This review summarizes the clinical and experimental studies on patients, mouse models, and in vitro cell cultures reporting erythropoietic changes upon malaria infection as well as factors accountable for the same. Inadequate erythropoietic response during malaria infection may be the collective effect of various mediators generated by host immune response as well as parasite metabolites. The interplay between various modulators causing the pathophysiology needs to be explored further. Globin gene expression profiling upon malaria infection should also be looked into as abnormal production of globin chains could be a possible contributor to ineffective erythropoiesis.

1. Introduction

During malaria infection, anemia is a common complication and causes mortality and morbidity in patients, especially children and pregnant women [1]. In the malaria endemic areas, the coexistence of other circumstances like parasitic infestations, iron, folate, and Vitamin B12 deficiency, E-B virus (Epstein-Barr virus) infection, and aberrant immune response is the important considerations for anemia. Inherited red cell disorders like α and β thalassemia, sickle cell anemia, enzyme deficiencies, and membrane defects also interplay with the infection [2]. World Health Organization (WHO) recommended haemoglobin levels to diagnose anemia at sea level are <13.0 g/dL and <12.0 g/dL for adult men (age 15 years and above) and adult nonpregnant women (age 15 years and above), respectively [3].

The pathophysiology of malarial anemia is said to be complex and multifactorial [4] dependent on properties of both host and parasite. It is not only due to hemolysis of infected as well as uninfected erythrocytes but also due to inability to replenish erythrocytes lost by hemolysis through inadequate erythroid response.

During infection, there is obvious loss of infected erythrocytes through parasite maturation but many uninfected cells are also destroyed due to antibody sensitization or other physiochemical membrane changes and increased reticuloendothelial activity in spleen. Suppression of erythropoiesis has been said to be additional factor contributing to worsening the condition. Ineffective erythropoiesis (active erythropoiesis with premature death of red blood cells, a decreased output of erythrocytes from the bone marrow) and dyserythropoiesis (defective development of erythrocytes, such as anisocytosis and poikilocytosis) during malaria infection are profusely discussed topic and numerous clinical and experimental studies have been undertaken to demonstrate the same. Despite that, mechanism still remains unclear.

In this review, we summarized the four different approaches used by researchers to understand the erythropoiesis in malaria infections such as clinical evaluation of patients, in vivo mice studies, in vitro culture studies, and gene expression profiling as well as factors proposed or found to cause inappropriate erythropoietic response during infection.

2. Method

A systematic literature search was performed and we summarized information on erythropoiesis on malaria infections and factors causing inadequate erythropoiesis. We searched for peer-reviewed articles published in English language in the PubMed and ScienceDirect databases.

We used search terms like malaria, erythropoiesis, ineffective erythropoiesis, dyserythropoiesis, and hemozoin in title, abstract, and keywords.

Total 1604 records were identified through database searches. Among those 1368 were excluded after reading titles, abstract, and keywords. Only peer-reviewed articles were included and conference abstracts, proceedings, and project reports were excluded. 255 full-text articles were assessed for the relevance to the subject of review and 76 were included in the main study.

3. Results

3.1. Ineffective Erythropoiesis and Dyserythropoiesis. A variety of abnormalities in the number, morphology, and function of blood and bone marrow cells were observed in human as well as murine *Plasmodium* species like *P. falciparum, P. vivax, P. chabundi, P. berghei,* and *P. yoelii* [5, 6].

3.1.1. Clinical Evaluation of Patients. Decreased production of erythroid cells was almost always found to be associated with dyserythropoiesis, that is, the production of morphologically defective cells which in functional terms results in ineffective erythropoiesis [4]. Light and electron microscope studies of marrow aspirates revealed morphological evidence of dyserythropoiesis in *P. falciparum* and *P. vivax* infected patients. Gambian patents infected with *P. falciparum* illustrated dyserythropoietic changes in the bone marrow [7]. Study on nine Thai *P. vivax* infected patients reported the presence of erythroblasts at various stages of degradation within the cytoplasm of macrophages [8]. Other changes as observed by light photomicrographs and electron micrographs included lymphocytosis in the bone marrow, appearance of giant metamyelocytes, macrophage hyperplasia, plasmacytosis, increased eosinophil granulocytopoiesis, reactive lymphocytes, monocytosis and mild neutrophilia in the peripheral blood, and increased number of megakaryocytes [8, 9]. Unlike *P. vivax* malaria, the microvasculature of the marrow was found to be obstructed by parasitized red cells in severe *P. falciparum* malaria [8]. Malarial anemia is characterized by the low reticulocytosis. It was first observed in 1939 by Vryonis [10] in acute malarial infections with *P. vivax* and *P. falciparum.* Srichaikul et al. [11] also reported

the absence of reticulocytosis during malarial infections in which hemolysis was observed indicating transient suppression of erythropoiesis. The inadequate erythroid response was observed in spite of elevated levels of erythropoietin. Kurtzhals et al. [12] studied three patient categories for reticulocytosis. He used RDW as a surrogate marker of release of young erythrocytes and reticulocytes. Initially RDW was low in all the three categories, severe malarial anaemia (SA), cerebral malaria (CM), and uncomplicated malaria (UM), in spite of markedly increased concentrations of erythropoietin (EPO). As parasites were removed after treatment, RDW increased dramatically.

The reticulocyte production index (RPI) is also used as marker in the diagnosis of anemia as well as in the determination of erythropoietic response. It is a standard measure of reticulocyte production that corrects for both the degree of anemia and the early release of reticulocytes from the bone marrow in anemic patients [13]. In the study of 106 Kenyan children, erythropoietic suppression (RPI < 2.0) was observed in significantly more number of children in each of the three groups categorized as mild malarial anemia (MA), moderate MA, and severe MA [14].

Similarly, in many studies, bone marrow inhibition was found to be correlated with the degree of parasitemia and could be reversed after clearance of parasites from blood. In the in vitro study of fifteen bone marrow cultures of *P. falciparum* patients, abnormalities were observed only during parasitemia [15]. Premature death of normoblasts, decreased normoblastic number, and cellular iron incorporation and defective haemoglobin synthesis were observed during development of the cultures. Dormer et al. [16] analysed erythroblast cell kinetics in five cases of acute *P. falciparum* malaria and noted changes in erythroblast morphology and reduced rate of erythroblast proliferation while Abdalla and Wickramasinghe [17] observed wide variation in the number of BFUe (burst forming unit) and CFUe (colony forming unit) in the bone marrow of Gambian children with falciparum malaria and moderate or severe anaemia. Significantly lower number of BFUe were noted in the patients who had parasitemia >1%. Similarly, in the study involving young Gambian children with *P. falciparum* malaria, the children who presented with chronic anemia (parasitemia <1%) demonstrated higher levels of erythroid hyperplasia and dyserythropoiesis [18]. Verhoef et al. [19] studied 328 Kenyan children with asymptomatic malaria and evaluated erythropoiesis by serum concentrations of erythropoietin and soluble transferrin receptor. Lower haemoglobin and higher serum concentrations of erythropoietin and transferrin receptors were detected during the malaria infection. Conversely, disappearance of malarial antigenemia resulted in increased hemoglobin concentrations and decreased concentrations of these serum indicators.

3.1.2. In Vivo Mice Studies. The above mentioned aspects of erythropoiesis were supported by the rodent malaria models which were proved to be useful in delineating the erythropoietic response followed by murine *Plasmodium* species. Several strains of *Plasmodium* can infect mice such as *P. chabaudi, P. berghei, P. yoelii,* and *P. vinckei.* Akin to the *P. falciparum*, *P. chabaudi* invades erythrocytes of all ages [20, 21] while *P. yoelii* has preference for reticulocytes [22] and hence may assist as a *P. vivax* model. Availability of differentially susceptible inbred mouse strains in which infections can be lethal and nonlethal improved the scope of murine models.

Maggio-Price et al. [23] experimentally infected rodents with *P. berghei* and attempted to characterize the erythropoietic response in terms of changes in marrow hematopoietic stem cells. Mice infected with *P. berghei* had dramatic decreases in bone marrow cellularity, erythroblasts, BFU-E, and CFU-E, 24 hours after infection. Similarly tissue culture studies of lethal (strain 17XL) *P. yoelii* infection in rodent showed decline in marrow BFU-E and marrow cellularity [24]. Erythropoietic responses during infection in resistant and susceptible mice were investigated during *P. chabaudi* AS infection [25]. It was observed that in vivo ^{59}Fe incorporation was significantly more depressed in bone marrow and more increased in the spleen in resistant mice during the period of anemia. The increase in splenic ^{59}Fe incorporation was a function of the size of the spleen. Chang and Stevenson [26] tried to investigate the mechanism of erythropoietic abnormalities by exploring upstream events of erythropoiesis affected by blood-stage *P. chabaudi* AS in mice treated with recombinant murine erythropoietin (EPO). It was found that suppression of EPO-induced proliferation of early EPOR-positive erythroid progenitors led to the impaired terminal maturation of TER119^{+} erythroblasts.

3.1.3. In Vitro Culture Studies. In the recent years, after the successful production of erythrocytes from the in vitro cultures of haematopoietic stem cells [27], the model system was being employed in the elucidation of complexity of malarial anemia. The kinetics of differentiation in in vitro erythropoiesis model system closely resembles that of erythroid cell maturation in the bone marrow and differentiation occurs in a relatively synchronous manner.

Panichakul et al. [5] in 2012 reported the inhibition of erythroid cell expansion and differentiation followed by exposure of *P. vivax* infected intact erythrocytes as well as lysates in culture system established by isolating haematopoietic stem cells from normal human cord blood. Inhibition of erythroid development was determined by reduction in the expression of glycophorin A and CD71 on the growing erythroid cells. Similar observations were observed in the experiments performed with different laboratory strains of *P. falciparum* using the same culture system (unpublished observations).

Expression of CD71, essential for uptake of iron bound to transferrin, is normally increased on maturing erythroblasts that require iron from haemoglobin synthesis as well as on other actively growing cells [28]. These findings suggests that impaired erythroblast maturation may be a consequence of decreased iron uptake by developing RBCs. Additional studies are required to address this possibility.

3.1.4. Gene Expression Studies. Transcriptional changes can be utilized as an important first step in understanding the host cell's adaptive response to infection by blood stage *Plasmodium*. Microarray analysis data of murine transcriptional responses during the infection revealed strongly suppressed erythropoiesis, starting early during infection, and highly upregulated transcription of genes that control host glycolysis, including lactate dehydrogenase [29]. Recently Tamez et al. [30] showed that exposure of *P. falciparum* to erythroid progenitors in vitro upregulated a set of genes which are associated with signalling, erythropoiesis, and erythroid cell development.

Gene expression profiling of growing erythrocytes could be an important key for understanding the pathophysiology of the disease. During the intraerythrocytic phase of its life cycle, malaria parasite matures within a cell in which haemoglobin is the single major cytosolic protein. Haemoglobin is the main amino acid reservoir available to the intraerythrocytic *Plasmodium*. The qualitative and quantitative changes in haemoglobin have been shown to inhibit the parasite growth in vitro [31, 32]. Being an important protein, it is important to check the expression profiling of globin genes which may help us to understand host parasite interactions and its potential contribution to both infection and disease.

Imbalance in α and β globin chains has been greatly discussed in cases of thalassemias [33–35]. Altered α/β globin gene expression ratio in such cases is an important indicator of ineffective erythropoiesis as well as disease severity [35, 36]. In 1975, Orkin et al. [37], working on murine erythroleukemic cell line, have reported differential expression of α and β globin genes during cellular differentiation. Substantial excess amount of α RNA was observed (α/β ratio ~3.7) early in induction, and the α/β RNA ratio progressively approached 1 as differentiation proceeds further. Studies are required to check if parasites or their products can affect the balance between productions of α and β globin chains in the erythroid progenitors. This extreme α/β anomaly may be the reason of severe ineffective erythropoiesis.

3.2. Factors Affecting Erythropoiesis. Various host and parasite mediators responsible for the erythropoietic changes during malaria infection have been documented in the literature, hemozoin crystals and cytokines being largely discussed.

3.2.1. Malaria Pigment Hemozoin (Hz) and Hemozoin Generated Products. Hemozoin is a by-product of heme detoxification by malaria parasites through biocrystallization process. As the parasite multiplies in host, hemozoin is continuously produced and released together with the merozoites and engulfed by macrophages, monocytes, neutrophils, and other immune cells such as dendritic cells (DCs) [38]. Hemozoin stimulates the secretion of biologically active 4-hydroxynonenal (4-HNE) through oxidation of membrane lipids. It also activates macrophages and DCs to produce inflammatory cytokines [39]. Hemozoin and other generated products are receiving increasing attention due to their role in host immune system modulation.

Dysregulation in the innate immune response is believed to be an important cause of impaired erythroid responses in children with severe malarial anemia. The ability of *P. falciparum* derived Hz to cause dysregulation in pro- and anti-inflammatory cytokines, growth factors, chemokines, and effector molecules has been studied extensively [40].

Dysregulation of innate inflammatory mediators is a result of phagocytosis of malarial pigment hemozoin by immune cells. During acute falciparum malaria in children, altered production of soluble immune mediators, such as nitric oxide (NO) and prostaglandin-E2 (PGE2), has been observed from peripheral blood mononuclear cells (PBMCs) [41, 42]. Recent findings in a murine model of malaria demonstrate that injection of Hz in BALB/c mice induces the expression of chemokines (Macrophage Inflammatory Protein-1, MIP-1α, MIP-1β, MIP-2, and Monocyte Chemoattractant Protein-1, MCP-1) [43]. Moreover experiments using PBMCs from healthy, malaria-naive adults also illustrated dysregulation in β-chemokine production by Hz [44].

Hemozoin has been shown to inhibit the erythroid development in vitro and in vivo. Hemozoin within the bone marrow and plasma levels of hemozoin in patients with malarial anemia were associated with reduced reticulocyte response [45]. Conflicting results have been reported regarding inhibition of erythropoiesis with or without apoptosis by hemozoin crystals. Lamikanra et al. [45] described inhibition of erythroid cell development in vitro by *P. falciparum* isolated hemozoin independently of inflammatory mediators. It was characterised by delayed expression of the erythroid markers and increased apoptosis of progenitor cells. In the absence of tumor necrosis factor (TNF), hemozoin inhibited erythroid development in vitro. Conversely, after addition of TNF, it has been found to be synergized with hemozoin to inhibit erythropoiesis [46]. Giribaldi et al. [47] investigated the possible role of hemozoin and 4-hydroxynonenal in malarial dyserythropoiesis. 4-HNE generated by monocytes as well as supernatants of HZ and HZ-fed monocytes had been shown to inhibit progenitor growth. In the in vitro experiments performed by Skorokhod et al. [48], growth of erythroid cells was inhibited without apoptosis during cocultivation with HZ or treatment with low micromolar 4-HNE.

After HZ/HNE treatment, expression of cell-cycle regulation proteins was investigated and the expressions of critical proteins, p53 and p21, were increased while the master transcription factor in erythropoiesis, GATA-1, was found to be reduced. The regulator protein of G_1-to-S-phase transition (retinoblastoma protein) was consequently hypophosphorylated. HZ and HNE inhibited protein expression of crucial receptors (R) in erythropoiesis, namely, transferrin R1, stem cell factor R, interleukin-3R, and erythropoietin R. Thus it was clear that HZ and HNE inhibited erythropoiesis by interfering with cell cycle and cell-cycle regulation proteins acted as targets for HZ and HNE in the inhibition process.

Hemozoin leads to the continuous targeting of the host innate immune system, leading to both pro- and anti-inflammatory responses; thus, currently, the potential application of hemozoin crystals for their use in vaccine as an adjuvant has been evaluated [49]. Both natural and synthetic forms of hemozoin are observed to possess adjuvant properties but used different innate immune receptors.

Further studies may provide deeper insights into the molecular mechanisms involved in immune responses to malarial infection.

3.2.2. Cytokines. Severe disease in both human and mouse seems to be dependent on the levels of proinflammatory and anti-inflammatory cytokines. The relative balance between pro- and anti-inflammatory cytokines determines the degree of malarial anemia [50–54]. Higher levels of proinflammatory cytokines during the acute phase of infection appear to limit disease progression, while an anti-inflammatory response appears to promote enhanced pathogenesis [51, 55–57].

Parasites and its byproducts elevate a strong inflammatory response by increasing TNFα and IFNγ. These cytokines can inhibit all stages of erythropoiesis [58–60]. In a study involving *P. vinckei*, appreciable erythrophagocytosis and dyserythropoiesis were observed in bone marrow preparations from TNF-treated mice and those with severe illness due to *P. vinckei* [61].

The potent anti-inflammatory cytokine, IL10, has been suggested as important factor to regulate TNFα levels. The low IL10/TNFα ratio has been associated with severe anemia in young children [52, 62]. Many other proinflammatory cytokines such as IL12, nitric oxide (NO), and migration inhibitory factor (MIF) have been implicated in pathophysiology of anemia. IL12 is considered to be a stimulator of erythropoiesis [63, 64]. It is found to enhance the numbers of erythroid burst (BFU-E) and colony forming units (CFU-E) in bone marrow and spleen cells significantly in vitro from normal and day 7 infected resistance and susceptible mice. Effect of NO on cell development was studied in an in vitro model of erythropoiesis, developed using CD34+ stem cells derived from peripheral blood. NO significantly inhibited erythroid cell proliferation and maturation by increased apoptosis of erythropoietin-stimulated CD34+ cells [65].

3.2.3. β-Chemokines. In addition to cytokines, the important mediators in malaria pathogenesis are chemokines. Chemokines are chemotactic cytokines having the ability to induce directed chemotaxis in nearby responsive cells. Chemokines are important for bridging innate and adaptive immune responses and regulating hematopoietic maturation [66, 67].

The chemokines expression profile has largely been studied for their potential role in regulating disease severity in malaria patients.

Ochiel et al. [44] determined circulating protein levels and transcript profiles of β-chemokines (Macrophage Inflammatory Protein 1 [MIP-1α, MIP-1β] and Regulated on Activation, Normal T-cell Expressed and Secreted [RANTES]) [68] and α-chemokine (Stromal cell Derived Factor 1 [SDF-1]) in plasma and PBMCs (peripheral blood mononuclear cells), respectively, in children with various degrees of *P. falciparum* malaria. Children with acute falciparum malaria showed dysregulation of β-chemokines characterized by elevated MIP-1α and MIP-1β and decreased RANTES at the mRNA and protein level. Significant reduction in circulating levels of RANTES was observed in healthy children with a history of severe malaria relative to those that previously experienced mild malaria indicating the protective role of RANTES against severe disease. Interestingly, transcriptional analysis of RANTES revealed that children with previous severe malaria had significantly higher RANTES mRNA expression than those with previous mild malaria. Similarly Were et al. [14] demonstrated the reduced circulating RANTES and peripheral blood mononuclear cell RANTES mRNA levels in Gabonese children with acute malaria (defined by hyperparasitemia and mild-to-moderate forms of anemia) [44].

RANTES is a specific chemoattractant for memory T cells and regulates inflammation by promoting leukocyte activation, angiogenesis, antimicrobial effects, and hematopoiesis [69]. It can promote migration of erythroid precursors into hematopoietic tissues [70] and prevent apoptosis of erythroid progenitors [71] suggesting that suppression of RANTES may lead to an ineffective erythropoietic response.

3.2.4. Monocyte Migration Inhibitory Factor (MIF).

Ingestion of parasite infected erythrocytes or malarial pigment (hemozoin) induces the release of macrophage migration inhibitory factor (MIF) from macrophages, a proinflammatory mediator. MIF has been thought to have intrinsic role in the development of the anemic complications and bone marrow suppression that are associated with malaria infection. At concentrations found in the circulation of malaria infected patients, MIF was found to suppress erythropoietin-dependent erythroid colony formation. Moreover, MIF synergized with known antagonists of hematopoiesis, tumor necrosis factor, and γ interferon [72]. MIF also caused inhibition of erythroid (BFU-E), multipotential (CFU-GEMM), and granulocyte-macrophage (CFU-GM) progenitor-derived colony formation [73].

Mouse studies regarding MIF demonstrated similar observations. MIF was detected in the sera of *P. chabaudi* infected BALB/c mice, and circulating levels correlated with disease severity [73]. However, infection of MIF knockout mice with *P. chabaudi* resulted in less severe anemia, improved erythroid progenitor development, and increased survival compared with wild-type controls [72]. It is therefore conceivable that neutralization of MIF may protect against bone marrow suppression to some extent.

Consistent with the role of MIF as erythropoietic suppressor, the elevated serum MIF levels were found in patients with severe malaria [50]; however decreased serum concentration was observed in Kenyan children with malaria [74]. It was demonstrate that, in children, hemozoin acquisition by monocytes was associated with low levels of peripheral blood MIF and increased severity of anemia.

Soluble factors of *Plasmodium* have also been studied for their effect on erythropoiesis. Cell-free conditioned media prepared from spleen cells of mice infected with *P. chabaudi* [75] as well as *P. berghei* and *P. vinckei* [76] were able to inhibit erythroid cell proliferation of splenic erythroid cells in vitro and this inhibition was not reversed by increasing the concentration of EPO.

These factors either individually or collectively generate an ineffective erythropoietic response. Understanding the interplay between these mediators would provide the insights into mechanism invoking inadequate erythropoiesis.

4. Conclusion

Inadequate erythropoiesis is the important pathophysiology of malarial anemia. Understanding the pathophysiology and associated host parasite interactions would provide deeper insights into immune mechanism involved in the malarial infection and would help in the development of therapeutic strategies to treat severe malarial anemia. The interplay between various modulators causing ineffective erythropoiesis needs to be explored further.

It is also important to check whether parasites or their products mount any transcriptional responses in globin genes and affect the balance among the globin chains that can be analyzed for their potential contribution to the ineffective erythropoiesis and dyserythropoiesis.

Conflict of Interests

The authors declare that there is no conflict of interests regarding the publication of this paper.

References

[1] B. M. Greenwood, "The epidemiology of malaria," *Annals of Tropical Medicine and Parasitology*, vol. 91, no. 7, pp. 763–769, 1997.

[2] K. Ghosh and K. Ghosh, "Pathogenesis of anemia in malaria: a concise review," *Parasitology Research*, vol. 101, no. 6, pp. 1463–1469, 2007.

[3] WHO, *Haemoglobin Concentrations for the Diagnosis of Anaemia and Assessment of Severity*, Vitamin and Mineral Nutrition Information System, World Health Organization, Geneva, Switzerland, 2011.

[4] R. E. Phillips and G. Pasvol, "Anaemia of *Plasmodium falciparum* malaria," *Baillière's Clinical Haematology*, vol. 5, no. 2, pp. 315–330, 1992.

[5] T. Panichakul, W. Payuhakrit, P. Panburana, C. Wongborisuth, S. Hongeng, and R. Udomsangpetch, "Suppression of erythroid development in vitro by *Plasmodium vivax*," *Malaria Journal*, vol. 11, article 173, 2012.

[6] N. Thawani, M. Tam, M.-J. Bellemare et al., "Plasmodium products contribute to severe malarial anemia by inhibiting erythropoietin-induced proliferation of erythroid precursors," *Journal of Infectious Diseases*, vol. 209, no. 1, pp. 140–149, 2014.

[7] S. Abdalla, D. J. Weatherall, S. N. Wickramasinghe, and M. Hughes, "The anaemia of *P. falciparum* malaria," *British Journal of Haematology*, vol. 46, no. 2, pp. 171–183, 1980.

[8] S. N. Wickramasinghe, S. Looareesuwan, B. Nagachinta, and N. J. White, "Dyserythropoiesis and ineffective erythropoiesis in *Plasmodium vivax* malaria," *British Journal of Haematology*, vol. 72, no. 1, pp. 91–99, 1989.

[9] S. N. Wickramasinghe and S. H. Abdalla, "Blood and bone marrow changes in malaria," *Baillière's Best Practice and Research in Clinical Haematology*, vol. 13, no. 2, pp. 277–299, 2000.

[10] G. Vryonis, "Observations in the parasitisation of erythrocytes by *Plasmodium vivax*, with special reference to reticulocytes," *American Journal of Hygiene*, vol. 30, article 41, 1939.

[11] T. Srichaikul, M. Wasanasomsithi, V. Poshyachinda, N. Panikbutr, and T. Rabieb, "Ferrokinetic studies and erythropoiesis in malaria," *Archives of Internal Medicine*, vol. 124, no. 5, pp. 623–628, 1969.

[12] J. A. L. Kurtzhals, O. Rodrigues, M. Addae, J. O. O. Commey, F. K. Nkrumah, and L. Hviid, "Reversible suppression of bone marrow response to erythropoietin in *Plasmodium falciparum* malaria," *British Journal of Haematology*, vol. 97, no. 1, pp. 169–174, 1997.

[13] G. R. Lee, *Anemia: General Aspects*, Lippincott Williams & Wilkins, Baltimore, Md, USA, 10th edition, 1999.

[14] T. Were, J. B. Hittner, C. Ouma et al., "Suppression of RANTES in children with *Plasmodium falciparum* malaria," *Haematologica*, vol. 91, no. 10, pp. 1396–1399, 2006.

[15] T. Srichaikul, T. Siriasawakul, and M. Poshyachinda, "Ferrokinetics in patients with malaria: haemoglobin synthesis and normoblasts in vitro," *Transactions of the Royal Society of Tropical Medicine and Hygiene*, vol. 70, no. 3, pp. 244–246, 1976.

[16] P. Dormer, M. Dietrich, P. Kern, and R. D. Horstmann, "Ineffective erythropoiesis in acute human *P. falciparum* malaria," *Blut*, vol. 46, no. 5, pp. 279–288, 1983.

[17] S. H. Abdalla and S. N. Wickramasinghe, "A study of erythroid progenitor cells in the bone marrow of Gambian children with falciparum malaria," *Clinical and Laboratory Haematology*, vol. 10, no. 1, pp. 33–40, 1988.

[18] S. H. Abdalla, "Hematopoiesis in human malaria," *Blood Cells*, vol. 16, no. 2-3, pp. 401–419, 1990.

[19] H. Verhoef, C. E. West, R. Kraaijenhagen et al., "Malarial anemia leads to adequately increased erythropoiesis in asymptomatic Kenyan children," *Blood*, vol. 100, no. 10, pp. 3489–3494, 2002.

[20] R. Carter and D. Walliker, "New observations on the malaria parasites of rodents of the Central African republic: *Plamodium vinkei* petteri subsp. Nov and *Plasmodium chabaudi* Landau, 1965," *Annals of Tropical Medicine and Parasitology*, vol. 69, no. 2, pp. 187–196, 1975.

[21] K. Chotivanich, R. Udomsangpetch, J. A. Simpson et al., "Parasite multiplication potential and the severity of Falciparum malaria," *Journal of Infectious Diseases*, vol. 181, no. 3, pp. 1206–1209, 2000.

[22] P. C. C. Garnham, R. G. Bird, J. R. Baker, S. S. Desser, and H. M. S. El-Nahal, "Electron microscope studies on motile stages of malaria parasites VI. The oöknete of *Plasmodium berghei yoelii* and its transformation into the early oocyst," *Transactions of the Royal Society of Tropical Medicine and Hygiene*, vol. 63, no. 2, pp. 187–194, 1969.

[23] L. Maggio-Price, D. Brookhoff, and L. Weiss, "Changes in hematopoietic stem cells in bone marrow of mice with *Plasmodium berghei* malaria," *Blood*, vol. 66, no. 5, pp. 1080–1085, 1985.

[24] L. Weiss, J. Johnson, and W. Weidanz, "Mechanisms of splenic control of murine malaria: tissue culture studies of the erythropoietic interplay of spleen, bone marrow, and blood in lethal (strain 17XL) *Plasmodium yoelii* malaria in BALB/c mice," *The American Journal of Tropical Medicine and Hygiene*, vol. 41, no. 2, pp. 135–143, 1989.

[25] G. S. Yap and M. M. Stevenson, "*Plasmodium chabaudi* AS: erythropoietic responses during infection in resistant and susceptible mice," *Experimental Parasitology*, vol. 75, no. 3, pp. 340–352, 1992.

[26] K.-H. Chang and M. M. Stevenson, "Malarial anaemia: mechanisms and implications of insufficient erythropoiesis during blood-stage malaria," *International Journal for Parasitology*, vol. 34, no. 13-14, pp. 1501–1516, 2004.

[27] T. Panichakul, J. Sattabongkot, K. Chotivanich, J. Sirichaisinthop, L. Cui, and R. Udomsangpetch, "Production of erythropoietic cells in vitro for continuous culture of *Plasmodium vivax*," *International Journal for Parasitology*, vol. 37, no. 14, pp. 1551–1557, 2007.

[28] P. Ponka and C. N. Lok, "The transferrin receptor: role in health and disease," *International Journal of Biochemistry and Cell Biology*, vol. 31, no. 10, pp. 1111–1137, 1999.

[29] A. C. Sexton, R. T. Good, D. S. Hansen et al., "Transcriptional profiling reveals suppressed erythropoiesis, up-regulated glycolysis, and interferon-associated responses in murine malaria," *Journal of Infectious Diseases*, vol. 189, no. 7, pp. 1245–1256, 2004.

[30] P. A. Tamez, H. Liu, A. Wickrema, and K. Haldar, "*P. falciparum* modulates erythroblast cell gene expression in signaling and erythrocyte production pathways," *PLoS ONE*, vol. 6, no. 5, Article ID e19307, 2011.

[31] G. Pasvol, "The interaction between sickle haemoglobin and the malarial parasite *Plasmodium falciparum*," *Transactions of the Royal Society of Tropical Medicine and Hygiene*, vol. 74, no. 6, pp. 701–705, 1980.

[32] C. R. Brockelman, B. Wongsattayanont, P. Tan-Ariya, and S. Fucharoen, "Thalassemic erythrocytes inhibit in vitro growth of *Plasmodium falciparum*," *Journal of Clinical Microbiology*, vol. 25, no. 1, pp. 56–60, 1987.

[33] R. F. Rieder and G. W. James III, "Imbalance in α and β globin synthesis associated with a hemoglobinopathy," *The Journal of Clinical Investigation*, vol. 54, no. 4, pp. 948–956, 1974.

[34] J.-Y. Han, R.-P. Zeng, G. Cheng, B. Hu, H. Li, and Y.-R. Lai, "Quantitative analysis of human globin gene expression in beta-thalassemia using real-time RT-PCR," *Yi Chuan*, vol. 27, no. 1, pp. 57–64, 2005.

[35] C. Chaisue, S. Kitcharoen, P. Wilairat, A. Jetsrisuparb, G. Fucharoen, and S. Fucharoen, "α/β-Globin mRNA ratio determination by multiplex quantitative real-time reverse transcription-polymerase chain reaction as an indicator of globin gene function," *Clinical Biochemistry*, vol. 40, no. 18, pp. 1373–1377, 2007.

[36] F. Maryami, R. Mahdian, S. Jamali et al., "Comparisons between RT-PCR, real-time PCR, and in vitro globin chain synthesis by α/β ratio calculation for diagnosis of α- from β-thalassemia carriers," *Archives of Iranian Medicine*, vol. 16, no. 4, pp. 217–220, 2013.

[37] S. H. Orkin, D. Swan, and P. Leder, "Differential expression of α and β globin genes during differentiation of cultured erythroleukemic cells," *The Journal of Biological Chemistry*, vol. 250, no. 22, pp. 8753–8760, 1975.

[38] P. Arese and E. Schwarzer, "Malarial pigment (haemozoin): a very active 'inert' substance," *Annals of Tropical Medicine and Parasitology*, vol. 91, no. 5, pp. 501–516, 1997.

[39] F. Martinon, A. Mayor, and J. Tschopp, "The inflammasomes: guardians of the body," *Annual Review of Immunology*, vol. 27, pp. 229–265, 2009.

[40] D. J. Perkins, T. Were, G. C. Davenport, P. Kempaiah, J. B. Hittner, and J. M. Ong'echa, "Severe malarial anemia: innate immunity and pathogenesis," *International Journal of Biological Sciences*, vol. 7, no. 9, pp. 1427–1442, 2011.

[41] C. C. Keller, J. B. Hittner, B. K. Nti, J. B. Weinberg, P. G. Kremsner, and D. J. Perkins, "Reduced peripheral PGE2 biosynthesis in *Plasmodium falciparum* malaria occurs through hemozoin-induced suppression of blood mononuclear

cell cyclooxygenase-2 gene expression via an interleukin-10-independent mechanism," *Molecular Medicine*, vol. 10, no. 1–6, pp. 45–54, 2004.

[42] C. C. Keller, P. G. Kremsner, J. B. Hittner, M. A. Misukonis, J. B. Weinberg, and D. J. Perkins, "Elevated nitric oxide production in children with malarial anemia: hemozoin-induced nitric oxide synthase type 2 transcripts and nitric oxide in blood mononuclear cells," *Infection and Immunity*, vol. 72, no. 8, pp. 4868–4873, 2004.

[43] M. Jaramillo, I. Plante, N. Ouellet, K. Vandal, P. A. Tessier, and M. Olivier, "Hemozoin-inducible proinflammatory events in vivo: potential role in malaria infection," *The Journal of Immunology*, vol. 172, no. 5, pp. 3101–3110, 2004.

[44] D. O. Ochiel, G. A. Awandare, C. C. Keller et al., "Differential regulation of β-chemokines in children with *Plasmodium falciparum* malaria," *Infection and Immunity*, vol. 73, no. 7, pp. 4190–4197, 2005.

[45] A. A. Lamikanra, M. Theron, T. W. A. Kooij, and D. J. Roberts, "Hemozoin (malarial pigment) directly promotes apoptosis of erythroid precursors," *PLoS ONE*, vol. 4, no. 12, Article ID e8446, 2009.

[46] C. Casals-Pascual, O. Kai, J. O. P. Cheung et al., "Suppression of erythropoiesis in malarial anemia is associated with hemozoin in vitro and in vivo," *Blood*, vol. 108, no. 8, pp. 2569–2577, 2006.

[47] G. Giribaldi, D. Ulliers, E. Schwarzer, I. Roberts, W. Piacibello, and P. Arese, "Hemozoin- and 4-hydroxynonenal-mediated inhibition of erythropoiesis. Possible role in malarial dyserythropoiesis and anemia," *Haematologica*, vol. 89, no. 4, pp. 492–493, 2004.

[48] O. A. Skorokhod, L. Caione, T. Marrocco et al., "Inhibition of erythropoiesis in malaria anemia: role of hemozoin and hemozoin-generated 4-hydroxynonenal," *Blood*, vol. 116, no. 20, pp. 4328–4337, 2010.

[49] C. Coban, M. Yagi, K. Ohata et al., "The malarial metabolite hemozoin and its potential use as a vaccine adjuvant," *Allergology International*, vol. 59, no. 2, pp. 115–124, 2010.

[50] S. C. Chaiyaroj, A. S. M. Rutta, K. Muenthaisong, P. Watkins, M. Na Ubol, and S. Looareesuwan, "Reduced levels of transforming growth factor-β1, interleukin-12 and increased migration inhibitory factor are associated with severe malaria," *Acta Tropica*, vol. 89, no. 3, pp. 319–327, 2004.

[51] D. Dodoo, F. M. Omer, J. Todd, B. D. Akanmori, K. A. Koram, and E. M. Riley, "Absolute levels and ratios of proinflammatory and anti-inflammatory cytokine production in vitro predict clinical immunity to *Plasmodium falciparum* malaria," *Journal of Infectious Diseases*, vol. 185, no. 7, pp. 971–979, 2002.

[52] C. Othoro, A. A. Lal, B. Nahlen, D. Koech, A. S. S. Orago, and V. Udhayakumar, "A low interleukin-10 tumor necrosis factor-α ratio is associated with malaria anemia in children residing in a holoendemic malaria region in western Kenya," *Journal of Infectious Diseases*, vol. 179, no. 1, pp. 279–282, 1999.

[53] D. J. Perkins, J. B. Weinberg, and P. G. Kremsner, "Reduced interleukin-12 and transforming growth factor-β1 in severe childhood malaria: relationship of cytokine balance with disease severity," *Journal of Infectious Diseases*, vol. 182, no. 3, pp. 988–992, 2000.

[54] D. Torre, F. Speranza, M. Giola, A. Matteelli, R. Tambini, and G. Biondi, "Role of Th1 and Th2 cytokines in immune response to uncomplicated *Plasmodium falciparum* malaria," *Clinical and Diagnostic Laboratory Immunology*, vol. 9, no. 2, pp. 348–351, 2002.

[55] L. Malaguarnera, R. M. Imbesi, S. Pignatelli, J. Simporè, M. Malaguarnera, and S. Musumeci, "Increased levels of interleukin-12 in *Plasmodium falciparum* malaria: correlation with the severity of disease," *Parasite Immunology*, vol. 24, no. 7, pp. 387–389, 2002.

[56] M. Musumeci, L. Malaguarnera, J. Simporè, A. Messina, and S. Musumeci, "Modulation of immune response in *Plasmodium falciparum* malaria: role of IL-12, IL-18 and TGF-β," *Cytokine*, vol. 21, no. 4, pp. 172–178, 2003.

[57] S. Winkler, M. Willheim, K. Baier et al., "Reciprocal regulation of Th1- and Th2-cytokine-producing T cells during clearance of parasitemia in *Plasmodium falciparum* malaria," *Infection and Immunity*, vol. 66, no. 12, pp. 6040–6044, 1998.

[58] K. L. Miller, J. C. Schooley, K. L. Smith, B. Kullgren, L. J. Mahlmann, and P. H. Silverman, "Inhibition of erythropoiesis by a soluble factor in murine malaria," *Experimental Hematology*, vol. 17, no. 4, pp. 379–385, 1989.

[59] D. Kwiatkowski, A. V. S. Hill, I. Sambou et al., "TNF concentration in fatal cerebral, non-fatal cerebral, and uncomplicated *Plasmodium falciparum* malaria," *The Lancet*, vol. 336, no. 8725, pp. 1201–1204, 1990.

[60] C. Dufour, A. Corcione, J. Svahn et al., "TNF-α and IFN-γ are overexpressed in the bone marrow of Fanconi anemia patients and TNF-α suppresses erythropoiesis in vitro," *Blood*, vol. 102, no. 6, pp. 2053–2059, 2003.

[61] I. A. Clark and G. Chaudhri, "Tumour necrosis factor may contribute to the anaemia of malaria by causing dyserythropoiesis and erythrophagocytosis," *British Journal of Haematology*, vol. 70, no. 1, pp. 99–103, 1988.

[62] J. A. L. Kurtzhals, V. Adabayeri, B. Q. Goka et al., "Low plasma concentrations of interleukin 10 in severe malarial anaemia compared with cerebral and uncomplicated malaria," *The Lancet*, vol. 351, no. 9118, pp. 1768–1772, 1998.

[63] K. Mohan and M. M. Stevenson, "Dyserythropoiesis and severe anaemia associated with malaria correlate with deficient interleukin-12 production," *British Journal of Haematology*, vol. 103, no. 4, pp. 942–949, 1998.

[64] K. Mohan and M. M. Stevenson, "Interleukin-12 corrects severe anemia during blood-stage *Plasmodium chabaudi* AS in susceptible A/J mice," *Experimental Hematology*, vol. 26, no. 1, pp. 45–52, 1998.

[65] G. A. Awandare, P. Kempaiah, D. O. Ochiel, P. Piazza, C. C. Keller, and D. J. Perkins, "Mechanisms of erythropoiesis inhibition by malarial pigment and malaria-induced proinflammatory mediators in an in vitro model," *American Journal of Hematology*, vol. 86, no. 2, pp. 155–162, 2011.

[66] H. E. Broxmeyer, "Regulation of hematopoiesis by chemokine family members," *International Journal of Hematology*, vol. 74, no. 1, pp. 9–17, 2001.

[67] J. W. Lillard Jr., U. P. Singh, P. N. Boyaka, S. Singh, D. D. Taub, and J. R. McGhee, "MIP-1α and MIP-1β differentially mediate mucosal and systemic adaptive immunity," *Blood*, vol. 101, no. 3, pp. 807–814, 2003.

[68] K. Bacon, M. Baggiolini, H. Broxmeyer et al., "Chemokine/chemokine receptor nomenclature," *Journal of Interferon and Cytokine Research*, vol. 22, no. 10, pp. 1067–1068, 2002.

[69] A. D. Luster, "The role of chemokines in linking innate and adaptive immunity," *Current Opinion in Immunology*, vol. 14, no. 1, pp. 129–135, 2002.

[70] D. E. Wright, E. P. Bowman, A. J. Wagers, E. C. Butcher, and I. L. Weissman, "Hematopoietic stem cells are uniquely

selective in their migratory response to chemokines," *Journal of Experimental Medicine*, vol. 195, no. 9, pp. 1145–1154, 2002.

[71] M. Majka, A. Janowska-Wieczorek, J. Ratajczak et al., "Numerous growth factors, cytokines, and chemokines are secreted by human CD34$^+$ cells, myeloblasts, erythroblasts, and megakaryoblasts and regulate normal hematopoiesis in an autocrine/paracrine manner," *Blood*, vol. 97, no. 10, pp. 3075–3085, 2001.

[72] M. A. McDevitt, J. Xie, G. Shanmugasundaram et al., "A critical role for the host mediator macrophage migration inhibitory factor in the pathogenesis of malarial anemia," *The Journal of Experimental Medicine*, vol. 203, no. 5, pp. 1185–1196, 2006.

[73] J. A. Martiney, B. Sherry, C. N. Metz et al., "Macrophage migration inhibitory factor release by macrophages after ingestion of *Plasmodium chabaudi*-infected erythrocytes: possible role in the pathogenesis of malarial anemia," *Infection and Immunity*, vol. 68, no. 4, pp. 2259–2267, 2000.

[74] G. A. Awandare, Y. Ouma, C. Ouma et al., "Role of monocyte-acquired hemozoin in suppression of macrophage migration inhibitory factor in children with severe malarial anemia," *Infection and Immunity*, vol. 75, no. 1, pp. 201–210, 2007.

[75] G. S. Yap and M. M. Stevenson, "Inhibition of in vitro erythropoiesis by soluble mediators in *Plasmodium chabaudi* AS malaria: lack of a major role for interleukin 1, tumor necrosis factor alpha, and gamma interferon," *Infection and Immunity*, vol. 62, no. 2, pp. 357–362, 1994.

[76] K. L. Miller, P. H. Silverman, B. Kullgren, and L. J. Mahlmann, "Tumor necrosis factor alpha and the anemia associated with murine malaria," *Infection and Immunity*, vol. 57, no. 5, pp. 1542–1546, 1989.

26

An Etiologic Profile of Anemia in 405 Geriatric Patients

Tabea Geisel,[1,2] **Julia Martin,**[1,2] **Bettina Schulze,**[3] **Roland Schaefer,**[4]
Matthias Bach,[3] **Garth Virgin,**[5] **and Jürgen Stein**[1,2,6]

[1] *Crohn Colitis Center Rhein-Main, 60594 Frankfurt/Main, Germany*

[2] *Institute of Nutritional Science, University of Giessen, 35392 Giessen, Germany*

[3] *St. Elisabethen Krankenhaus, 60487 Frankfurt/Main, Germany*

[4] *Krankenhaus Sachsenhausen, Teaching Hospital of the J. W. von Goethe University Frankfurt/Main, 60594 Frankfurt/Main, Germany*

[5] *Vifor Pharma Deutschland GmbH, 81379 Munich, Germany*

[6] *Department of Gastroenterology and Nutritional Medicine, Krankenhaus Sachsenhausen, Teaching Hospital of the J. W. von Goethe University Frankfurt/Main, 60594 Frankfurt/Main, Germany*

Correspondence should be addressed to Jürgen Stein; j.stein@em.uni-frankfurt.de

Academic Editor: Donald S. Silverberg

Background. Anemia is a common condition in the elderly and a significant risk factor for increased morbidity and mortality, reducing not only functional capacity and mobility but also quality of life. Currently, few data are available regarding anemia in hospitalized geriatric patients. Our retrospective study investigated epidemiology and causes of anemia in 405 hospitalized geriatric patients. *Methods.* Data analysis was performed using laboratory parameters determined during routine hospital admission procedures (hemoglobin, ferritin, transferrin saturation, C-reactive protein, vitamin B12, folic acid, and creatinine) in addition to medical history and demographics. *Results.* Anemia affected approximately two-thirds of subjects. Of 386 patients with recorded hemoglobin values, 66.3% were anemic according to WHO criteria, mostly (85.1%) in a mild form. Anemia was primarily due to iron deficiency (65%), frequently due to underlying chronic infection (62.1%), or of mixed etiology involving a combination of chronic disease and iron deficiency, with absolute iron deficiency playing a comparatively minor role. *Conclusion.* Greater awareness of anemia in the elderly is warranted due to its high prevalence and negative effect on outcomes, hospitalization duration, and mortality. Geriatric patients should be routinely screened for anemia and etiological causes of anemia individually assessed to allow timely initiation of appropriate therapy.

1. Introduction

Iron deficiency is the most prevalent nutritional deficiency worldwide. This metal ion is an essential element in a variety of physiological processes in human beings, including the production of energy in the brain. Iron is also an enzymatic cofactor in the synthesis of neurotransmitters and myelin and is well known for being especially important as a means of oxygen transportation [1]. The main consequence of iron deficiency is anemia, a common condition and significant problem in the older population. However, many physicians continue to neglect the significance of anemia as a serious clinical condition in the elderly [2]. While decreased hemoglobin levels were previously largely considered a normal consequence of aging, there is now evidence that anemia is associated with an increased risk for morbidity and mortality [3, 4]. According to hemoglobin (Hb) cut-off levels defined by the World Health Organization (WHO) (<12 g/dL for females, <13 g/dL for males) [5], anemia is present in 10% of women and 11% of men over the age of 65, increasing to 20% of women and 26% of men over 85 [6]. An even higher prevalence is seen in hospitalized patients, of whom approximately 40–50% have been found to be anemic [7]. The primary consequences of anemia, even mild anemia in which hemoglobin values are only marginally reduced (>9.5 g/dL), are the impairment of functional capacities and a reduced quality of life [8–10]. Furthermore, in elderly persons, anemia can impair physical performance and mobility, thus increasing the risk of falls. An association between anemia in older adults and mortality has been observed in several studies, even in the absence of concomitant illness. In elderly patients, anemia is often overlooked, despite the fact that it has been shown to have potentially serious consequences [2–5, 10].

Data describing the prevalence and causes of anemia in hospitalized geriatric populations are rare and incongruent. Our aim was therefore to determine the epidemiology and etiology of anemia in a hospitalized geriatric population in Germany.

2. Methods

2.1. Study Design. In this German study, all patients who were admitted between March 2010 and March 2011 to the Geriatric Clinic of the St. Elisabethen Krankenhaus in Frankfurt, Germany, and whose medical records were available were included. The data was analyzed retrospectively.

Patients included in the study were aged 65 years or over. The presence of anemia was defined according to criteria issued by the WHO: hemoglobin (Hb) <12 g/dL for females and <13 g/dL for males. Hb values on admission were available for 386 of the 405 patients (95.3%) and three grades of anemia severity were differentiated: severe (Hb < 8 g/dL), moderate (Hb 8 to <9.5 g/dL), and mild (Hb ≥ 9.5 g/dL). In addition, patient data were assessed for routinely determined levels of serum iron (in 92.6% of patients), serum ferritin (95.6%), transferrin saturation (TSAT) (99.0%), vitamin B_{12} (91.9%), folic acid (88.1%), CRP (96.8%), and serum creatinine (99.51%).

2.1.1. Definition of Anemia Classification

Anemia Associated with Iron Deficiency. Patients with Hb levels under 12 g/dL (women) and 13 g/dL (men) and a TSAT value <20% were considered to have anemia associated with iron deficiency. Three subcategories were defined.

  (i) Anemia related to absolute iron deficiency (iron deficiency anemia, IDA) was characterized by a decreased serum ferritin level (<30 μg/mL) in combination with low serum CRP levels (≤0.5 mg/dL).

  (ii) Anemia caused by inflammation (AI) was defined by high ferritin levels (>100 μg/mL) and increased CRP (≥0.5 mg/dL).

  (iii) Patients with ferritin levels between 30 μg/mL and 100 μg/mL and high CRP levels (≥0.5 mg/dL) were classified as having mixed anemia (IDA/AI).

Anemia due to Factors Other Than Iron Deficiency. Patients with Hb levels under 12 g/dL (women) and 13 g/dL (men) and a TSAT value ≥ 20% were considered to have anemia caused by factors other than iron deficiency. Four subcategories were defined.

  (i) Anemia secondary to cobalamin deficiency was diagnosed if the serum level was <150 pg/mL.

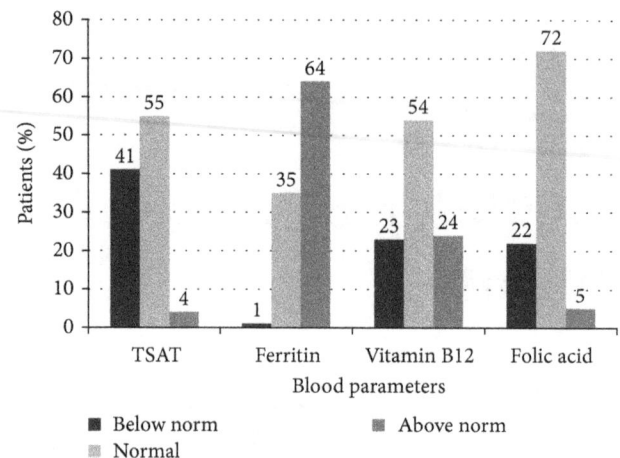

FIGURE 1: Anemia-related laboratory parameters at time of admission (TSAT = transferrin saturation).

  (ii) Anemia secondary to folic acid deficiency was diagnosed if the serum level was <2 μg/L.

  (iii) Anemia of chronic renal insufficiency (CRI) was classified by creatinine values >1.2 mg/dL in females and >1.5 mg/dL in males [11–13].

  (iv) Anemia secondary to other etiologies was defined as unexplained anemia (UA) [6]. See Figure 1.

2.2. Statistical Analysis. The primary objective of this study was to determine the prevalence of anemia and of different etiological subtypes of anemia in a hospitalized geriatric patient population.

Descriptive statistics were attained through the calculation of arithmetical means, standard deviations, and minimum and maximum values of all data. To test the significance of all categorical variables, the Chi-squared test (Pearson) was performed. Arithmetical means were calculated with t-tests for dependent and independent samples, and correlations were determined using the Spearman Rho method. All outcomes with a minimum of $P < 0.05$ were considered significant. Missing values were disregarded in all statistical tests. All statistical analyses were performed using IBM SPSS Statistics 20SPSS statistical software.

3. Results

During the period studied, 405 patients (116 men and 289 women) who were admitted to the geriatric clinic had medical records available and were therefore included in the study. The average age was 83.6 ± 6.9 years (range 65–101 years). The patients were divided into three observational groups according to age: 65 to 75 years, 76 to 85 years, and over 85 years of age, representing 12.10%, 36.79%, and 51.11% of the study population, respectively.

The most frequent main causes of hospitalization in this geriatric patient group were fractures (39.4%, $n = 150$), cardiovascular disease (18.4%, $n = 70$), and disturbances of gait and mobility (16.8%, $n = 64$). Other reasons for

TABLE 1: Anemia subtypes according to main reason for hospitalization.

	All patients $n = 368$ $n (\%^*)$	All anemic patients $n = 241$ $n (\%^{*1})$	IDA $n (\%^{*1})$	IDA/AI $n (\%^{*1})$	AI $n (\%^{*1})$	B_{12}/folic acid deficiency $n (\%^{*1})$	Renal anemia $n (\%^{*1})$	UA $n (\%^{*1})$
Fractures	150 (40.76)	110 (43.90)	0 (0)	9 (8.18)	31 (28.18)	8 (7.27)	10 (9.09)	52 (47.27)
Cardiovascular disease	70 (19.02)	40 (57.14)	3 (7.50)	6 (15.00)	15 (37.50)	3 (7.50)	7 (17.50)	6 (15.00)
Disturbance of gait and mobility	64 (17.39)	26 (40.63)	1 (3.85)	5 (19.23)	3 (11.54)	2 (7.69)	5 (19.23)	10 (38.46)
Digestive tract diseases	15 (4.08)	13 (86.67)	1 (7.69)	2 (15.38)	4 (30.77)	2 (15.38)	4 (30.77)	0 (0)
Disorders of the musculoskeletal apparatus	14 (3.80)	13 (92.86)	0 (0)	1 (7.69)	3 (23.08)	3 (23.08)	6 (46.15)	0 (0)
Neoplasma	14 (3.80)	10 (71.43)	0 (0)	1 (10)	6 (60.00)	2 (20)	1 (10)	0 (0)
Infectious diseases	9 (2.45)	7 (77.78)	1 (14.29)	2 (28.57)	2 (28.57)	1 (14.29)	1 (14.92)	0 (0)
Injuries	9 (2.45)	4 (44.44)	0 (0)	2 (50.00)	0 (0)	1 (25.00)	1 (25)	0 (0)
Other reasons	23 (6.25)	18 (78.26)	1 (5.56)	3 (16.67)	4 (22.22)	2 (11.11)	4 (22.22)	4 (22.22)
		241 (100)	7 (2.90^{*2})	31 (12.86^{*2})	68 (28.22^{*2})	24 (9.96^{*2})	39 (16.18^{*2})	72 (29.88^{*2})

*Relating to all hospitalized patients.
^{*1}Relating to all anemic patients with this diagnosis.
^{*2}Relating to all anemic patients.

TABLE 2: Iron parameters in all patients subdivided into age groups.

	Number of patients		Mean ± SD		Median		Min.		Max.	
	Female	Male	Female	Male	Female	Male	Female	Male	Female	Male
Hb (g/dL)										
65–75 years	33	21	11.67 ± 3.01	11.84 ± 2.05	11.5	11.6	9	8.5	19.5	16.5
76–85 years	97	59	11.58 ± 2.24	11.91 ± 1.81	11.6	11.4	8.1	9.1	19.7	16.2
>85 years	149	29	11.30 ± 2.0	11.94 ± 1.97	11.4	12.4	8.1	8.9	16.9	16.2
Serum iron (mg/dL)										
65–75 years	32	19	3.53 ± 1.93	5.05 ± 3.08	3	5	1	1	8	9
76–85 years	97	57	4.15 ± 2.36	4.26 ± 2.117	4	5	1	1	9	8
>85 years	142	27	4.7 ± 2.38	3.85 ± 2.37	5	4	1	1	9	8
Serum ferritin (μg/L)										
65–75 years	35	22	184.14 ± 206.62	371.36 ± 232.83	116	314	29	41	1131	905
76–85 years	94	58	262.38 ± 263.06	336.71 ± 284.13	201.5	253	18	56	2026	1435
>85 years	149	27	262.38 ± 263.06	336.56 ± 291.14	212	216	7	38	1352	1250
TSAT (%)										
65–75 years	36	22	18.64 ± 12.35	18.18 ± 9.39	15	18.5	4	4	60	35
76–85 years	100	61	20.44 ± 12.39	21.44 ± 11.61	18	20	3	6	87	67
>85 years	153	30	19.62 ± 10.03	20.97 ± 14.41	17	18	5	6	52	79
CRP (mg/dL)										
65–75 years	35	22	4.77 ± 6.29	1.47 ± 1.85	2.3	0.65	0.2	0.2	28.7	7.4
76–85 years	127	82	4.77 ± 6.29	2.19 ± 4.02	1.7	0.95	0	0.2	28.7	30
>85 years	151	28	3.88 ± 6.08	1.7 ± 0.7	1.9	0.7	0	0	49	9.8

admission were digestive tract diseases (3.9%, $n = 15$), disorders of the musculoskeletal apparatus (3.7%, $n = 14$), neoplasms (3.7%, $n = 14$), infectious diseases (2.4%, $n = 9$), and injuries (2.4%, $n = 9$), with a further 6.0% ($n = 23$) admitted for other reasons.

Table 1 shows the distribution of these conditions according to specific anemia subtypes. On average, the patients had eight additional diagnoses concurrent to the primary diagnosis, and mean duration of stay in the clinic of all study subjects was 22 days. The main demographic characteristics of the patients are summarized in Table 2.

Of those hospitalized patients whose Hb values at admission were available ($n = 386$), 66.3% (74.8% of men and 62.9% of women) were anemic. There was no correlation between age and Hb level. While only four patients (1.5%) were found to be severely anemic, 37 (13.5%) had moderate anemia and the remaining 85.1% were categorized as having mild anemia.

The total number of patients diagnosed with anemia was 237, of whom 154 (65.0%) were defined as having iron deficiency anemia, with TSAT values <20%. Absolute IDA was found in only 7 (4.6%) of these patients, while 33 (21.4%) had a combination of IDA and AI. The majority of patients with IDA ($n = 95$, 61.7%) were diagnosed with AI, indicated by high CRP and ferritin levels.

Decreased levels of vitamin B_{12} or folic acid were determined as the cause of anemia in 30 patients (5.9% and 6.8%, resp.). In a further 46 (19.4%) study subjects, anemia was found to be the result of chronic renal insufficiency. The remaining patients fell into none of these categories and were therefore classified as having "unexplained anemia."

The mean serum ferritin level of 315.7 μg/L fell within the normal reference range. Serum ferritin values were, however, increased in the majority of study subjects (64%), while 35% were found to have normal serum ferritin levels.

4. Discussion

Anemia is a common condition in the elderly, especially in hospitalized geriatric patients, and is known to be associated with increased morbidity and mortality. The present study was specifically aimed at investigating the epidemiology and etiology of anemia in a hospitalized geriatric population. Blood samples were retrospectively analyzed for the purpose of the study.

The most striking conclusion drawn is the high prevalence of anemia across the board in elderly patients admitted to hospital owing to a wide range of different disorders. Two-thirds of the patients studied were found to be anemic on admission. Although one other study, also focusing on geriatric inpatients, has shown a similar prevalence of anemia [7], most research involving elderly subjects has found the prevalence to be lower [6, 10, 14]. This discrepancy may be accountable to the fact that, in contrast to the current study with its population of hospitalized elderly patients, most other studies have examined ambulant patients or older people in the community [15, 16]. Geriatric persons with health problems severe enough to result in hospital admission are more likely than the geriatric population as a whole to suffer from acute infection and also to have an increased risk of blood loss due to surgery. Thus, hospitalized patients are at a higher risk of developing anemia [17]. Anemia was found in most cases to be mild, with an Hb level > 10 g/dL, in accordance with previously published results [6, 18]. However, even mild anemia is frequently associated with negative outcomes with regard to mortality and morbidity in the elderly [2, 19] and should therefore not be accepted as a normal physiological response to the aging process. Furthermore, the etiological origins of anemia must be determined in all cases in order to facilitate the choice and implementation of effective therapy. It might be seen as a limitation of the present study that reasons for hospital admission were not taken into account. However, we

deliberately chose to include all geriatric patients admitted to our clinic, independent of grounds for hospitalization, in order to gain a broader perspective on the prevalence and causes of anemia in elderly patients.

No statistically significant correlation was detected between patients' age and Hb values. This is not in keeping with results of previous research, which have suggested an age-related decrease in Hb levels [6]. Again, this may relate to the specific elderly population included, since all study subjects had serious health issues (and thus, presumably, an increased risk of anemia), whereas in the geriatric population as a whole, the prevalence of serious illness increases with age. Thus, in terms of general state of health, the older the hospitalized patients are, the more representative they can be considered to be of the general population in that age group. As a consequence, what might be considered an innate "bias" of our population towards seriously ill patients (in comparison to studies involving nonhospitalized geriatric persons) is not independent of age, but probably more pronounced in the context of the younger geriatric population.

Determination of the underlying cause of anemia in geriatric persons is complicated by comorbidity and polypharmacy, which are particularly common among the elderly [5]. This must also be taken into account when classifying and comparing the results.

Nonetheless, anemia in the elderly can generally be categorized into four major types: anemia related to nutrient deficiencies (iron, cobalamin, and folic acid), anemia related to chronic inflammation, anemia due to renal insufficiency, and unexplained anemia [6].

Of 237 patients considered to be anemic, 154 (65.0%) had TSAT values <20% and were therefore diagnosed with iron deficiency anemia. In terms of the classification of anemia, the most common etiological subtypes were anemia of inflammation or a mixed form resulting from AI and IDA. Only a few studies have investigated the etiologic profile of anemia in hospitalized patients in the age range from 65 to 101 years [7, 14]. Comparing our results to previous studies is complicated by differences in anemia classification. However, inflammation seems to be the predominant cause of anemia in the observed population, with nutritive factors playing only a limited role [14]. In elderly persons, the causes of anemia vary depending on their clinical setting. AI and IDA are, however, the most common forms of anemia both in community-dwelling and in hospitalized geriatric patients [14]. In our study, IDA was less prevalent than expected in light of results obtained in prior studies.

Only 4.6% of our study subjects with iron deficiency-associated anemia were found to have absolute iron deficiency anemia (IDA), in comparison to 17% in previous reports [6, 20]. A possible explanation for this discrepancy might be the higher mean age (83.6 years) of our patients compared to populations of similar studies, whose mean ages were between 77 and 80 years [13, 21]. Furthermore, we had a high number of comorbidities in our study population. A recent study with a comparable prevalence of comorbidities disclosed an IDA rate of 31% [7].

Sixty-two percent of patients with iron deficiency-related anemia were diagnosed with AI. Petrosyan et al. reported a similar prevalence rate (60%) of AI in a comparable study population [7]. Prevalence rates in community-dwelling elderly persons, however, may be considerably lower. For example, the NHANES (National Health and Nutrition Examination Survey) III demonstrated a prevalence of 24% for this type of anemia in a community-dwelling elderly population [6]. Considerable differences in prevalence may be accountable to the setting (community-dwelling elderly, nursing home residents, or hospital patients), variations in mean age of the study population, and the resultant respective variations in the number of comorbidities and chronic conditions. While AI predominantly occurs as a consequence of chronic or long-term illness or infection, it is also associated with malignancy and inflammatory disorders. These are conditions whose prevalence increases with advancing age and which are more likely to be encountered in a hospitalized setting. Since fractures were the most frequent main cause of hospitalization in our study population, these patients came into the rehabilitation ward. Since an increase in inflammation parameters (CRP and ferritin) is to be expected under these circumstances, this represents an additional explanation for the high prevalence of AI in our study [22]. Studies of noninstitutionalized older persons have demonstrated higher and lower prevalences of IDA and AI, respectively [21, 23].

In our study, anemia of mixed etiology resulting from iron deficiency and chronic inflammation was also analyzed. Thirty-three patients (21.43%) were found to have combined IDA and AI.

Anemia due to deficiencies of vitamin B_{12} or folic acid was found in 5.91% and 6.75% of patients, respectively. Other studies showed higher prevalence rates of 10–20% for cobalamin and 21% for folic acid deficiency [7, 24, 25]. Guralnik et al. determined anemia secondary to folic acid or cobalamin deficiency in 14% of their elderly population [6]. However, comparison of these results is of limited value, as different diagnostic criteria were used.

Anemia of chronic renal insufficiency (CRI) was defined by creatinine values >1.2 mg/dL in females and >1.5 mg/dL in males. Forty-seven (19.41%) of the elderly patients assessed were found to have CRI-related anemia. While previous studies have reported a prevalence of 8–17.5% for anemia resulting from renal insufficiency, most of these studies used a glomerular filtration rate (GFR) of <30 mL/min as the defining criterion for chronic kidney disease [7, 26, 27]. While GFR is indeed considered a better parameter for the diagnosis of chronic renal insufficiency, the present study, due to its retrospective design, was only able to assess chronic renal illness on the basis of the available creatinine values. The results of the studies are therefore not directly comparable.

The patients that fell into none of the given etiological subgroup categories were therefore classified as having unexplained anemia. Possible underlying mechanisms for unexplained anemia include physiological changes such as higher circulating levels of proinflammatory cytokines, myelodysplasia, decreased androgen levels, and a decrease in the proliferative capacity of bone marrow stem cells [6, 28].

Our study has strengths and limitations. The most limiting factor is the retrospective design of the study. Consequently, only those laboratory parameters which were collected as clinical routine on admission were available to be assessed.

Important strengths of the study are the large study population ($n = 405$), the wide spectrum of reasons for admission and of underlying disease or condition, and the use of a variety of different iron and inflammation parameters as assessment criteria for the classification of different causes of anemia.

Conclusive evidence from a large number of studies has confirmed that adequate treatment of iron deficiency significantly improves rates of mortality and morbidity in patients suffering from a wide range of conditions, including chronic heart failure [29, 30], coronary heart disease [31], chronic kidney disease [32, 33], cancer [34, 35], and rheumatoid arthritis [36, 37]. Nevertheless, screening and treatment of ID continue to be widely neglected in the routine management of geriatric patients. There is clearly a need for greater awareness of the high prevalence of anemia in the elderly and of its significance in terms of poorer outcomes, prolonged hospital stays, and increased mortality. Our study underlines the importance of routine screening and individual assessment of the etiological causes of anemia in geriatric patients, allowing the timely initiation of optimal and appropriate therapy. In addition, the perioperative administration of intravenous iron is advisable in order to reduce anemia-related complications and minimize transfusion requirements.

Rather than relying on a single biomarker, screening should include a range of parameters including TSAT, serum ferritin, and CRP. A new generation of intravenous iron preparations allows rapid single-session doses of up to 1,000 mg, thus offering an excellent option for effective treatment and prevention of iron deficiency in all patients, including the elderly [38]. Dosage can be calculated using standard calculation methods such as the Ganzoni formula.

Abbreviations

AI:	Anemia of inflammation
CRI:	Chronic renal insufficiency
CRP:	C-reactive protein
GFR:	Glomerular filtration rate
IDA:	Iron deficiency anemia
NHANES:	National Health and Nutrition Examination Survey
TSAT:	Transferrin saturation
UA:	Unexplained anemia
WHO:	World Health Organization.

Conflict of Interests

Tabea Geisel, Julia Martin, and Bettina Schulze have no conflict of interests.

Authors' Contribution

All authors contributed to the concept and design of the work and to the acquisition and interpretation of data. Tabea

Geisel drafted the paper. All authors revised the paper for important intellectual content and approved the final version for publication.

Acknowledgments

The sponsor's role was limited to financial support only. The sponsor took no active part in data collection, data analysis, data interpretation, or paper preparation. The authors would like to thank Janet Collins for proof reading and language support. Garth Virgin is an employee of Vifor Pharma Deutschland GmbH. Roland Schaefer has acted as a consultant for Vifor Pharma Deutschland GmbH. Matthias Bach has received speaker honoraria for Vifor Pharma Deutschland GmbH. Jürgen Stein has received speaker honoraria and is a member of the board of Vifor Pharma Deutschland GmbH.

References

[1] R. R. Crichton, S. Wilmet, R. Legssyer, and R. J. Ward, "Molecular and cellular mechanisms of iron homeostasis and toxicity in mammalian cells," *Journal of Inorganic Biochemistry*, vol. 91, no. 1, pp. 9–18, 2002.

[2] A. R. Nissenson, L. T. Goodnough, and R. W. Dubois, "Anemia: not just an innocent bystander?" *Archives of Internal Medicine*, vol. 163, no. 12, pp. 1400–1404, 2003.

[3] S. D. Denny, M. N. Kuchibhatla, and H. J. Cohen, "Impact of anemia on mortality, cognition, and function in community-dwelling elderly," *American Journal of Medicine*, vol. 119, no. 4, pp. 327–334, 2006.

[4] B. W. J. H. Penninx, M. Pahor, R. C. Woodman, and J. M. Guralnik, "Anemia in old age is associated with increased mortality and hospitalization," *Journals of Gerontology A*, vol. 61, no. 5, pp. 474–479, 2006.

[5] World Health Organization, "Nutritional Anemia: Report of a WHO Scientific Group," *Technical Report Series*, vol. 405, pp. 1–40, 1968.

[6] J. M. Guralnik, R. S. Eisenstaedt, L. Ferrucci, H. G. Klein, and R. C. Woodman, "Prevalence of anemia in persons 65 years and older in the United States: evidence for a high rate of unexplained anemia," *Blood*, vol. 104, no. 8, pp. 2263–2268, 2004.

[7] I. Petrosyan, G. Blaison, and E. Andrés, "Anaemia in the elderly: an aetiologic profile of a prospective cohort of 95 hospitalised patients," *European Journal of Internal Medicine*, vol. 23, pp. 524–528, 2012.

[8] A. A. Lash and S. M. Coyer, "Anemia in older adults," *Medsurg Nursing*, vol. 17, no. 5, pp. 298–305, 2008.

[9] D. R. Thomas, "Anemia and quality of life: unrecognized and undertreated," *Journals of Gerontology A*, vol. 59, no. 3, pp. 238–241, 2004.

[10] W. P. J. den Elzen, J. M. Willems, R. G. J. Westendorp, A. J. M. De Craen, W. J. J. Assendelft, and J. Gussekloo, "Effect of anemia and comorbidity on functional status and mortality in old age: results from the Leiden 85-plus Study," *Canadian Medical Association Journal*, vol. 181, no. 3-4, pp. 151–157, 2009.

[11] G. Weiss and L. T. Goodnough, "Anemia of chronic disease," *New England Journal of Medicine*, vol. 352, no. 10, pp. 1011–1059, 2005.

[12] C. Gasche, A. Berstad, R. Befrits et al., "Guidelines on the diagnosis and management of iron deficiency and anemia in inflammatory bowel diseases," *Inflammatory Bowel Diseases*, vol. 13, no. 12, pp. 1545–1553, 2007.

[13] E. Joosten, W. Pelemans, M. Hiele, J. Noyen, R. Verhaeghe, and M. A. Boogaerts, "Prevalence and causes of anaemia in a geriatric hospitalized population," *Gerontology*, vol. 38, no. 1-2, pp. 111–117, 1992.

[14] M. Tettamanti, U. Lucca, F. Gandini et al., "Prevalence, incidence and types of mild anemia in the elderly: the "Health and Anemia" population-based study," *Haematologica*, vol. 95, no. 11, pp. 1849–1856, 2010.

[15] E. M. Inelmen, M. D'Alessio, M. R. A. Gatto et al., "Descriptive analysis of the prevalence of anemia in a randomly selected sample of elderly people living at home: some results of an Italian multicentric study," *Aging*, vol. 6, no. 2, pp. 81–89, 1994.

[16] M. E. Salive, J. Cornoni-Huntley, J. M. Guralnik et al., "Anemia and hemoglobin levels in older persons: relationship with age, gender, and health status," *Journal of the American Geriatrics Society*, vol. 40, no. 5, pp. 489–496, 1992.

[17] E. A. Price, R. Mehra, T. H. Holmes, and S. L. Schrier, "Anemia in older persons: etiology and evaluation," *Blood Cells, Molecules, and Diseases*, vol. 46, no. 2, pp. 159–165, 2011.

[18] R. Eisenstaedt, B. W. J. H. Penninx, and R. C. Woodman, "Anemia in the elderly: current understanding and emerging concepts," *Blood Reviews*, vol. 20, no. 4, pp. 213–226, 2006.

[19] L. Ferrucci, J. M. Guralnik, S. Bandinelli et al., "Unexplained anaemia in older persons is characterised by low erythropoietin and low levels of pro-inflammatory markers," *British Journal of Haematology*, vol. 136, no. 6, pp. 849–855, 2007.

[20] B. J. Anía, V. J. Suman, V. F. Fairbanks, and L. J. Melton III, "Prevalence of anemia in medical practice: community versus referral patients," *Mayo Clinic Proceedings*, vol. 69, no. 8, pp. 730–735, 1994.

[21] A. A. Merchant and C. N. Roy, "Not so benign haematology: anaemia of the elderly," *British Journal of Haematology*, vol. 156, no. 2, pp. 173–185, 2012.

[22] P. P. Vinha, A. A. Jordão Jr., J. A. Farina Jr., H. Vannucchi, J. S. Marchini, and S. F. D. C. da Cunha, "Inflammatory and oxidative stress after surgery for the small area corrections of burn sequelae," *Acta Cirurgica Brasileira*, vol. 26, no. 4, pp. 320–324, 2011.

[23] O. J. Kirkeby, S. Fossum, and C. Risoe, "Anaemia in elderly patients. Incidence and causes of low haemoglobin concentration in a city general practice," *Scandinavian Journal of Primary Health Care*, vol. 9, no. 3, pp. 167–171, 1991.

[24] L. C. Pennypacker, R. H. Allen, J. P. Kelly et al., "High prevalence of cobalamin deficiency in elderly outpatients," *Journal of the American Geriatrics Society*, vol. 40, no. 12, pp. 1197–1204, 1992.

[25] R. Carmel, R. Green, D. S. Rosenblatt, and D. Watkins, "Update on cobalamin, folate, and homocysteine," *Hematology*, vol. 2003, pp. 62–81, 2003.

[26] A. S. Artz and M. J. Thirman, "Unexplained anemia predominates despite an intensive evaluation in a racially diverse cohort of older adults from a referral anemia clinic," *Journals of Gerontology A*, vol. 66, no. 8, pp. 925–932, 2011.

[27] B. Terrier, M. Resche-Rigon, E. Andres et al., "Prevalence, characteristics and prognostic significance of anemia in daily practice," *QJM*, vol. 105, no. 4, Article ID hcr230, pp. 345–354, 2012.

[28] L. Ferrucci, R. D. Semba, J. M. Guralnik et al., "Proinflammatory state, hepcidin, and anemia in older persons," *Blood*, vol. 115, no. 18, pp. 3810–3816, 2010.

[29] M. Kapoor, M. D. Schleinitz, A. Gemignani, and W. C. Wu, "Outcomes of patients with chronic heart failure and iron deficiency treated with intravenous iron: a meta-analysis," *Cardiovascular & Hematological Disorders-Drug Targets*, vol. 13, pp. 35–44, 2013.

[30] E. A. Jankowska, S. von Haehling, S. D. Anker, I. C. Macdougall, and P. Ponikowski, "Iron deficiency and heart failure: diagnostic dilemmas and therapeutic perspectives," *European Heart Journal*, vol. 34, pp. 816–829, 2013.

[31] N. S. Belousova, S. A. Il'ina, G. É. Chernogoriuk, and L. I. Tiukalova, "The influence of correction of iron metabolism and erythron characteristics in mild iron deficiency states on clinical manifestations of coronary heart disease," *Klinicheskaia Meditsina*, vol. 90, pp. 41–46, 2012.

[32] G. Wong, K. Howard, E. Hodson, M. Irving, and J. C. Craig, "An economic evaluation of intravenous versus oral iron supplementation in people on haemodialysis," *Nephrology Dialysis Transplantation*, vol. 28, pp. 413–420, 2013.

[33] D. W. Coyne, T. Kapoian, W. Suki et al., "Ferric gluconate is highly efficacious in anemic hemodialysis patients with high serum ferritin and low transferrin saturation. Results of the Dialysis Patients' Response to IV Iron with Elevated Ferritin (DRIVE) study," *Journal of the American Society of Nephrology*, vol. 18, no. 3, pp. 975–984, 2007.

[34] A. Gafter-Gvili, B. Rozen-Zvi, and L. Vidal, "Intravenous iron supplementation for the treatment of chemotherapy-induced anaemia—systematic review and meta-analysis of randomised controlled trials," *Acta Oncologica*, vol. 52, pp. 18–29, 2013.

[35] H. T. Steinmetz, "The role of intravenous iron in the treatment of anemia in cancer patients," *Therapeutic Advances in Hematology*, vol. 3, pp. 177–191, 2012.

[36] E. Bloxham, V. Vagadia, K. Scott et al., "Anaemia in rheumatoid arthritis: can we afford to ignore it?" *Postgraduate Medical Journal*, vol. 87, no. 1031, pp. 596–600, 2011.

[37] W.-S. Chen, C.-Y. Liu, H.-T. Lee et al., "Effects of intravenous iron saccharate on improving severe anemia in rheumatoid arthritis patients," *Clinical Rheumatology*, vol. 31, no. 3, pp. 469–477, 2012.

[38] W. Y. Qunibi, "The efficacy and safety of current intravenous iron preparations for the management of iron-deficiency anaemia: a review," *Arzneimittel-Forschung*, vol. 60, no. 6 a, pp. 399–412, 2010.

Permissions

All chapters in this book were first published in ANEMIA, by Hindawi Publishing Corporation; hereby published with permission under the Creative Commons Attribution License or equivalent. Every chapter published in this book has been scrutinized by our experts. Their significance has been extensively debated. The topics covered herein carry significant findings which will fuel the growth of the discipline. They may even be implemented as practical applications or may be referred to as a beginning point for another development.

The contributors of this book come from diverse backgrounds, making this book a truly international effort. This book will bring forth new frontiers with its revolutionizing research information and detailed analysis of the nascent developments around the world.

We would like to thank all the contributing authors for lending their expertise to make the book truly unique. They have played a crucial role in the development of this book. Without their invaluable contributions this book wouldn't have been possible. They have made vital efforts to compile up to date information on the varied aspects of this subject to make this book a valuable addition to the collection of many professionals and students.

This book was conceptualized with the vision of imparting up-to-date information and advanced data in this field. To ensure the same, a matchless editorial board was set up. Every individual on the board went through rigorous rounds of assessment to prove their worth. After which they invested a large part of their time researching and compiling the most relevant data for our readers.

The editorial board has been involved in producing this book since its inception. They have spent rigorous hours researching and exploring the diverse topics which have resulted in the successful publishing of this book. They have passed on their knowledge of decades through this book. To expedite this challenging task, the publisher supported the team at every step. A small team of assistant editors was also appointed to further simplify the editing procedure and attain best results for the readers.

Apart from the editorial board, the designing team has also invested a significant amount of their time in understanding the subject and creating the most relevant covers. They scrutinized every image to scout for the most suitable representation of the subject and create an appropriate cover for the book.

The publishing team has been an ardent support to the editorial, designing and production team. Their endless efforts to recruit the best for this project, has resulted in the accomplishment of this book. They are a veteran in the field of academics and their pool of knowledge is as vast as their experience in printing. Their expertise and guidance has proved useful at every step. Their uncompromising quality standards have made this book an exceptional effort. Their encouragement from time to time has been an inspiration for everyone.

The publisher and the editorial board hope that this book will prove to be a valuable piece of knowledge for researchers, students, practitioners and scholars across the globe.

List of Contributors

Mulugeta Melku
Department of Hematology, School of Biomedical and Laboratory Sciences, College of Medicine and Health Sciences, University of Gondar, 6200 Gondar, Ethiopia

Zelalem Addis
Department of Medical Microbiology, School of Biomedical and Laboratory Sciences, College of Medicine and Health Sciences, University of Gondar, 6200 Gondar, Ethiopia

Meseret Alem
Department of Immunology and Molecular Biology, School of Biomedical and Laboratory Sciences, College of Medicine and Health Sciences, University of Gondar, 6200 Gondar, Ethiopia

Bamlaku Enawgaw
Department of Hematology, School of Biomedical and Laboratory Sciences, College of Medicine and Health Sciences, University of Gondar, 6200 Gondar, Ethiopia

Leeniyagala Gamaralalage Thamal Darshana and Deepthi Inoka Uluwaduge
Medical Laboratory Sciences Unit, Department of Allied Health Sciences, Faculty of Medical Sciences, University of Sri Jayewardenepura, Gangodawila, Nugegoda 10250, Sri Lanka

Anneke B. Oostra, Aggie W. M. Nieuwint, Hans Joenje and Johan P. de Winter
Department of Clinical Genetics, VU University Medical Center, Van der Boechorststraat 7, 1081 BT Amsterdam, The Netherlands

Jéssica Barbieri
Regional University of Northwestern Rio Grande do Sul (UNIJUÍ), Ijuí, RS, Brazil

Paula Caitano Fontela
Program in Respiratory Sciences, the Federal University of Rio Grande do Sul (UFRGS), Porto Alegre, RS, Brazil

Matias Nunes Frizzo
Department of Life Sciences, the Regional University of Northwestern Rio Grande do Sul (UNIJUÍ), Rua do Comércio No. 3000, Bairro Universitário, 98700 000 Ijuí, RS, Brazil
Cenecista Institute for Higher Education, Rua Dr. João Augusto Rodrigues 471, 98801 015 Santo Ângelo, RS, Brazil

Yana Picinin Sandri
Program in Integral Attention to Health (PPGAIS-UNIJUI/UNICRUZ), Ijuí, RS, Brazil
Cenecista Institute for Higher Education, Rua Dr. João Augusto Rodrigues 471, 98801 015 Santo Ângelo, RS, Brazil

Carine Eloise Prestes Zimmermann
Program in Pharmacology of the Health Sciences Center,The Federal University of Santa Maria (UFSM), RS, Brazil
Cenecista Institute for Higher Education, Rua Dr. João Augusto Rodrigues 471, 98801 015 Santo Ângelo, RS, Brazil

Emanelle Kerber Viera Mallet
Cenecista Institute for Higher Education, Rua Dr. João Augusto Rodrigues 471, 98801 015 Santo Ângelo, RS, Brazil

Eliane Roseli Winkelmann
Program in Integral Attention to Health (PPGAIS-UNIJUI/UNICRUZ), Ijuí, RS, Brazil
Department of Life Sciences, the Regional University of Northwestern Rio Grande do Sul (UNIJUÍ), Rua do Comércio No. 3000, Bairro Universitário, 98700 000 Ijuí, RS, Brazil

Levi Makala and Betty S. Pace
Department of Pediatrics, Georgia Health Sciences University, Augusta, GA 30912, USA

Jung-Mo Ahn
Department of Chemistry, University of Texas at Dallas, Richardson, TX 75083, USA

Salvatore Di Maro
Department of Pharmacological and Toxicological Chemistry, University of Naples Federico II, 80100 Naples, Italy

Tzu-Fang Lou
Department of Molecular and Cell Biology, University of Texas at Dallas, TX 75080, USA

Sharanya Sivanand
Department of Developmental Biology, University of Texas Southwestern Medical Center, Dallas, TX 75390, USA

Najim Ameziane, Stefan Dentro, Lianne Kerkhoven, Hans Joenje, Josephine C. Dorsman, Johan J. P. Gille, Erik A. Sistermans and Johan P. de Winter
Department of Clinical Genetics, VU University Medical Center, Van der Boechorststraat 7, 1081 BT Amsterdam, The Netherlands

Daoud Sie and Bauke Ylstra
Department of Pathology, VU University Medical Center, De Boelelaan 1117, 1081 HV Amsterdam, The Netherlands

Yavuz Ariyurek
Leiden Genome Technology Center, Center for Human and Clinical Genetics, Leiden University Medical Center, Einthovenweg 20, 2333 ZC Leiden, The Netherlands

Aysel Vehapoglu, Ayşegul Dogan Demir, Selcuk Uzuner and Mustafa Atilla Nursoy
Department of Pediatrics, School of Medicine, Bezmialem Vakif University, 34093 Istanbul, Turkey

Gamze Ozgurhan
Department of Pediatrics, Suleymaniye Obstetrics and Gynecology Hospital, 34010 Istanbul, Turkey

Serdar Turkmen
Department of Biochemistry, Istanbul Training and Research Hospital, 34098 Istanbul, Turkey

Arzu Kacan
Department of Pediatrics, Istanbul Training and Research Hospital, Istanbul, Turkey

Robert M. Kalicki, Stefan Farese and Dominik E. Uehlinger
Department of Nephrology, Hypertension and Clinical Pharmacology, Inselspital Bern, University Hospital and University of Bern, Freiburgstrasse 15, 3010 Bern, Switzerland

Martin Jones and Ann Rose
Department of Medical Genetics, University of British Columbia, Vancouver, BC, Canada V6T 1Z4

Mohamed El Missiry, Mohamed Hamed Hussein, Sadaf Khalid, Cornelio Uderzo and Lawrence Faulkner
Cure2Children Foundation, Via Marconi 30, 50131 Florence, Italy

Sarah Khan, Fatima Itrat and Naila Yaqub
Children's Hospital Pakistan Institute of Medical Sciences, Islamabad, Pakistan

Judith H. E. Verhagen-Oldenampsen, Jurgen R. Haanstra, Paulina M. H. van Strien, Marijke Valkhof and Ivo P. Touw
Department of Hematology, Erasmus Medical Center, Dr Molewaterplein 50, 3015 GE Rotterdam, The Netherlands

Marieke von Lindern
Department of Hematopoiesis, Sanquin Research and Landsteiner Laboratory, AMC/UvA, Plesmanlaan 125, 1066 CX Amsterdam, The Netherlands
Department of Hematology, Erasmus Medical Center, Dr Molewaterplein 50, 3015 GE Rotterdam, The Netherlands

Gabriel Costa Osanan, Cezar Alencar De Lima Rezende, Henrique Vitor Leite and Antônio Carlos Vieira Cabral
Department of Gynecology and Obstetrics, Federal University of Minas Gerais, Brazil

Zilma Silveira Nogueira Reis
Obstetrics and Gynaecology Department, Universidade Federal de Minas Gerais (UFMG), Avenida Professor Alfredo Balena, 190, Funcionários, Belo Horizonte, 30.130.100 Minas Gerais, Brazil
Department of Gynecology and Obstetrics, Federal University of Minas Gerais, Brazil

Tiago Lanfernini Ricardo Coelho
Federal University of Minas Gerais, Brazil

Rukmini B. Govekar, Poonam D. Kawle and Surekha M. Zingde
Advanced Centre for Treatment, Research and Education in Cancer, Tata Memorial Centre, Kharghar, Navi Mumbai 410610, India

Suresh H. Advani
Department of Medical Oncology, Jaslok Hospital and Research Centre, Mumbai 400026, India

Chelsea Jenkins, Jenny Kan and Maureen E. Hoatlin
Department of Biochemistry and Molecular Biology, Oregon Health and Science University, 3181 SW Sam Jackson Parkway, Portland, OR 97239, USA

Khaled M. Musallam
Department of Internal Medicine, American University of Beirut Medical Center, Beirut 1107 2020, Lebanon

Luca A. Lotta and Flora Peyvandi
Angelo Bianchi Bonomi Haemophilia andThrombosis Center, Department of Medicine and Medical Specialties, IRCCS Ca' Granda Foundation Maggiore Policlinico Hospital, University of Milan, 20122 Milan, Italy

Pier M. Sfeir and Faek R. Jamali
Division of General Surgery, Department of Surgery, American University of Beirut Medical Center, Beirut 1107 2020, Lebanon

Frits R. Rosendaal
Departments of Clinical Epidemiology and Thrombosis & Hemostasis, Leiden University Medical Center, 2333 ZA Leiden, The Netherlands

Toby Richards
Division of Surgery and Interventional Science, University College London Hospital, London WC1E 6AU, UK

Donat R. Spahn
Institute of Anesthesiology, University Hospital and University of Zurich, 8006 Zurich, Switzerland

Kaivan Khavandi
King's College London British Heart Foundation Centre, The Rayne Institute, St. Thomas' Hospital, King's Health Partners AHSC, London SE1 7EH, UK

Iskandar Barakat
Department of Medicine, Staten Island University Hospital, New York, NY 10305, USA

Benjamin Demoss
Department of Internal Medicine, Emory University School of Medicine, Atlanta, GA 30322, USA

Nahid Ashjazadeh, Sajad Emami, Peyman Petramfar and Ehsan Yaghoubi
Shiraz Neuroscience Research Center, Department of Neurology, Shiraz University of Medical Sciences, Shiraz, Iran

Mehran Karimi
Hematology Research Center, Shiraz University of Medical Sciences, Shiraz, Iran

LamiaMustafa Al-Naama
Department of Biochemistry and Haemoglobinopathy Units, College of Medicine, University of Basrah, Basrah, Iraq

Meaad Kadum Hassan
Department of Paediatrics and Haemoglobinopathy Units, College of Medicine, University of Basrah, Basrah, Iraq

Muhannad Maki Abdul Karim
Department of Biochemistry, College of Medicine, University of Basrah, Basrah, Iraq

Charlotte Hodson and Helen Walden
Protein Structure and Function Laboratory, Lincoln's Inn Fields Laboratories, London Research Institute, Cancer Research UK, 44 Lincoln's Inn Fields, London WC2A 3LY, UK

Raden Tina Dewi Judistiani, Lani Gumilang and Se ita Aryuti Nirmala
Public Health Department, Faculty of Medicine, Universitas Padjadjaran, Sumedang, West Java, Indonesia

Setyorini Irianti
Obstetric and Gynecology Department, Dr. Hasan Sadikin Hospital, Bandung, West Java, Indonesia

Deni Wirhana
Obstetric and Gynecology Department, Waled Regency Public Hospital, Cirebon, West Java, Indonesia

Irman Permana and Liza Sofjan
Department of Child Health, Waled Regency Public Hospital, Cirebon, West Java, Indonesia

Hesty Duhita
Obstetric and Gynecology Department, Syamsudin SH Public Hospital, Sukabumi, West Java, Indonesia

Lies Ani Tambunan and Jeffry Iman Gurnadi
Obstetric and Gynecology Department, Cibabat General Hospital, Cimahi, West Java, Indonesia

Umar Seno
Obstetric and Gynecology Department, Kota Bandung General Hospital, Bandung, West Java, Indonesia

Tetty Yuniati, Budi Setiabudiawan and Reni Ghrahani
Department of Child Health, Faculty of Medicine, Universitas Padjadjaran, Sumedang, West Java, Indonesia

Agnes Rengga Indrati
Clinical Pathology Department, Faculty of Medicine, Universitas Padjadjaran, Sumedang, West Java, Indonesia

Yunia Sribudiani
Department of Biochemistry and Molecular Biology, Faculty of Medicine, Universitas Padjadjaran, Sumedang, West Java, Indonesia

Irene Ule Ngole Sumbele, Sharon Odmia Sama and Germain Sotoing Taiwe
Department of Zoology and Animal Physiology, University of Buea, Buea, Cameroon

Helen Kuokuo Kimbi
Department of Medical Laboratory Sciences, University of Bamenda, Bamenda, Cameroon

Oseni Bashiru Shola and Fakoya Olatunde Olugbenga
Department of Biomedical Sciences, Faculty of Basic Medical Sciences, College of Health Sciences, Ladoke Akintola University of Technology, Ogbomosho 210214, Oyo State, Nigeria

Adamu Kenea, Efrem Negash and Lemi Bacha
Faculty of Public Health and Medical Sciences, Mettu University, Mettu, Ethiopia

Negash Wakgari
Department of Midwifery, College of Medicine and Health Sciences, Hawassa University, Hawassa, Ethiopia

Kemal N. Kawo
Department of Statistics, Madda Walabu University, Robe, Ethiopia

Zeytu G. Asfaw
School of Mathematical and Statistical Sciences, Hawassa University, Hawassa, Ethiopia

Negusse Yohannes
Department of Statistics, Dilla University, Dilla, Ethiopia

Vrushali A. Pathak
Department of Haematogenetics, National Institute of Immunohaematology (ICMR), KEM Hospital, Parel, Mumbai 400012, India

Kanjaksha Ghosh
Surat Raktadan Kendra & Research Centre, Udhna Khatodara Urban Health Centre, Udhna Magdalla Road, Surat, Gujrat 395002, India

Tabea Geisel and Julia Martin
Crohn Colitis Center Rhein-Main, 60594 Frankfurt/Main, Germany
Institute of Nutritional Science, University of Giessen, 35392 Giessen, Germany

Bettina Schulze and Matthias Bach
St. Elisabethen Krankenhaus, 60487 Frankfurt/Main, Germany

Roland Schaefer
Krankenhaus Sachsenhausen, Teaching Hospital of the J.W. von Goethe University Frankfurt/Main, 60594 Frankfurt/Main, Germany

Garth Virgin
Vifor Pharma Deutschland GmbH, 81379 Munich, Germany

Jürgen Stein
Department of Gastroenterology and Nutritional Medicine, Krankenhaus Sachsenhausen, Teaching Hospital of the J.W. von Goethe University Frankfurt/Main, 60594 Frankfurt/Main, Germany
Crohn Colitis Center Rhein-Main, 60594 Frankfurt/Main, Germany
Institute of Nutritional Science, University of Giessen, 35392 Giessen, Germany

Index